Handbook of Cardiac Anesthesia and Perioperative Care

Handbook of Cardiac Anesthesia and Perioperative Care

A Demythologized Approach

John D. Wasnick, M.D.

Attending Anesthesiologist, Cardiac Anesthesia Group, North Texas Anesthesia Consultants, Dallas

Butterworth–Heinemann

Boston•Oxford•Johannesburg•Melbourne•New Delhi•Singapore

Recognizing the importance of preserving what has been written, Butterworth–Heinemann prints its books on acid-free paper whenever possible.

 Butterworth–Heinemann supports the efforts of American Forests and the Global ReLeaf program in its campaign for the betterment of trees, forests, and our environment.

Library of Congress Cataloging-in-Publication Data

Wasnick, John D.
    Handbook of cardiac anesthesia and perioperative care : a demythologized approach / John D. Wasnick.
        p.   cm.
    Includes bibliographical references and index.
    ISBN 0-7506-9748-2
    1. Anesthesia in cardiology. 2. Cardiac intensive care.
    I. Title.
        [DNLM: 1. Anesthesia--methods. 2. Heart Surgery. 3. Heart--drug effects. 4. Critical Care.   WO 245 W319h 1997]
    RD87.3.H43W37 1997
    617.9'67412--DC21
    DNLM/DLC
    for Library of Congress   97-26004
                                                                          CIP

British Library Cataloguing-in-Publication Data
A catalogue record for this book is available from the British Library.

The publisher offers special discounts on bulk orders of this book.
For information, please contact:
Manager of Special Sales
Butterworth–Heinemann
313 Washington Street
Newton, MA 02158-1626
Tel: 617-928-2500
Fax: 617-928-2620

For information on all Butterworth–Heinemann publications available, contact our World Wide Web home page at: http://www.bh.com

10 9 8 7 6 5 4 3 2 1

Printed in the United States of America

Contents

Preface

Myths have been fixtures of the Western tradition since before the time of Homer. When we entered medical school and, later, residency, we expected to have little time for such literary diversion. To our surprise and disdain, we found that new myths were being written in nearly every cardiac surgery operating room on an almost daily basis. Institutional techniques, protocols, and drugs acquired an almost god-like reverence during the course of routine clinical care. Indeed, the phrase, "the way we do it" began to have an all too familiar and, frankly, annoying ring.

Of course, when these myriad ways of doing anesthesia were enshrined, a different paradigm for the specialty was operative. At that time, anesthesia was a "hot" field, with Alpha Omega Alpha graduates flocking to our ever-expanding residencies. New technologies, the role of the anesthesiologist as intensivist, and the growing need for anesthesia care made the specialty most attractive.

Today, trends are considerably different. Technologically based, specialty-centered practice has been chastened by the limitations of capitation. Our residencies go unfilled. Recent anesthesia residency graduates find themselves unable to locate employment as they go from fellowship to fellowship. Although anesthesiology today faces a surplus of physician graduates, it is not inconceivable that in years to come we will experience a shortfall. As residency positions go unfilled, an unfortunate shortage of competent, well-trained anesthesiologists may occur.

In such an environment, anesthesiologists would need to be as clinically flexible as possible. No longer would they be able to simply adhere to "the way." Anesthesiologists must be prepared to provide anesthetic care with what is available in a given setting. Pharmaceuticals and other technologies once deemed essential may no longer be so valued, as dictated by fiscal constraints. *Handbook of Cardiac Anesthesia and Perioperative Care* has been written to address a time of future limitations. My goal is to provide a cardiac anesthesia resource that avoids absolutes to the degree possible. It is principally structured to assist the anesthesiologist who infrequently provides cardiac care. Indeed, anesthesiologists who have been away from cardiac anesthesia for some time may find this an ideal brief refresher before returning to community cardiac anesthesia practice.

In creating this text, principles based on Aristotelian ideas regarding the ways of human understanding have been adopted. Aristotle posits that knowledge may be conceptualized as *theoria, poiesis,* and *praxis. Theoria* is the result of reflective thought. *Poiesis* is the acquisition of certain skills. Last, *praxis* is an understanding acquired through active engagement. Although this text will, to a degree, review theoretical concerns and technical skills, it is this text's primary purpose to provide a *praxis* understanding of our work. There are many fine, exhaustive texts of cardiac anesthesia and some very practical handbooks already available as well. So why this book? Why *praxis?* In essence, I hope to take the reader into the operating room along with me, just as I go every working day to provide cardiac anesthesia care. Along the way, I hope to strike down myths and legends and find a flexible approach to problems as faced by cardiac anesthesiologists in the course of daily practice. I avoid rigid protocols and excessive theoretical modeling. Practicing physicians, I believe, don't rely on either approach, and certainly neither do I.

The text begins and ends where cardiac anesthesia takes place: in the operating room and the intensive care unit, respectively. Starting with straightforward bypass patients, we will progressively meet increasingly complex cases. At all times, discussions are practical, flexible, and engaging. Forgive me if, at times, a ray of cynicism shines through. So then, let us meet our patients as we discover a flexible approach to cardiac anesthesia. One promise is made from the start: All of the patients in this book will live and none will file suit. If only real life practice were as promising.

JDW

Acknowledgments

Many people assisted with the preparation of this text. I especially wish to thank Karen Bohannon, who prepared the manuscript. Juan Carlos Reynoso, medical photographer, and Linka Behn, medical artist, also were of great help. Jana Friedman and Susan Pioli of Butterworth–Heinemann and Dana Tackett of Silverchair Science + Communications were very patient with me as I reworked this text. I am grateful to them for seeing this through to publication.

Last, I wish to thank Wendy, Basil, and Cosmo for putting up with many late nights and lost weekends. This text is dedicated to my many patients for allowing me the opportunity to practice medicine.

Handbook of Cardiac Anesthesia and Perioperative Care

I

Management of Otherwise Healthy Patients for Coronary Artery Bypass

Introduction

Now that you have chosen to practice cardiac anesthesia, where should you begin? Whether you find yourself as a resident, fellow, or established practitioner returning to cardiac practice, careful case selection will make your initial experience confidence building. The so-called otherwise healthy patient for coronary artery bypass may rank among the world's great oxymorons. Nevertheless, there are many unfortunate patients whose sole medical problem is angina that is unresponsive to medical or invasive cardiology therapy. Often, these patients have suffered no damage to the myocardium and generally are free of other organ system deficiencies. Although you may have little choice in your patient selection, a good praxis understanding of cardiac anesthesia first begins with a carefully guided development of your anesthesia skills. In other words, as we encounter patients and apply our knowledge and skills, it is far better to start out conservatively and then advance in patient difficulty. Too often, individuals are pushed beyond their level of expertise too quickly, only to find themselves and more importantly their patients in jeopardy. When such occurrences happen, surgeons and other institutional authorities come to believe that only certain anointed individuals possess skills to care for the sickest of patients. Although we do not deny that individual physicians may vary in their abilities, carefully matching physician and patient can allow the cardiac anesthesia novitiate to gradually take charge of the most difficult cases. Mismatching a patient and physician only leads to surgeons and institution retreating to reliance on institutional protocols and to the belief that only select individuals have the ability to provide anesthetic care. Such

3

rigidity, we believe, can only weaken the position of anesthesiologists in general while aggrandizing the reputations of a few.

To assist in managing the so-called otherwise healthy patient, Section I provides a comprehensive guide to the routine coronary artery bypass patient from start to finish. This provides a basic framework by which the rudimentary aspects of anesthesia care may be comprehended. By no means is this a cookbook approach to every patient. Only your own judgment can dictate what is proper for a given patient. Rather, we present a guide by which the essence of anesthesia decision making is distilled, leaving the academic and scientific details to be more comprehensively treated by many other fine texts.

So then, let us meet our first patient. Mr. XY is a 64-year-old man with minimal past history. During the past 3 months the patient has developed progressive exertional angina. There is no history of myocardial infarction. Cardiac catheterization revealed three-vessel disease with significant stenosis of the left anterior descending artery, circumflex artery, and the right coronary artery. Medical management has consisted of nitrate therapy and a calcium antagonist. He is scheduled for a three-vessel coronary artery bypass with left internal mammary artery.

Here we have a typical example of a so-called otherwise healthy patient for bypass. Indeed, the information provided previously is probably all that will be given to you as the anesthesiologist when you contact Mr. XY in the first place. Most likely, a patient with this history will be admitted on the morning of surgery, so your opportunity to contact Mr. XY and build what constitutes the 1990s version of the physician–patient relationship occurs primarily over the telephone in the immediate preoperative period. With the limited time to get to know the patient, what do we need to know about Mr. XY and how are we going to help navigate him through what will be for us a routine case, but for him one of the great stressors of his life? That is our goal in providing a praxis understanding: What do we need to know to get the patient through the procedure safely?

1

What the Anesthesiologist Needs to Know About the Coronary Artery Bypass Patient

Using the long-held notion that the anesthesiologist is the internist of the operating room, the cardiac anesthesiologist by extension has perpetuated the myth that the anesthesiologist is, in fact, the cardiologist of the operating room. Although it is true that a cardiac anesthesiologist will benefit from as extensive a background in cardiology as possible, it must never be forgotten that the anesthesiologist's main purpose in the operating room is not to be an internist or a cardiologist. Anesthesia alone carries responsibilities and a knowledge base without having to identify ourselves as some lesser operating room variant of a medical subspecialist. That point being made, however, it is important for the anesthesiologist to have a certain knowledge of cardiology so to maximally assist our patients.

Risk Factors

As an anesthesiologist, your need to know the risk factors for coronary disease are primarily self-serving. Namely, how do we avoid coronary artery disease in ourselves? After all, the patient is already here for bypass surgery, so the anesthesiologist is not likely to be able to effect any immediate life-style changes. Nevertheless, there are risk factors that can affect anesthesia management, and it is from this perspective, and this perspective alone, that we must identify the risks of coronary artery disease and assess their impact on how we provide anesthetic care.

Smoking

The coronary artery bypass (CAB) patient, even if otherwise healthy, may well have significant pulmonary disease as a consequence of excessive tobacco use. Often this information is not provided in any detail when the anesthesiologist is given patient information. Therefore, it is important to be as alert as possible to the presence of chronic obstructive pulmonary disease and bronchospasm in the CAB population deemed otherwise healthy. The anesthetic implications of pulmonary disease are discussed more fully in Chapter 2.

Diabetes Mellitus

The patient with juvenile-onset diabetes would hardly qualify as being otherwise healthy, considering the vast potential for debilitating nephropathy, retinopathy, and neuropathy, as well as other complications in this patient population. The patient with adult-onset diabetes mellitus presents a different scenario. Patients with adult-onset diabetes frequently have poor outpatient blood sugar control. Often they develop significant hyperglycemia associated with electrolyte and acid-base disturbances perioperatively. As such, it is useful to identify the patient with adult-onset diabetes preoperatively. Also, the adult-onset diabetic may be significantly overweight, resulting in potentially difficult airway and ventilatory management as a consequence of redundant pharyngeal tissue and restrictive lung disease, respectively. Last, autonomic dysfunction in patients with diabetic neuropathy may lead to cardiovascular collapse in the perioperative period as well as place the patient at risk for silent myocardial ischemia and infarction.

Hypertension

Again, as an anesthesiologist, there is little for us to do in correcting long-standing hypertension. Nevertheless, this risk factor for coronary

Table 1-1. Determinants of Essential and Secondary Hypertension

Essential hypertension
   Stress
   Diet
   Genetic factors
Secondary hypertension
   Pheochromocytoma
   Renal vascular disease
   Primary aldosteronism
   Cushing's syndrome
   Thyrotoxicosis

artery disease does present one or two challenges to consider as we approach the routine CAB patient. Hypertension may be considered either essential or secondary. The causes of both types of hypertension are listed in Table 1-1.

Although we would expect patients to have been identified and treated for hypertension by the time the anesthesiologist contacts them, we must nevertheless be aware of how hypertension may affect our anesthetic management. Anesthetic considerations focus on both the hypertension and the treatments for hypertension.

Untreated hypertension can lead to blood pressure lability perioperatively. As a consequence, patients are at risk for myocardial ischemia and ventricular dysfunction. The consequences of perioperative hypertension include myocardial ischemia, ventricular failure, pulmonary edema, aortic dissection, and intracerebral hemorrhage.

Antihypertensive therapy can lead to difficulties for the anesthesiologist perioperatively as well. Table 1-2 presents common antihypertensive therapies along with their associated adverse effects in general and those of concern to the anesthesiologist in particular. As seen in Table 1-2, patients taking antihypertensive medications have an increased likelihood of hypotension at the time of anesthesia induction. Nevertheless, the overwhelming majority of patients who are encountered will have been on antihypertension and anti-ischemia therapy for some time. It is best to continue therapy through the perioperative period to avoid potential ischemia and other complications during surgery that result from the withdrawal of antihypertensive medications.

Table 1-2. Common Antihypertensive Agents and Their Adverse Effects of Concern to the Anesthesiologist

Drug	Action	Adverse Effect
Methyldopa	Stimulates alpha receptors; decreases release of norepinephrine; decreases peripheral resistance	Orthostatic hypotension
Clonidine	Alpha$_2$ agonist; decreases release of norepinephrine; decreases renin release; decreases peripheral resistance	Orthostatic hypotension and acute hypertensive crisis on drug withdrawal
Beta blockers (propranolol, esmolol, metoprolol, atenolol)	Antagonizes effects of catecholamines at beta receptors; produces decreased heart rate and decreased cardiac output	Bronchospasm; bradycardia; hypotension
Angiotensin-converting enzyme inhibitors (enalapril, captopril)	Inhibits conversion of angiotensin I to angiotensin II; decreases aldosterone production; decreases vascular tone	Acute renal failure; orthostatic hypotension
Calcium antagonist (nifedipine, diltiazem)	Inhibits Ca^{2+} uptake in smooth muscle; decreases peripheral resistance	Reflex tachycardia; hypotension

Other Risk Factors

A family history of coronary artery disease, hyperlipidemia, and a seemingly daily increasing number of genetic markers all contribute to the development of coronary disease in given patients. Of course, these factors, unlike those previously highlighted, have little consequence to our role as anesthesiologists. We must always first and foremost concentrate on those risk factors that affect anesthetic management.

Table 1-3. Myocardial Ischemia: A Problem of Supply and Demand*

Determinants of Decreased Myocardial Oxygen Supply	Determinants of Increased Myocardial Oxygen Demand
Decreased blood oxygen content	Tachycardia
Reduction of coronary blood flow secondary to vasospasm, hypotension, and tachycardia	Increased myocardial contractility
Increased left ventricular pressure	Increased volume load to the heart
Fixed vascular obstruction	Increased myocardial wall tension Increased obstruction to ventricular outflow

*Ischemia results from either decreased oxygen supply or increased oxygen demand. Myocardial oxygen supply does not equal myocardial oxygen demand.

Mechanisms of Ischemia and Infarction

Having reviewed those risk factors that commonly bring patients to us, we must now address our patient, Mr. XY. Like many other patients, he has no history other than angina. We must conclude from the start that he presents as a consequence of a familial propensity toward vascular disease. However unfortunate our patient may be, his being otherwise healthy works in his favor. It is hoped that, not only will he do better from a surgical standpoint, but perhaps from an anesthetic standpoint as well.

But before we become too complacent, we must never forget our reason for encountering Mr. XY. He has angina and thus myocardial infarction is a threat. We must always ask what we as anesthesiologists can do that might hurt our patients. Therefore, an understanding of the mechanisms of ischemia and infarction is necessary to assist us in preventing perioperative ischemia and possibly infarction and death as a consequence of our anesthetic manipulations.

Although perhaps too easily stated as an imbalance in myocardial oxygen supply and demand, this model succinctly expresses the problem of myocardial ischemia (Table 1-3).

Considering the myriad causes of imbalance in the supply and demand equation, the opportunities for the anesthesiologist to disturb or correct this relationship are indeed great. Obviously, there is little the anesthesiologist can do that can alter fixed coronary lesions. After all, that is why the patient is in surgery. Nevertheless, the other determinants can be altered for better or worse in the course of manipulations conducted by the anesthesiologist.

The oxygen content of blood is determined by the concentration of serum hemoglobin and the blood oxygen saturation. Inadequate oxygenation obviously leads to myocardial ischemia, along with ischemia of other organ systems. Of course, this should hardly be revelatory to anyone at this stage in practice. Certainly, the anesthesiologist is not going to permit the patient to be deoxygenated. Similarly, it is unlikely that the anesthesiologist would permit the serum hemoglobin level to decrease to such a level so as to produce decreased blood oxygen content capable of producing myocardial ischemia. Nevertheless, patients refusing blood products may find themselves in such a situation (see Chapter 20 concerning Jehovah's Witnesses). More directly under the anesthesiologist's control are factors relating to cardiac performance that lead to inadequate myocardial oxygen supply.

Although coronary blood flow is autoregulated over a wide range of mean arterial pressures, in the presence of fixed lesions the ability of autoregulation of blood flow to compensate for vascular obstruction is minimal. Therefore, decreased systemic perfusion can lead to decreased coronary perfusion, resulting in decreased myocardial oxygen supply.

Likewise, as much of left coronary blood flow occurs during diastole, increases of left ventricular end-diastolic pressure can reduce oxygen supply to the heart. Tachycardia decreases diastolic time, which can lead to inadequate delivery of oxygenated blood to the myocardium.

Thus, the implications to the anesthesiologist caring for Mr. XY are clear. Should our anesthetic manipulations lead to tachycardia, hypotension, and hypoxemia, we put the patient at risk for ischemia. The classic cardiology consultation tells us to avoid hypoxemia and hypotension. Of course, when we receive such advice we generally simply say, "Thank you." As patronizing as such advice may be, it is essentially accurate based on the determinants of myocardial oxygen supply.

The anesthesiologist may also perturb the balance between oxygen supply and demand by altering the myocardial oxygen demand.

Increased myocardial contractility (as a consequence of autonomic stimulation) increases oxygen demand. Inadequate anesthesia leading to catecholamine release provides an example of an anesthesia-related precipitant of myocardial ischemia. Likewise, exogenously administered catecholamines may also contribute to myocardial oxygen demand. Increased myocardial wall tension also contributes to an increased need for myocardial oxygen supply. The LaPlace relationship directly relates ventricular wall tension to ventricular volume and pressure and indirectly to myocardial wall thickness. Although knowledge of such proportions is useful for examination purposes, anesthesiologists do not think in terms of this relationship in clinical practice. Rather, clinicians understand that increased intracavitary pressures and volumes lead to varying degrees of increased myocardial oxygen requirements. As discussed later in this text, providing Mr. XY with a nondistended, contracting heart will prove to be one goal of successful anesthesia management.

Ultimately, inadequate oxygen supply in the setting of uncompensated demand leads Mr. XY and those like him to suffer myocardial ischemia, infarction, or both. Myocardial infarction represents nothing less than individual myocyte death. Although mechanisms of cellular injury and cellular death are, of course, central to the future of medicine, they do not necessarily come to mind in the operating room. Perhaps as research progresses, we will discover that, indeed, such mechanisms should receive greater attention and, indeed, represent the future of both cardiology and cardiac anesthesia. For the present, however, the anesthesiologist should recall that as cellular myocardial adenosine triphosphate (ATP) concentrations decline, the various energy-dependent processes that lead to cellular and extracellular ion concentrations become dysfunctional. An elevated intracellular ionic calcium level further leads to a diminution in ATP formation and further disruption of cellular integrity. Although the anesthesiologist may not now directly practice molecular medicine per se, such a rudimentary understanding does caution against the indiscriminate use of calcium chloride perioperatively.

When examining myocardial ischemia and infarction at the level of the organ systems, it is clear that impairment of both systolic function and energy-dependent diastolic relaxation occurs with oxygen deprivation. The development of myocardial ischemia and infarction can produce any number of symptoms and signs (Table 1-4).

Of course, by the time we contact Mr. XY, the patient's angina should already be well under some form of medical control. Nevertheless, as we shall see, occasionally a patient is taken to surgery emergently after acute myocardial infarction. In this circumstance, the patient may not have been stabilized medically prior to our encounter with him or her. It is always preferable for the patient to have been stabilized medically before being taken for coronary artery revascularization. Still, even in those patients who are allegedly medically managed, the anesthesiologist may frequently encounter the patient having an

Table 1-4. Signs and Symptoms of Myocardial Ischemia

Chest pressure (angina)
Jaw or arm discomfort
Tachypnea
Diaphoresis
Nausea and vomiting
Syncope
Dysrhythmia
Hypotension
Shock
Pulmonary edema

acute episode of myocardial ischemia, infarction, or both. It is not unusual while on preoperative rounds to find a patient who demonstrates acute ischemia. Therefore, it is important that the practicing anesthesiologist be capable of identifying and initiating therapy for myocardial ischemia and infarction.

Brief Review of Tests of Cardiac Function

In addition to recognizing the classic and nonclassic symptoms of perioperative myocardial ischemia, the anesthesiologist in practice must have a basic understanding of the results of electrocardiography, myocardial enzyme studies, radionucleotide scans, and echocardiography in the diagnosis of perioperative ischemia and infarction.

Electrocardiographic changes reflect the varying intracellular ion concentrations associated with the development of ischemia and infarction. T-wave inversions, ST-segment elevations, ST-segment depressions, premature ventricular contractions, and Q waves herald possible myocardial ischemia, injury, and cellular death. Figure 1-1 provides some sample electrocardiographic changes associated with myocardial ischemia and infarction.

Myocardial enzymes are released at the time of cell death and provide markers of myocardial infarction. Creatine kinase–MB (CK–MB) band is specific for the myocardium. CK–MB levels increase several hours after myocardial infarction, peaking at 24 hours and then return-

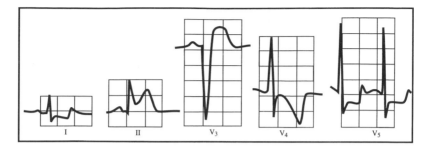

Figure 1-1. *Electrocardiographic changes associated with myocardial ischemia and infarction. (Modified from WJ Hoffman, JD Wasnick [eds]. Postoperative Critical Care of the Massachusetts General Hospital [2nd ed]. Boston: Little, Brown, 1992;143.)*

ing to normal over the ensuing 3-day postinfarction period. A CK–MB band of greater than 5% of total creatine kinase is considered diagnostic of myocardial infarction. Another marker, lactate dehydrogenase (LD) is present in five differing isozymes throughout the body. A ratio of LD1 to LD2 of more than 1 is considered diagnostic of myocardial infarction. LD1 elevation may remain increased for up to 2 weeks after myocardial infarction. Last, cardiac-specific troponin assay detects very small myocardial infarctions. Although the anesthesiologist generally will not be the one to make the diagnosis of myocardial infarction, it is nevertheless important to recognize that increases in myocardial enzyme concentrations may reflect an acute myocardial infarction in the immediate preoperative period. It is important to note myocardial enzyme concentration, especially in patients who are recently admitted with chest pain and are scheduled for surgery. The discovery of a myocardial infarction in the perioperative period may complicate patient management during the course of surgical revascularization.

Nuclear medicine may also be employed to assist in the diagnosis of myocardial ischemia and infarction. Table 1-5 briefly presents such tests and their applications.

Stress echocardiography, dobutamine, or dipyridamole-induced pharmacologic stress testing, along with advances in computerized tomography all may be used in screening patients for coronary vascular disease prior to invasive study.

At present, an anesthesiologist's awareness of the necessity of these tests is primarily for the sake of completeness to distinguish the physician anesthetist first and foremost from other practitioners. Although

Table 1-5. Nuclear Medicine Scans and Assessment of Myocardial Perfusion and Infarction

Study Type	Description
Technetium 99 pyrophosphate	Technetium 99 pyrophosphate concentrates in infarcted myocytes; it is used to detect myocardial infarction 2–3 days after cell death.
Gated blood pool scans	Nucleotide-labeled red blood cells provide an image of ventricular function and wall motion.
Thallium/exercise tolerance test	Thallium is delivered to perfused myocardium. Areas of myocardial ischemia and infarction appear as defects. Thallium redistributes to ischemic areas after recovery from pharmacologically or exercise-induced stress.

we are currently not called on to assess or evaluate such diagnostic dilemmas as whether the patient has had a myocardial infarction or if the patient needs cardiac catheterization, it should be remembered that the emphasis in anesthesia practice in the next century may compel the practitioner to be ever more the perioperative physician. Even though current patients such as Mr. XY present to us previously diagnosed with a particular condition, we can only begin to speculate on what the anesthesiologist's role may be in the coming decades. Indeed, nonintensivist anesthesiologists may be expected in the ensuing years to take even greater responsibility for the total perioperative management of the patient as part of their comprehensive duties.

Review of Medical Therapy for Myocardial Ischemia and Infarction

Like the overwhelming majority of patients, it is hoped that Mr. XY has already been stabilized on a medical regimen when he presents to the anesthesiologist. The medical interventions prior to the anesthesiologist's assumption of patient care may range from sublingual nitroglycerin to multiple catheterizations, angioplasty, and previous treatments with the latest "clot buster." The patients may or may not be prescribed any number of anticoagulants, anti-ischemics, and antiplatelet therapies. Because our patients generally present to us after having been evaluated and treated by our cardiology colleagues, we must first ask two pivotal questions: First, what were the cardiologist's goals in treating this patient? Second, how well did the cardiologist succeed (namely, why is the patient coming to surgery now)?

So then, what are the cardiologist's goals, and by extension our own, in treating the ischemic patient? We previously noted that ischemia was the result of an imbalance between myocardial oxygen supply and myocardial oxygen demand. Restoration of that balance is therefore paramount in the therapy and prevention of myocardial ischemia. Obviously, had Mr. XY developed ischemia as a consequence of decreased blood oxygen content, hypotension, or medically induced tachycardia, those causative factors would have been readily corrected. Rather, in our patient population, obstruction of coronary blood flow remains the primary agent responsible for an imbalance between oxygen supply and demand in the myocardium. How the cardiologist chooses to restore blood flow certainly affects perioperative management. Had Mr. XY waited until he had developed myocardial infarction, it is likely that he would have experienced possibly one or two interventions designed to restore blood flow to the ischemic myocardium.

Thrombolytic Therapy

The development of thrombus at the site of coronary atheromas provides the insult generally leading to myocardial injury and infarction. Thrombolytic therapy attempts to restore blood flow to injured myocardium so to minimize the extent of myocardial damage. The benefit of thrombolytic therapy has been questioned if initiated from 4 to 6 hours after myocardial infarction. Nevertheless, the possibility of improved oxygen delivery to so-called stunned, noninfarcted myocytes continues to lengthen the window by which institution of thrombolytic therapy is commenced. Intravenously administered tissue plasminogen activator and streptokinase constitute the mainstay of the "clot buster" armamentarium. Streptokinase has been associated with allergic reactions. Table 1-6 presents the contraindications and complications of intravenous thrombolytic therapy. After blood flow is restored, heparin anticoagulation is generally initiated.

Cardiac Catheterization and Angioplasty

Although angioplasty after thrombolytic therapy may not always be efficacious, patients with residual ischemia and chest discomfort are occa-

Table 1-6. Contraindications and Complications of Intravenous Thrombolytic Therapy

Contraindications
    Coagulopathy
    Stroke
    Intracranial lesions (aneurysm, arteriovenous malformation)
    Recent surgery
    Gastrointestinal bleeding
    Genitourinary bleeding
Complications
    Hypersensitivity reactions
    Reperfusion arrhythmias
    Coagulopathy
    Bleeding

sionally taken to the catheterization laboratory for an attempt to reopen occluded vessels. Chapter 12 describes anesthesia management for coronary angioplasty, both electively and in the emergency situation.

Impact of Medical Therapy on Anesthesia Management

Had our patient Mr. XY been so unfortunate as to develop a myocardial infarction, it is likely it would have been some time (days to weeks) before he would be taken electively to surgery. Of course, patients do not always have simple, straightforward myocardial infarctions. In fact, those patients with recent myocardial infarctions that anesthesiologists are likely to encounter will have already been treated with thrombolytic therapy, angioplasty, or both. In general, should such patients appear for surgery, their situation is often complicated by ventricular dysfunction leading to shock, by dysrhythmias, and by coagulopathy. Section II describes management of this type of patient in great detail. The practical message found herein is that if patients present to the anesthesiologist immediately after a myocardial infarction for which thrombolytic therapy, angioplasty, or both have failed, they must be considered as being in great jeopardy should emergency CAB be necessary.

Table 1-7. Nitrate Therapy in the Angina Patient

Route of Drug Delivery	Dose
Sublingual	0.3–0.6 mg (tablet or spray)
Oral (isosorbide dinitrate)	2.5–10 mg
Intravenous	50 μg/minute, increased as needed

Specific Medical Therapy for Myocardial Ischemia

Fortunately for anesthesiologists, the majority of our patients do not present directly from the catheterization laboratory with an acute infarction, having failed thrombolytic therapy. Rather, many patients are just like our typical patient, Mr. XY, an individual with coronary artery disease who has been managed medically for some time, but now has increasingly unstable angina. Many of Mr. XY's cohorts have undergone angioplasty in the past year or two. Others have experienced an uncomplicated myocardial infarction previously followed by several years of successful medical management. Medical management of the angina patient centers once again on maintaining a delicate balance between myocardial oxygen supply and demand.

Nitrates

At the very least, the overwhelming majority of patients such as Mr. XY will have readily administered nitroglycerin tablets, sprays, paste, and patches. Nitrates are vasodilators that principally decrease intraventricular volume and as a consequence intraventricular pressure. In this manner, they reduce myocardial oxygen demand and generally improve coronary perfusion pressure. Nitroglycerin may also be considered a coronary vasodilator. Nitrates may be administered sublingually (0.4-mg tablets), sublingually, by spray, topically, and orally. Patients admitted to the hospital may frequently be managed with intravenous nitroglycerin. Oral and topical nitrates are typically a part of an anti-ischemia regimen for the angina patient. Table 1-7 provides a guide to nitrate therapy. Associated adverse effects include headache, hypotension, methemoglobinemia, and ventilation/perfusion mismatch secondary to impairment of hypoxic pulmonary vasoconstriction.

Table 1-8. Comparative Effects of Calcium Channel Blockers

	Nifedipine	Nicardipine	Nimodipine	Diltiazem	Verapamil
Decreased blood pressure	+++	+++	+++	+++	+++
Coronary vasodilation	+++	+++	+++	++	++
Increased heart rate	++	++	++	±	±
Venous capacitance	0	0	0	0	0
Decreased inotropy	+	0	+	++	+++
Decreased atrioventricular conduction	0	0	0	+++	+++

0 = negligible effect; + = greater effect; ± = greater or lesser effect.
Source: Modified from WJ Hoffman, JD Wasnick (eds). Postoperative Critical Care of the Massachusetts General Hospital (2nd ed). Boston: Little, Brown, 1992.

Calcium Antagonists

Calcium channel blockers frequently find their way into anti-ischemia regimens due to their ability to affect the myocardial oxygen supply and demand balance. To varying degrees, calcium antagonists produce vasodilation, thereby reducing ventricular volume and myocardial wall tension. Likewise, decreased myocardial contractility associated with certain calcium channel blockers (i.e., diltiazem, verapamil), along with calcium channel antagonist induced bradycardia may reduce myocardial oxygen demand (Table 1-8). Adverse reactions seen in patients taking calcium antagonists include bradycardia, ventricular failure, reflex tachycardia, and hypotension. The continuing use of calcium antagonists remains the subject of ongoing investigation regarding their role in anti-ischemia therapy. Nevertheless, it is likely that patients such as Mr. XY will present having been administered some form of calcium antagonist (Table 1-9).

Table 1-9. Routine Dosage of Calcium Antagonists

Drug	Dosage
Nifedipine	10–20 mg PO q8h
Verapamil	80 mg PO q8h up to 480 mg/qd
Diltiazem	30–90 mg PO q6h up to 360 mg/qd

Table 1-10. Beta Blockers Likely To Be Encountered by the Anesthesiologist

Drug	Dose	Property
Atenolol	50–100 mg PO qd	Long-acting, cardioselective
Metoprolol	100–200 mg PO qd (divided)	Long-acting, cardioselective
Propranolol	100–240 mg PO qd (divided)	Nonselective
Labetalol	200–400 mg PO bid	Nonselective beta blockade, minimal alpha blockade

Beta Blockers

Beta blockers remain an essential component of both anti-ischemia and antihypertension therapy. Patients presenting for CAB are frequently being treated with beta blockade. The list of beta blockers available is seemingly endless and the choice of drug depends on $beta_1$-receptor (myocardial) selectivity as well as ease of dosage. As with other mainstays of anti-ischemia therapy, beta blockers affect the balance between myocardial oxygen supply and demand. By inhibiting catecholamine action at $beta_1$-receptors, myocardial contractility and heart rate are reduced. As a consequence, oxygen demand is decreased. Beta blocker–induced bradycardia may likewise improve oxygen delivery as a consequence of increasing diastolic time. Of course, these benefits may be offset by decreased myocardial contractility and the resulting decrease in cardiac output.

$Beta_2$-receptor blockade can impair $beta_2$-mediated peripheral vasodilation and bronchodilation.

Beta-blockade therapy is an essential component of treatment for myocardial infarction. Improved survival after myocardial infarction occurs in patients treated by beta blockade primarily as a consequence of beta blockers' antiarrhythmogenicity as well as by decreasing myocardial oxygen demand (Table 1-10). Adverse effects of beta blockers include hypotension, ventricular failure, bronchospasm, bradycardia, and fatigue.

Summary

Having now reviewed common medical therapy for ischemia prophylaxis, there may be the tendency to attempt to adjust a patient's medical management perioperatively. Anesthesiologists often worry about the interaction of myocardial depressants such as calcium antagonists and beta blockers when coupled with the depressant effects of anesthetic agents. As such, anesthesiologists frequently attempt to remove such therapy preoperatively. Additionally, anesthesiologists suffering from unchecked ego attempt to alter medical therapy perioperatively because they believe that they, and not the cardiologist, know what is best for the patient. Both courses of action can lead to difficulties for both the physician and patient in the perioperative period. In general, it is prudent to continue all anti-ischemia medications perioperatively. This is especially true because the patient, such as Mr. XY, will often be coming to the hospital from home and is, as such, outside of our immediate medical management. Although anecdotal experiences are simply that, many anesthesiologists can recall at least one occasion when surgery was canceled because an outpatient died on the way to the hospital on the morning of surgery. Clearly, had the anesthesiologist attempted to alter medical therapy in the immediate perioperative period, such manipulations could have led to accusations and medicolegal jeopardy. Therefore, it is surely best to avoid any significant adjustment in medical therapy in the immediate perioperative period.

Often it is wise when contacting the outpatient CAB patient the night before surgery to inquire as to whether the patient has experienced any angina symptoms that day. If the patient gives any indication of increased angina, it is advisable to instruct the patient to go to the hospital and contact the primary caregiver. It is never wise to alter medical therapy over the telephone.

Should we be fortunate enough to find our patient in the hospital, therapy can be better controlled. Nevertheless, it remains advisable not to adjust medical therapy without first consulting the cardiologist, surgeon, or both. Although such adjustments may be indicated, any adverse outcome resulting from an anesthesiologist's action outside of the immediate preoperative period will be subject to interspecialty criticism.

So What's Wrong with Mr. XY Anyway?

Like all patients who find their way to cardiac surgery, somewhere along the way Mr. XY and others like him have undergone a left-sided heart catheterization. Although as anesthesiologists we do not need to be particularly adroit at the interpretation of catheterization films, we should use such films and the reports generated by them to alert us to some potential concerns relating to our management in the perioperative period.

The presence of significant occlusions of the left main coronary artery should immediately indicate the tenuous nature of the patient's condition. Such disease signifies that the left ventricle is at jeopardy in the event of myocardial ischemia or infarction. These patients present particular challenges from anesthesia induction up to the time of cardiopulmonary bypass. Coronary stenosis of approximately 50% may be considered significant. Varying combinations of lesions of the circumflex and left anterior descending arteries similarly can put patients at great risk for myocardial infarction. From a practical standpoint, knowledge of the extent and number of lesions is critical to anesthesia management. First, by knowing the severity of the lesions (i.e., left main stenosis), we are better prepared for sudden hemodynamic collapse and the need for institution of bypass emergently. Second, should several bypass grafts be planned, we can expect a relatively longer time for the cardiopulmonary bypass (especially if performed by a particularly slow surgeon). Longer periods of cardiopulmonary bypass and the increased requirements for cardioplegia result in increased volume delivery to the patient intraoperatively, with resulting hemodilution. If this is expected, the availability of blood products should be closely confirmed. Also, we can expect potentially greater difficulty in weaning the patient from cardiopulmonary bypass (see Chapter 6) should prolonged bypass time be required. Last, the presence of occlusive disease throughout the vascular system may imply that no clear location exists for the surgeon to attach bypass grafts due to the occlusion. In this setting, potentially time-consuming coronary endarterectomies may be indicated, further prolonging the bypass and thereby increasing postbypass difficulties (see Chapter 6). Such difficulties include coagulopathy, platelet consumption, ventricular dysfunction, and ventilatory insufficiency. Figure 1-2 presents angiographic views of normal and diseased coronary vasculature.

Ventriculography outlines the left ventricular cavity, providing an assessment of ventricular wall motion and left ventricular function.

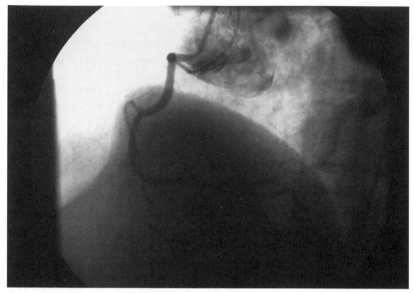

A

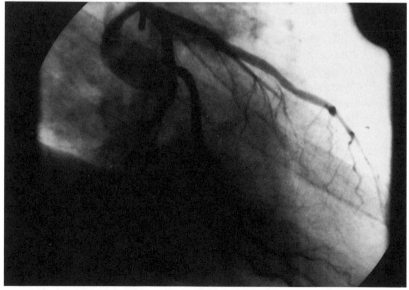

B

Figure 1-2. *(A) The right coronary artery. (B) The left coronary arterial system. (C) The right coronary artery with lesions. (D) The left coronary anatomy with lesions.*

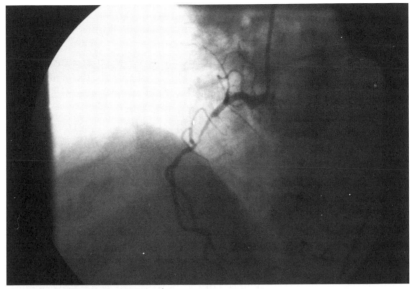

C

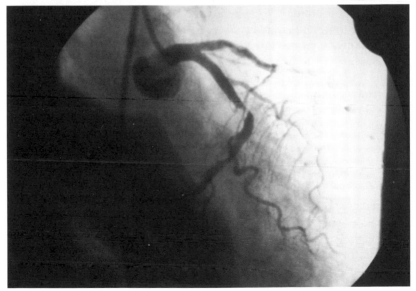

D

Areas of wall motion abnormality are identified, as are ventricular aneurysms. Mitral insufficiency is characterized. Figure 1-3 presents typical ventriculograms.

As we shall see in Chapter 6, adequacy of ventricular function is a strong predictor of perioperative mortality and morbidity. Knowledge of left ventricular function is imperative in planning anesthetic management. Measurement of intracavitary pressures similarly assists in assessment of left ventricular function. Increased left ventricular end-diastolic pressure (higher than 15 mm Hg) may well indicate ventricular dysfunction. Valvular lesions and the pressure gradients associated with them also affect ventricular dysfunction and are discussed in Chapter 14.

Having briefly examined the course that has led our patient to the operating room, we will now spend a few moments and look at exactly how surgery itself will unfold. After all, specialty anesthesia is first and foremost just plain old anesthesia. This does not imply that anesthesia consists of just using either the big syringe or the little syringe. This type of anesthesia is not fundamentally different from any other type of anesthesia either. So what then makes cardiac anesthesia different? The chapters that follow attempt to examine that question. But first and foremost, we believe that the myriad activities that surround the surgery and perfusion teams may lead trainees and those who practice cardiac anesthesia less frequently to become distracted by the tubes, tension, and ego that permeate such environments. Also, established anesthesiologists in our experience often fail to explain to trainees what the surgical team is doing. Therefore, to assist in identifying what our surgical colleagues are up to, we review the operative procedure step by step photographically.

Brief Overview of Coronary Artery Bypass

Following is a discussion of the CAB procedure; Chapter Appendix 1 provides a step-by-step, visual depiction of the the process.

Induction and intubation are completed after venous access and arterial monitoring are established. Next central access is achieved, and the pulmonary artery flotation catheter is passed. Bladder catheterization is also completed. Prophylactic antibiotics are administered. The sternum is prepared and the incision made. The assistant harvests the vein from the saphenous system while the surgeon frequently dissects the internal mammary artery. A radial artery may also be taken as a bypass conduit. The pericardium is next incised and the heart exposed. After

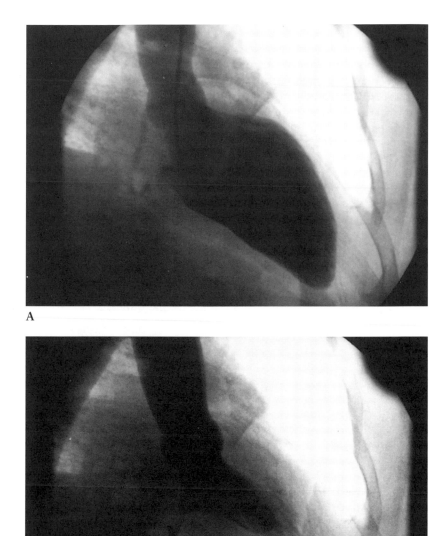

A

B

Figure 1-3. *A ventriculogram at end diastole (A) and at end systole (B).*

heparinization, the aorta cannula is placed, which will return oxygenated blood from a bypass circuit. The venous cannula is next positioned. Once adequate anticoagulation is confirmed, the surgeon releases clamps on the venous cannula and cardiopulmonary bypass is commenced. Aortic cardioplegia cannula and coronary sinus catheters are placed to provide anterograde and retrograde cardioplegia, respectively. The aorta is cross clamped, eliminating the flow of blood to the heart. Cardioplegia is infused and the heart arrested. Distal anastomosis is then completed. The cross clamp is removed, and the proximal anastomosis is then attached. The patient is next weaned from bypass. The bypass cannulas are removed and anticoagulation reversed. The sternum is closed and the surgery completed.

What a wonderful world it would be if such operations were always to go as smoothly as in our pictorial presentation. They don't, but then again why not start with anything but a perfect case done by perfect surgeons and, of course, lest we forget, perfect anesthesiologists. As we continue through this section, we examine more closely how anesthesiologists can help or hinder the progress of surgery such as that outlined.

Appendix 1:
Coronary Artery Bypass

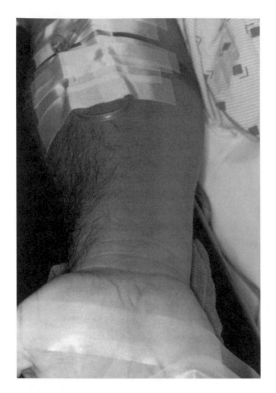

Figure 1A-1. *Intravenous A-line position.*

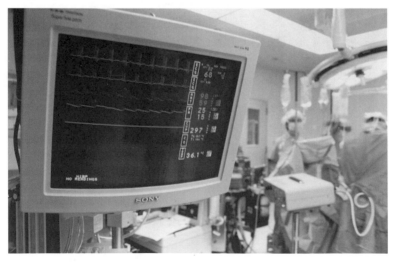

Figure 1A-2. *Hemodynamic monitoring at induction and intubation.*

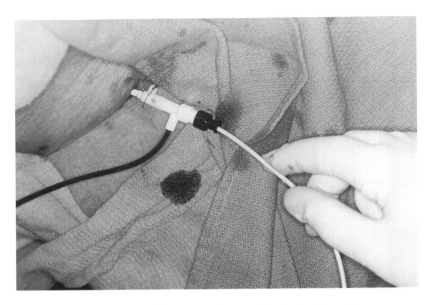

Figure 1A-3. *Swan-Ganz placement after antibiotic administration.*

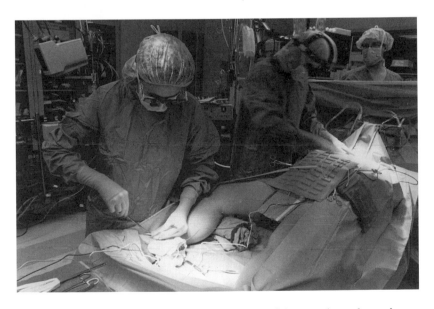

Figure 1A-4. *Sternal preparation and bypass graft harvest from the saphenous vein system.*

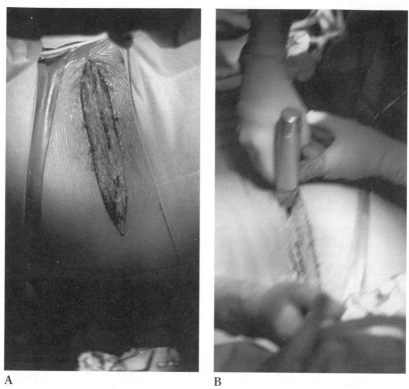

A   B

Figure 1A-5. *(A) Skin incision. (B) Sternal saw is used to open the chest through median sternotomy incision.*

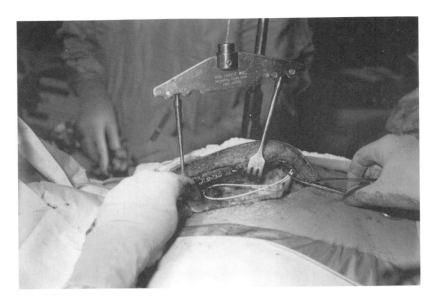

Figure 1A-6. *Mammary artery harvest.*

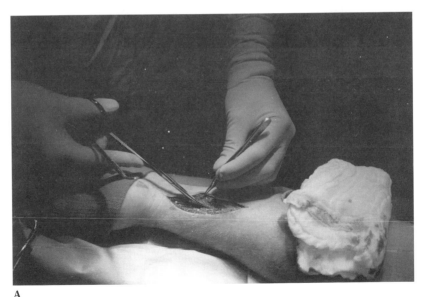

A

Figure 1A-7. *(A) Beginning radial artery harvest.*

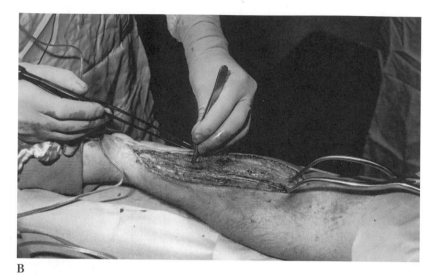

B

Figure 1A-7. *Continued. (B) Radial artery exposed.*

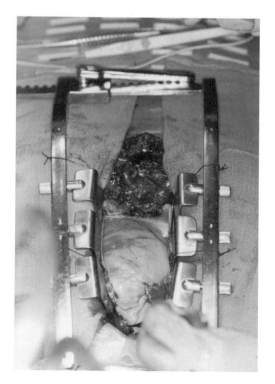

Figure 1A-8. *Pericardial resection and exposure of the heart with a sternal retractor.*

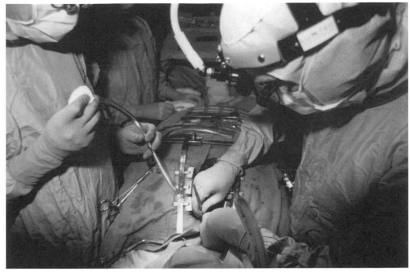

A

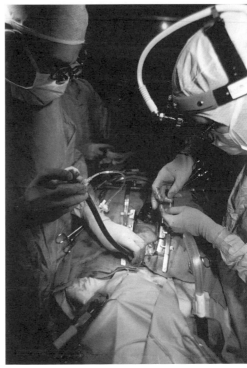

Figure 1A-9. *Aorta cannulation. (A) The surgeon opens the aorta for placement of the cannula. (B) Aortic blood returns to the aortic perfusion cannula.*

B

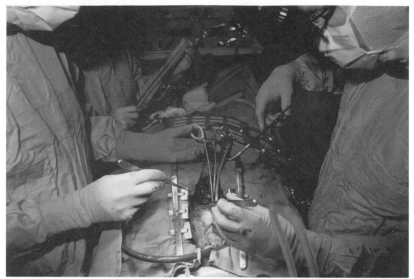

A

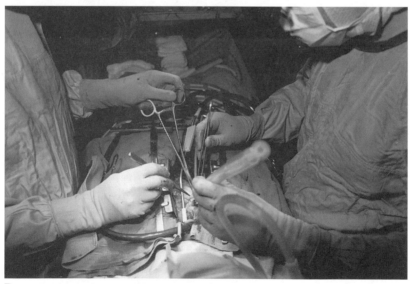

B

Figure 1A-10. *Venous cannulation. (A) Atrial cannulation sutures are placed in the right atrium. (B) Venous drainage cannula is placed. (C) Aortic and venous cannulas are attached to lines to connect to the cardiopulmonary bypass machine.*

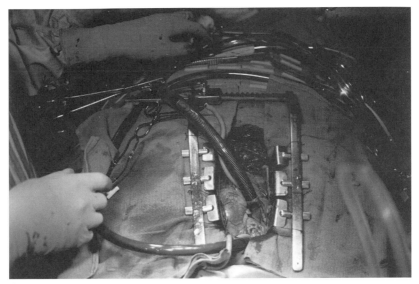

C

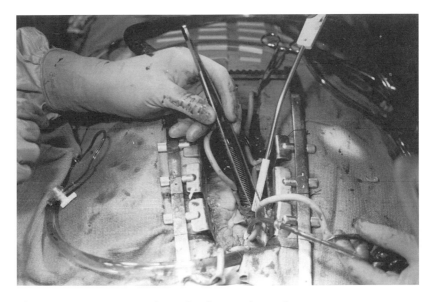

Figure 1A-11. *Anterograde cardioplegia catheter placement.*

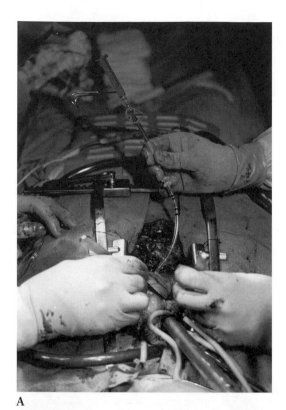

Figure 1A-12. *Coronary sinus cannulation. (A) Retrograde cardioplegia catheter. (B) Retrograde cardioplegia catheter placed in the coronary sinus.*

A

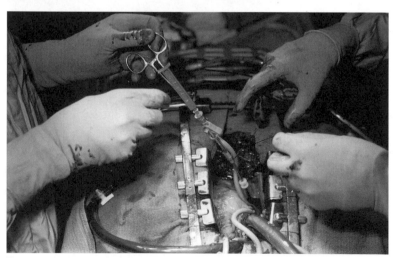

B

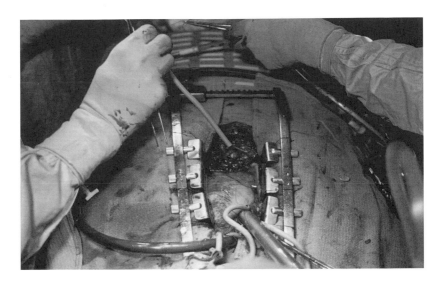

Figure 1A-13. *Initiation of cardiopulmonary bypass.*

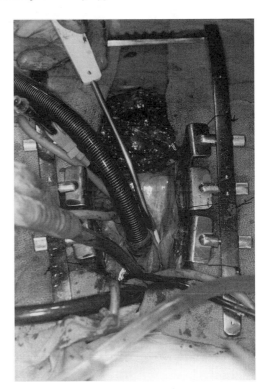

Figure 1A-14. *The heart before cardioplegia and the application of cross clamp.*

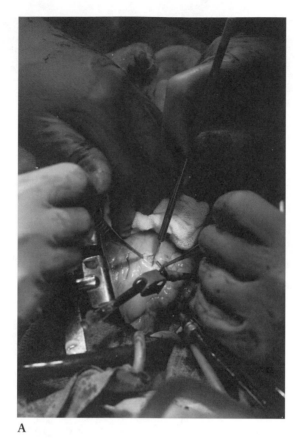

A

Figure 1A-15. *Distal anastomosis. (A) Site for distal anastomosis identified. (B) Bypass graft prepared.*

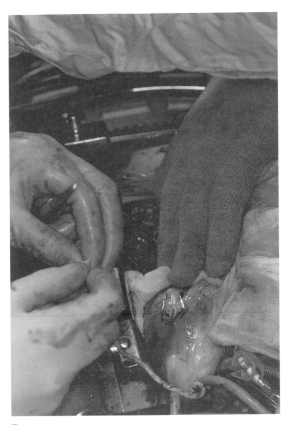

B

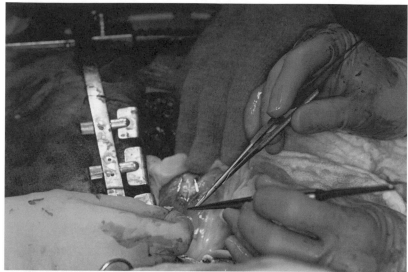

C

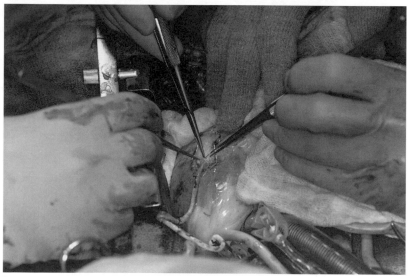

D

Figure 1A-15. *Continued. (C) Graft attached to distal anastomotic site (I). (D) Graft attached to distal anastomotic site (II). (E) Distal graft attachment completed.*

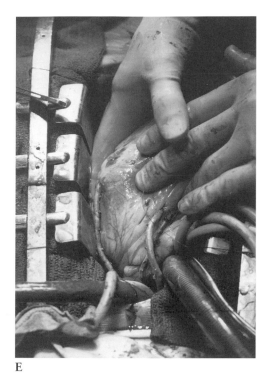

E

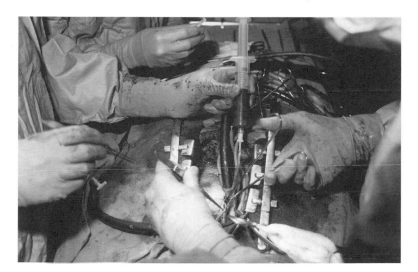

Figure 1A-16. *Proximal anastomosis.*

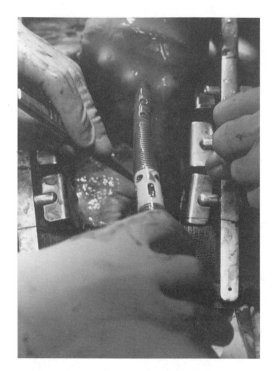

Figure 1A-17. *Venous cannula out after patient successfully weaned from cardiopulmonary bypass.*

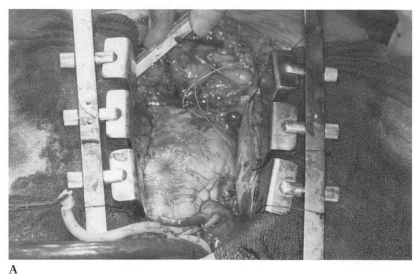

A

Figure 1A-18. *Arterial cannula out. (A) Arterial cannula in place in aorta.*

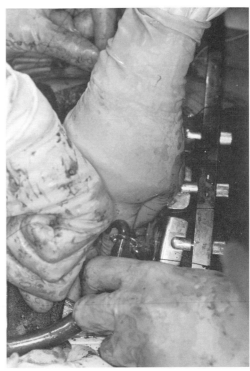

Figure 1A-18. *(B) Arterial cannula withdrawn by surgeon. (C) Cannula removed; the proximal graft anastomosis visible.*

B

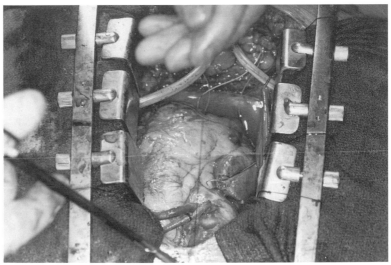

C

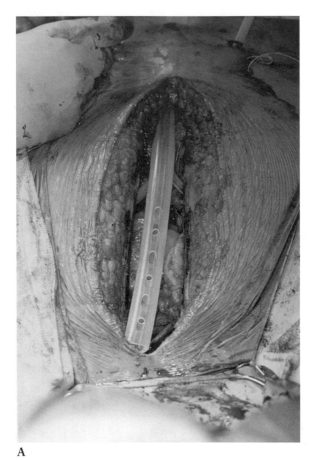

A

Figure 1A-19. *The chest before sternal wire placement. (A) Mediastinal chest tube in position. (B) Sternal wires being placed. (C) Sternal wires ready for chest closure.*

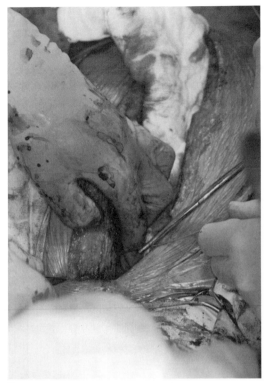

B

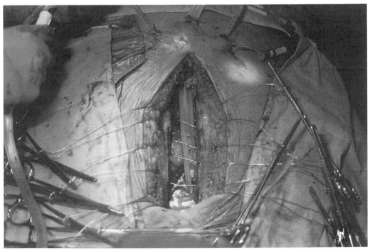

C

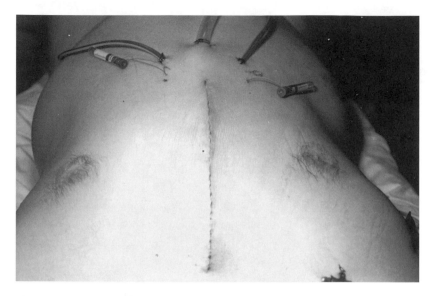

Figure 1A-20. *Closed chest. Epicardial pacemaker wires contained in test tube bottles.*

2

Preoperative Visit

Is the Patient Otherwise Healthy?

Now that we have reviewed the circumstances that might lead Mr. XY and those like him to our attention, we can begin to assess him as a candidate for anesthesia. Remember, his cardiologist and surgeons have already declared him a candidate for surgery. What they most assuredly have not considered are the specific concerns that we might have as anesthesiologists. Therefore, we submit that we should not be overly concerned with their decision making either. Nevertheless, as we shall see, it is prudent to be on guard for those events and conditions that might be beneficial to the patient if we should choose to delay a case. Therefore, in bringing our otherwise healthy patient to surgery, we must first ask, is the patient otherwise healthy? To answer this, we turn to our anesthesia history and physical examination (such as they are). Unfortunately, our opportunities to conduct a history and physical examination may be quite limited. With same-day cardiac surgery now quite routine, the time with which to conduct a patient interview is limited. We recommend that if you have no prescreening anesthesia clinic, the history be obtained by telephone the day before surgery. This will give you time to locate all records should you happen on a patient with some horrible anesthesia complication that the patient will no doubt be eager to recount to you. The physical examination, such as it is, can be readily completed on the morning of surgery, along with review of laboratory studies and other pertinent tests.

Anesthesia History

We are principally responsible for the patient's anesthesia management. We begin our contact with the patient with a simple, but very telling question, "Have you ever had anesthesia before?" Yes, of course, we are interested in their chest pain and their medical regimen, but we need to know what anesthesia encounters the patient has had in the past. How well did the patient tolerate our intervention? In particular, we are interested to know if other anesthesiologists had difficulty completing endotracheal intubation. We are constantly surprised by how many individuals are given such messages to relate to their future doctors by concerned and honest anesthesiologists. When we hear such information, we take this message quite seriously. We never presume that we will be so much more skillful than our predecessors at completing endotracheal intubation. Rather, we attempt to locate previous anesthesia records and, pending our physical examination, execute our plan for management of the difficult airway in the cardiac surgical patient (see Chapter 3).

Similarly, we prompt the patient for any allergic reactions and the character of those allergic responses. In particular, we are interested in the exact nature of those adverse reactions, especially to medicines that are likely to be encountered in the perioperative period. Often we are told of an "allergy to all 'caines,'" namely lidocaine, which, in fact, is not an allergy at all, but simply recollection of anesthesia toxicity. So-called morphine allergies often are, in fact, the result of histamine release that occurs after intravenous injection. True anaphylactic reactions are relatively uncommon; however, we obviously take all measures to prevent these occurrences. Last, we attempt to elicit from the patient some expression as to their emotional response to their upcoming anesthesia and surgery. This provides a good opportunity to get some sense of the patient's personality to better assess his or her needs. Should the patient express fear of loss of control, then we can adjust our interactions so as to be maximally empowering to the patient. On the other hand, if the patient expresses pure fright, perhaps a more sympathetic approach is beneficial. Of course, only experience in individual practice can determine the best interaction to undertake with a given patient. In general, we follow the dictates of what we call the three F's: friendly, formal, and formidable. In essence, we are friendly in a way that retains the formal professional nature of the doctor–patient relationship. At all times, however, we never lose sight of the fact that the patient is about to experience a formidable challenge. We also make certain the family and friends of the patient are likewise aware of the keen challenge both to the patient and the physician of cardiac surgery. A plain-speaking approach is our best protection against being involved in potential litigation (see Chapter 20).

Pulmonary History

After completing the general anesthesia history, we next focus our attention on those organ systems that might directly affect our anesthesia management. Although our patient may be labeled as being otherwise healthy, as we noted in Chapter 1, tobacco use is a clear risk factor for coronary artery disease. Similarly, tobacco use's contribution to pulmonary disease is not fully documented. The patient should be questioned as to continued tobacco use, wheezing, mucus production, dyspnea, orthopnea. We ask each patient if he or she has ever been admitted to the emergency room with breathing difficulties. If the patient has had hospitalization secondary to pulmonary disease, we inquire as to the need for ventilatory assistance or tracheostomy. We ask about a history of corticosteroid use and bronchodilator therapy and arrange for the continuation of those treatments through the perioperative period. We additionally acquire a history of deep vein thrombosis and pulmonary embolism. Should such a history be obtained, we avoid the use of antifibrinolytic therapy intraoperatively. Although we are generally concerned with the presence of chronic obstructive pulmonary disease, we must also be cognizant of the presence of restrictive pulmonary disease as well. Patients with connective tissue disease may well present with pulmonary restriction. Similarly, by account of their size, the massively obese are at increased risk for restrictive pulmonary disease. Should such patients be encountered, they should be carefully questioned in regard to any symptoms suggestive of respiratory insufficiency. These patients, in general, will need to be advised of the likelihood of a prolonged period of postoperative respiratory assistance.

Cardiac History

Because our patients are fully evaluated regarding cardiac function by catheterization study and echocardiography, there may be little new information to gain by any extensive cardiac history gathering. Nevertheless, a few points are worth noting. First, it is useful to have the patient characterize his or her angina pain. Not only will this description alert you to the particular symptomatology should the patient develop angina in the perioperative period, but it will also give you the opportunity to tell the patient to inform you should he or she develop any chest discomfort while you are caring for the patient. Second, we ask if those symptoms have occurred with greater frequency in the day or so leading up to our phone call or meeting the patient. Generally, patients have been stabilized on a medical regimen prior to being admitted for surgery. Nevertheless, we often find patients developing unstable angina or crescendo angina up through the night of surgery. If you call a patient and are told that he or she is having chest pain, it is important to emphasize that the patient should contact an ambulance and the appropriate surgeon or cardiologist be notified. One should never, as an anesthesiologist, attempt to treat angina over the phone. Regrettably, patients do not often recognize that their symptomatology has changed, and occasionally surgery is canceled because the patient has died simply as a consequence of not being in the hospital or responding to chest discomfort at the time of surgery. Third, it is important to question the patient as to whether he or she has experienced any sustained chest pain or any new symptoms since being evaluated by the primary care givers. Fresh myocardial infarction, the development of pulmonary edema, and so forth may increase the risk of surgery, and should the patient's history warrant it, myocardial enzyme studies or other tests may need to be obtained to rule out an infarction in the immediate preoperative period. If they remain otherwise stable, patients with recent myocardial infarction might benefit from medical stabilization before proceeding to surgery.

Similarly, we inquire about a history of arrhythmias and the new onset of palpitations. Rhythm disturbances can complicate the perioperative course. Should we identify a new onset atrial fibrillation, supraventricular tachycardias, or ventricular arrhythmias, we can arrange for cardiology consultation and rhythm stabilization prior to elective coronary bypass. Last, we remind the patient to continue antianginal, antiarrhythmic, and antihypertensive regimens throughout the perioperative period. In general, we continue all such medications throughout the hospital course leading up to surgery. Although many medications may adversely interact with anesthetics, we nonetheless prefer to continue the current medical regimen and adjust our anesthetic technique as needed to respond to any deleterious impact that anti-ischemic or antianginal therapy might present.

History of Renal Disease

For those patients not requiring hemodialysis and peritoneal dialysis, a history of renal disease may be difficult to illicit. Although hypertension, anemia, and electrolyte and acid–base imbalances may herald the presence of renal disease, in general, it is a diagnosis made by laboratory evidence. Those patients who present with an elevated serum creatinine level (more than 1.7 mg per dl) have an increased risk of perioperative renal dysfunction. Patients currently being treated with dialysis need to be managed perioperatively in close consultation with a nephrologist. Generally, dialysis is planned the day before surgery and perhaps again for the day after surgery to correct any electrolyte or fluid imbalances that occur as a consequence of potassium-laden cardioplegia and the volume load incumbent with cardiopulmonary bypass.

From an anesthesiology perspective, drugs completely dependent on the kidney for excretion should probably be avoided. Excess potassium should likewise be avoided in any perioperative infusion of intravenous fluid. Patients with arterial venous shunts should be recognized so that their arms can be carefully padded and protected to prevent any injury to the shunt perioperatively.

History of Hepatic Disease

Unless our patient appears icteric, we may be tempted simply to avoid obtaining any history of hepatic injury in general or alcoholism in particular. We recommend that inquiry be made as to alcohol consumption because heavy alcohol use frequently results in increased anesthesia requirements as a consequence of cross tolerance. Additionally, because the hospitalized patient will not be able to access the beverage of choice, we can be prepared to provide adequate benzodiazepine supplementation to prevent or treat the development of alcoholic withdrawal. As with the risks of perioperative ischemia, tachycardia resulting from alcoholic withdrawal would certainly be potentially deleterious to those patients at risk for coronary ischemia. Additionally, the delirious patient may go into withdrawal in the intensive care unit, where tubes and other cannulas may be readily disrupted by the thrashing patient. Many hospitals have liquor and other spirits available on the hospital formulary and we recommend that those patients who are at risk for alcoholic withdrawal be provided with the appropriate prophylaxis.

While obtaining a history related to alcoholism, it is also convenient to politely inquire about other substance abuse. In particular, intravenous drug abuse is of concern, not only because of the increased risk of human immunodeficiency virus infection (HIV) (although, of course, we employ universal precautions on all patients), but because vascular access may prove to be particularly difficult.

Patients occasionally give us a history of having hepatitis. Rarely is the patient able to identify the infectious agent by type. As such, universal precautions remain a cornerstone of cardiac anesthesia practice. Whether hepatitis occurs as a consequence of alcohol ingestion, an infectious agent, right ventricular failure, or another toxin, the anesthesiologist must carefully assess what effects hepatic dysfunction may have on anesthesia management. Such liver dysfunction may affect anesthetic management in the following ways: (1) coagulopathy, secondary to depleted coagulation factors; (2) esophageal varices complicating transesophageal echocardiography probe placement; (3) encephalopathy, although it is hoped that an encephalopathic patient would not be scheduled for elective heart surgery; (4) renal dysfunction, with the risk of hepatorenal syndrome; (5) bacterial peritonitis, not that a patient with peritonitis would be an operative candidate; and (6) arteriovenous shunting leading to inadequate oxygen delivery.

Although patients with hepatic failure resulting in encephalitis or hepatic renal syndrome would not be considered candidates for coronary artery bypass, cardiac patients with only alcoholic and viral hepatitis and cirrhosis are nonetheless often taken to coronary bypass surgery. The diseased liver may be more sensitive to perioperative hypoperfusion, which can lead to postoperative hepatic dysfunction with its myriad complications.

History of Hematologic Disorders

Generally, the surgeon or cardiologist will have identified any specific problems with the coagulation or hematologic status of the patient. Sickle cell disease, thalassemia, von Willebrand's disease, as well as the hemophilias, will generally have been identified long before our contact with the patient. Close communication with the patient's hematologist will assist in providing for red cell, platelet, and factor transfusions as necessary depending on the patient's primary hematologic disease state.

Close history taking may reveal that the patient has continued aspirin therapy or warfarin (Coumadin) up to the day of surgery, neces-

Table 2-1. Hematologic Disorders of Note to the Cardiac Anesthesiologist

Hemophilia A: X-linked recessive disorder leading to decreased factor VIII (procoagulant)

Symptoms: hemarthroses and ecchymoses

Therapy: factor VIII replacement via cryoprecipitate or factor concentrate

Hemophilia B: X-linked recessive disorder leading to decreased factor IX (procoagulant)

Symptoms: hemarthroses and ecchymoses

Therapy: factor IX replacement

von Willebrand's disease: Autosomal dominant disorder leading to decreased von Willebrand's factor

Symptoms: epistaxis and prolonged surgical bleeding

Therapy: factor VIII; von Willebrand's factor replacement through cryoprecipitate; DDAVP (0.3–0.4 µg/kg)

Sickle-cell disease: hemoglobin S causes red cells to sickle at low oxygen saturation

Therapy: avoid hypothermia, hypoxemia, vasoconstriction; exchange transfusion

Symptoms: Organ ischemia, splenic infarction, stroke

---

sitating assessment of bleeding time as well as prothrombin and partial thromboplastin times. If the patient is maintained on heparin therapy perioperatively, there is a possibility of resistance to heparin when providing suitable anticoagulation for cardiopulmonary bypass (see Chapter 5). Additionally, heparin-induced thrombocytopenia may necessitate platelet transfusion postbypass.

On a practical note, a review of the hematology history may first and foremost alert the anesthesiologist to check that a blood sample has been drawn for cross match should blood products be required. Although correcting hematology disorders preoperatively rests squarely on the hematologist, cardiologist, and surgeon, it is nonetheless important that the anesthesiologist be vigilant that those problems that might lead to hemorrhage be identified preoperatively and appropriately treated. Table 2-1 briefly describes some hematologic disorders and outlines appropriate preoperative therapies.

Fortunately, our patient has a simple history free of the numerous complicating factors discussed previously. Nevertheless, a quick history can identify a number of problems that complicate anesthesia as well as surgery. Thus, to the degree possible, identification of those problems can ease anesthetic management and after all, that is our goal.

Preoperative Physical Examination and Laboratory Review

Let's be frank: We have never heard of anesthesiologists teaching physical diagnosis in medical school. Perhaps some of you have, but in general, the physical examination is not considered the anesthesiologist's overarching strength. Of course, this does not mean that physical diagnosis is not important to the cardiac anesthesiologist. Indeed, a careful, directed, time-efficient physical examination relating to those things essential to the anesthesiologist must be performed as a matter of patient safety. As such, we do not have to transform ourselves into clones of Osler. Rather, we need to construct an examination relevant to our role as anesthesiologists in general and cardiac anesthesiologists in particular. Obviously before engaging in any physical examination it is worthwhile to check the vital signs. One can never be sure what a patient might be up to. Once the vital signs are considered to be acceptable and the patient is considered alive and stable, then proceed to the rest of the examination.

Airway, Airway, Airway

How redundant, how true, what more need be said than airway, airway, airway? There is nothing as relatively important as ease of airway management. So there is much truth in repeating the simple word *airway*, as it bespeaks a primary concern in the cardiac anesthesia patient as with any general anesthetic patient. (Approaches to airway management are discussed in Chapter 3.) We do not like bad airways any more than anyone else, and so we attempt early on to identify those individuals who are themselves, and by extension put us, at risk because of potentially difficult airway management. Although the history may often reveal previous intubation difficulties, we are especially concerned in the physical examination with the identification of the potentially difficult airway in patients who have not previously required general anesthesia.

Initial Assessment

As clinical anesthesiologists, we begin our airway assessment as soon as we say hello to the patient. For that matter, many anesthesiologists assess airways on all sorts of people as they just pass by on the street. Seeing a receding chin often evokes commentaries from a group of anesthesiologists such as, "I would hate to have to intubate that person," or something to that effect. What may be a passing comment among professional colleagues is, nonetheless, a useful instinct when assessing the airway preoperatively. Use that instinct because it may save you and, in particular, the patient, grave difficulty. So as you encounter your patient, you are, in fact, making an airway assessment based on your experience.

Specific Considerations in Airway Assessment

Although your own clinical experience may be your best guide to assessing the difficulty of airway management, there are a number of specific concerns that most anesthesiologists would probably regard as difficult for airway management. These include the following items.

Limited Mouth Opening

For obvious reasons, if a patient cannot open his or her mouth, oral intubation is not generally possible. In particular, beware of anyone who claims that once under anesthesia his or her jaw will relax; it often will not. Should such patients be encountered, awake airway management should be planned as described in Chapter 3.

Receding Chin (Micrognathia)

Although one can assess the distance between the jaw and the hyoid bone or look at the dangling uvula as an assurance that a receding chin does not lead to too anterior a larynx, no method is foolproof. Although we do look to see the tonsillar pillars and the uvula as a quick check of intubation ease and also attempt to assess a number of fingerbreadths between the chin and the hyoid bone, these assessments merely complement our experience of having intubated many, many patients. Although trainees will not have the experience as a resource, they will quickly develop that instinct by which they may detect when the patient is at risk for a particularly difficult intubation.

Should the jaw appear to be so micrognathic that intubation appears difficult, we arrange for fiberoptic examination by an otolaryngologist to document the laryngeal anatomy. If we conclude, after ear, nose, and throat consultation, that intubation would be virtually impossible, we proceed with the awake intubation for cardiac surgery as described in Chapter 3. Of note, male patients with receding chins frequently grow large beards to cosmetically compensate for their micrognathia. Special consideration is warranted when such patients are encountered to be certain that the airway has been closely assessed to confirm intubation ease.

Obesity and Muscular Neck

Massively obese patients are relatively common in the cardiac surgery operating room. In addition to countless other problems, the morbidly obese frequently present considerable airway management difficulties. Redundancy in pharyngeal tissues, poor mouth opening, and difficulty in head positioning make these patients particularly susceptible to the dangers of failed airway management. Only experience can dictate when a given patient might require awake intubation secondary to morbid obesity. Many of these patients, in fact, have relatively normal jaws, heads, and chests, with the bulk of their weight concentrated in the lower extremities and an enormous abdomen. Of course, the massively obese often present with signs of pulmonary restriction and a decreased functional residual capacity. As such, they readily desaturate after induction of anesthesia. Thus, when morbidly obese patients present for cardiac surgery, if there is any doubt about securing an airway, these patients are recommended to undergo awake intubation for cardiac surgery, described in Chapter 3.

Range of Motion

As the population ages, more and more patients come to surgery well into their 80s and 90s. These individuals may well have varying degrees of cervical stenosis and a limited range of motion in their necks. All patients should be assessed for range of motion and asked if they develop any paresthesias or other signs and symptoms with such movement. Also, it is wise to notice how a patient's head is positioned on the pillow in the room prior to surgery. Many patients simply cannot extend or flex their heads and must remain in a relative sniffing position. As with other airway difficulties, patients with limited range of motion must be considered for awake intubation, described in Chapter 3.

Teeth

As the population ages, fewer patients come to surgery with their own teeth. We, obviously, identify loose teeth and the overall care of the teeth in our preoperative assessment. Occasionally, we have identified dental abscesses in patients scheduled for valvular surgery, necessitating cancellation and extraction of loose dentition. In general, if teeth are loose, we prefer to have them removed prior to elective surgery, rather than engaging in dental practice ourselves. Dental extraction at the time of surgery as a consequence of anesthetic manipulation is never desirable. Not only does knocking out a tooth require explanation postoperatively, it tends to cast doubt on the competency of the anesthesia team. As intubation is such a visible part of what anesthesiologists do, dental injury becomes a source of discussion and belittlement of the anesthesiologist on the part of the operating room team. Therefore, to avoid both practicing dentistry and being the subject of operating room discussion, we prefer to have a dentist remove loose teeth prior to surgery. Also, remember that should loose teeth appear postoperatively, intubation is not in and of itself the cause of that missing or loose tooth. Many patients awaken biting down on bite blocks, oral airways, and endotracheal tubes, potentially resulting in dental injury. Thus, there are many other possible causes of dental injury in the perioperative period and it is important that anesthesiologists document the dental condition to avoid accusations regarding loose dentition.

Pulmonary Assessment

The pulmonary examination need not be overly detailed. Nevertheless, we do auscultate the lungs and, most important, observe the pattern of breathing.

Pattern of Breathing

Patients with rapid, shallow breathing patterns are of special concern. Firstly, tachypnea (respiratory rate of more than 30 per minute) is a sign of potential respiratory collapse. Should such patterns be encountered, consider if the patient may be experiencing acute pulmonary edema, infection, pneumothorax, or another adverse event requiring immediate evaluation and action. On the other hand, certain patients may simply present with severe obstructive or restrictive pulmonary disease with abnormal breathing patterns. Pursed lip breathing, clubbing, and use of accessory muscles are all signs of ventilatory impairment. Although we would hope that any acute pathology would have been corrected by the patient's medical team before surgery, many patients with significant lung disease nonetheless find their way to anesthesia and surgery with varying degrees of preoperative pulmonary therapy having been completed.

Auscultation

The lungs are auscultated to ensure bilateral breath sounds. Should rales or wheezing be present, both pulmonary and cardiac sources are considered. Again, should we encounter signs significant for an acute event, we should make certain that appropriate medical therapy is initiated. Patients coming to surgery electively should generally be free of bronchospasm and rales. In other words, we prefer patients not to be in ventricular failure or suffering asthma or other pulmonary pathology if we can help it. Of course, often we must work with a patient as he or she presents, and certainly patients with pulmonary disease are not unusual in the cardiac surgical operating room. Most important, we need to be certain in elective circumstances that the patient is in the best possible respiratory condition.

Tests of Pulmonary Function

Often patients appear accompanied by pulmonary function tests (PFTs) ordered by one of their primary doctors. Although reports of these studies are often laden with varying calculations, anesthesiologists need to determine very little from them. Additionally, if the decision has been already made to take the patient to surgery, poor pulmonary function is generally regarded as an afterthought to be dealt with in the intensive care unit. Of course, such an attitude does occasionally lead to patients who remain postoperatively dependent on ventilation for some time. Nonetheless, cardiac disease often predominates to such a degree that impaired pulmonary function is relegated to a secondary consideration.

So what do we need to be aware of regarding PFTs? Generally, the forced expiratory volume in a 1 second (FEV_1) and the forced vital capacity (FVC) are of primary interest. Significant reduction in FEV_1 compared with FVC, or a FEV_1/FVC, of less than 70% is often indicative of obstructive disease. Restrictive disease is characterized by a FVC of less than 80% of predicted and a FEV_1/FVC of more than 80%. Patients may complain of dyspnea as the FEV_1 is reduced. A calculated FEV_1 of 800 cc is considered the low mark by which patients may be considered candidates for pneumonectomy. These reports also include a flow volume curve to demonstrate airway obstruction and many other measures of pulmonary assessment that may be measured or calculated. However, the information we require may be obtained from the FEV_1/FVC, and that information will basically tell us that the patient is suffering from

Table 2-2. Mechanisms of Hypoxemia and Hypercarbia

Hypoxemia

   Hypoventilation

   Ventilation-perfusion mismatch (adult respiratory distress syndrome, pulmonary edema)

   Shunt (areas of lung perfused but not ventilated)

   Diffusion difficulties (inadequate oxygen diffusion across the pulmonary capillary membrane; not a significant contribution in general to hypoxemia)

Hypercarbia

   Increased carbon dioxide production (malignant hyperthermia, thyrotoxicosis, increased carbohydrate intake secondary to hyperalimentation)

   Decreased carbon dioxide ventilation (hypoventilation secondary to drugs, central nervous system injury, iatrogeny)

pulmonary disease that may complicate both the intraoperative and postoperative courses. So now we, the surgeon, and the internist know that the patient has bad lungs, but what does this change? Most likely the patient has little choice but to proceed with surgical revascularization. Ventilatory management in such situations comes as an afterthought after the surgery has been completed. Of course, if the patient has obstructive disease, we can be prepared with bronchodilators in the operating room if needed, particularly if PFT results show improvement with bronchodilator therapy. Likewise, if restriction is present we can apply positive end-expiratory pressure as necessary, intraoperatively. Still, it is in the postoperative period when such respiratory difficulties generally become manifest. These are described in Chapter 15.

One additional piece of information found on PFT results is a report on the patient's room air arterial blood gas (ABG). An arterial oxygen tension (PaO_2) level of less than 60 mm Hg and an arterial carbon dioxide tension ($PaCO_2$) level of more than 50 mm Hg for a patient breathing room air should suggest considerable respiratory impairment. Table 2-2 reviews physiologic mechanisms of hypoxemia and hypercarbia. Table 2-3 considers commonly employed measurements in assessing pulmonary function, and Table 2-4 presents both normal and abnormal measures of pulmonary function of note to us in the perioperative period.

These formulas are presented as a resource should you be reading this text as a resident or in preparation for examination. Information

Table 2-3. Calculations to Assess Pulmonary Function

Dead space: volume of gas not participating in gas exchange expressed as a ratio of dead space volume to total lung volume (V_D/V_T):

$$\frac{V_D}{V_T} = \frac{PaCO_2 - PeCO_2}{PaCO_2}$$

where $PeCO_2$ = measured expired CO_2 tension, and $PaCO_2$ = arterial carbon dioxide tension. Normal is 0.25–0.40.

Shunt: a measure of blood flow shunted from right to left without oxygenation expressed as a ratio of shunted flow ($\dot{Q}s$) over total blood flow ($\dot{Q}T$):

$$\frac{\dot{Q}s}{\dot{Q}T} = \frac{CcO_2 - CaO_2}{CcO_2 - CvO_2}$$

where CcO_2 = pulmonary capillary oxygen content determined by PAO_2 from alveolar gas equation, CaO_2 = arterial oxygen content, and CvO_2 = mixed venous oxygen content. Normal shunt fraction is 2–5%.

Blood oxygen content: a measure of oxygen content of blood CaO_2 = (1.39 cc O_2/Hgb) (gHgb/dl blood) (SaO_2) + PaO_2 (0.003 cc O_2/mm Hg/dl blood) CcO_2 and CvO_2 are calculated using appropriate saturations.

Alveolar gas equation: estimates alveolar oxygen tension:

$$PAO_2 = PIO_2 - \frac{PaCO_2}{R}$$

where PAO_2 = alveolar oxygen tension, PIO_2 = (P barometric – PH_2O) × FIO_2, $PaCO_2$ = arterial CO_2 tension, and R = respiratory quotient.

---

can be distilled from these equations that will alert us to possible post-operative difficulties regarding a patient's ventilation. In particular, if preoperative PFT results appear marginal, we warn the patient and family members of the risk of prolonged intubation. By this action, we attempt to protect ourselves from the frequent charge of family members and surgeons alike that anesthesia, per se, has resulted in the patient's requiring extensive postoperative ventilation. Should we determine that postoperative ventilation will be in excess of that of the average patient, we include such information as part of the informed consent (see Chapter 20).

In conclusion, should patients exhibit signs of acute exacerbations of pulmonary disease, we advise optimizing the condition with corticosteroids, bronchodilators, and so forth as guided by the pulmonologist. If, however, patients are to be taken to surgery with impaired pul-

Table 2-4. Bedside Tests of Pulmonary Function

Test	Norm	Intubate/Ventilate
Respiratory rate	12–20	>35
Vital capacity (ml/kg)	65–75	<15
Negative IF (cm H_2O)	75–100	<25
FEV_1 (ml/kg)	50–60	<10
PaO_2 (mm Hg)	75–100 (room air)	<70 (mask oxygen)
$PaCO_2$ (mm Hg)	35–45	>55*
VD/VT	0.25–0.40	>0.60

FEV_1 = 1-sec. forced expiratory volume; PaO_2 = arterial oxygen tension; $PaCO_2$ = arterial carbon dioxide tension; VD/VT = ratio of dead space to tidal volume; IF = inspiratory force.
*Except with chronic hypercapnia.
Source: Modified from H Pontoppidan, et al. Acute respiratory failure in the adult. N Engl J Med 1972;287:690.

monary function, we proceed after a frank discussion with the patient and family regarding the possibility of ventilatory difficulties. Generally, we do not frequently need tracheostomy and protracted ventilator care in most patients. Still, these are possible outcomes in patients presenting with poor pulmonary function for surgery.

Cardiovascular Evaluation

Generally, the physical examination of the cardiovascular system should be completed in some detail by the surgical team. Nonetheless, a few simple points are worth noting. Vital signs are helpful when examining a patient. After all, the patient may be hypotensive, tachycardic, or manifesting new arrhythmias right as we enter the room. We auscultate the heart to assess rhythm and to listen to murmurs, which no doubt have been diligently recorded by our cardiology colleagues. Most important, we assess pulses for possible sites of arterial cannulation. Some patients have been catheterized previously through the brachial artery. These patients may have diminished radial pulses. Others may present with subclavian stenosis, similarly reducing radial pulse intensity. If we encounter a decreased radial pulse, we inform the surgical team. This is essential because the surgical team might be planning to take internal mammary arteries as a graft. Should stenosis be present, these grafts might provide inadequate flow. Of course, we expect the surgical team will have already done this, but it nevertheless is helpful to remind them from time to time. We also auscultate the carotid arteries to detect bruits that may have been missed by previous examiners. Otherwise, additional anesthesia evaluation of the cardiovascular system adds little to what has been previously completed by the surgical and cardiology teams. Laboratory and other tests of cardiac functions have been previously discussed.

Neurologic Evaluation

Cardiopulmonary bypass is regrettably associated with varying degrees of neurologic injury. Embolization can result in injuries ranging from impaired mental functioning on neuropsychological examination to frank stroke with profound deficits. Unfortunately, because some patients will not awaken from anesthesia at the same level of neurologic functioning they were at when they were taken to surgery, a brief neurologic assessment is required. In general, this can be done simply by close observation without even requiring the patient to participate in a neurologic examination per se. Five areas need to be assessed to have a rough idea of a patient's baseline neurologic status.

1. *Motor.* Are there any gross defects? Is a tremor present? Parkinsonism can be found in elderly patients, resulting in unexpected dysautonomia, in which case we should avoid dopamine antagonists.

2. *Mental status.* Is the patient oriented at his or her neurologic baseline? If not, why not? Is the patient sedated too heavily? Are chronic subdural hematomas present?

3. *Recall.* Can the patient remember information? Often this is difficult to assess in the very aged patient.

4. *Identification of objects.* Can the patient phonate, identify, and speak correctly?

5. *Pupil size and vision.* Are the patient's visual fields intact? What are the pupillary responses? Has the patient had previous cataract surgery?

In essence, we briefly look to see what the patient's level of neurologic functioning is before we administer anesthesia. If a patient is not oriented preoperatively, he or she most certainly will not be postoperatively. It is always wise to have recorded baseline neurologic function preoperatively for comparison postoperatively. Unfortunately, many elderly patients suffer psychosis in the intensive care unit and are disoriented during hospitalization. In general, if motor skills, sensory functions, and responsiveness to commands appear to be grossly intact, we consider these patients to be at baseline and proceed with surgery. Although admission to the intensive care unit may already have sufficiently disoriented the patient, an intact examination should generally rule out any significant preoperative neurologic pathology. Strokes resulting from embolization as a consequence of cardiac catheterization may occur at any time perioperatively. In general, we avoid heavy sedation preoperatively to be able to assess neurologic functioning up to the time of surgery.

Other Laboratory Testing

It is generally wise to review the laboratory section of the patient's chart to see if anything has been missed. Patients may be found to have previously unreported irregularities in blood sugar concentration, resulting in possible glucose intolerance perioperatively. Anemia and coagulation difficulties may also be noted at this time. Patients may be noted to have elevated prothrombin times and partial thromboplastin times as a consequence of warfarin or heparin administration. Previously unknown anemia may reflect hemorrhage as a consequence of hematoma at the catheterization site or gastrointestinal bleeding as a consequence of anticoagulation in patients with gastrointestinal lesions. Hypokalemia may contribute to perioperative ventricular ectopy, especially after the institution of mechanical ventilation and the likelihood of some degree of respiratory alkalosis during anesthesia.

Elevation in cardiac enzyme levels signaling recent myocardial infarction has previously been mentioned. Elevated liver function test results may indeed be indicative of hepatic dysfunction and increased risk of perioperative liver injury. Although we consider all patients at risk for transmitting hepatitis and HIV, occasionally laboratory results will be provided for these diseases as well, which may provide for an additional degree of circumspection and precaution.

Premedication

How often have we been told that the best premedication is a well-informed patient who has had all of his or her questions answered by an informed and caring anesthesiologist? That is a myth, you say? Perhaps, but still this appears one maxim of anesthesia that experience does seem to support. If only the other anesthetic myths were as true. In reality, we must remember two things when we consider premedication of the cardiac patient. First, the patient wants surgery. After all, this is no elective procedure to improve cosmesis or sports performance. This is, theoretically at least, a lifesaving procedure. Thus, the patient wants to work with us to help him or her. Therefore, if we explain what we are doing, many will readily cooperate the best they can, especially during intravenous and arterial line placement, which can become uncomfortable. Second, we must remember that these patients have coronary disease and are at risk for perioperative decompensation. As we have previously noted, tachycardia and hypertension can contribute to perioperative ischemia. Thus, if patients are particularly anxious, they may precipitate an ischemic event. However, if we overly sedate patients, leading to hypotension or hypercarbia, we may elicit ischemia or arrhythmias as well, which may be equally dangerous. Therefore, what are we to do about premedication?

Clearly, there are some patients who are so distraught that it is not possible to work with him or her in the preoperative period without some degree of sedation. In general, we favor sedation with readily reversible agents should complications ensue. Diazepam (2.5–10.0 mg orally) administered on call to surgery provides a good starting dose, depending on a patient's size, drug history, and overall condition. Such a dose serves two functions: (1) Anxiolysis will be beneficial, and (2) many patients expect premedication and this most certainly fulfills their expectation. As such, they develop confidence in the anesthesia team and the surgeons that they have not been forgotten as they await surgery. This is especially important for patients arriving for same day surgery. However, do not premedicate any patient until you have completed your preoperative visit and have obtained appropriate informed consent.

Unfortunately, considering the current medicolegal environment, premedication is an area where anesthesiologists may become vulnerable. Should any adverse event occur after the administration of premedication, the patient and surgeon alike will quickly try to assign blame. For example, if the patient falls from the bed, the premedication and the anesthesiologist will be blamed. If the patient suffers ischemia, arrhythmias, stroke, or any of 1,000 other occurrences, somehow, someone will attempt to ascribe the difficulty to the anesthesiologist and the premedication, no matter how outrageous the claim may be. Thus, never premedicate the patient without first seeing that individual give informed consent and checking how the patient will tolerate such premedication.

Once we have contacted the patient and are able to devote our attention to him or her, intravenous midazolam (0.5–2.0 mg intravenously) may be administered with appropriate monitoring (electrocardiography, arterial oxygen saturation). Although premedication schemes may vary from institution to institution, we believe other combinations present greater difficulties than the simple mechanism outlined previously. Morphine sulfate (5–10 mg) and scopolamine (0.3 mg) have been used to provide analgesia and amnesia. Although this is effective, it does require an injection, which can be both painful and lead to hematoma formation in anticoagulated patients. Droperidol is avoided, especially in elderly patients, who may have some degree of parkinsonism. Butyrophenones' blockade of postsynaptic dopamine receptors makes them less desirable in patients who may have parkinsonism. Additionally, vasodilation as a consequence of $alpha_1$-adrenergic receptor blockade may lead to hypotension and ischemia in patients with obstructions to ventricular outflow (i.e., aortic stenosis or idiopathic hypertrophic subaortic stenosis). Figure 2-1 provides a simple guide by which premedication can be determined and administered.

Preoperative Disorientation

Last, be careful of the patient who appears disoriented in the preoperative period. Patients may suffer a stroke after cardiac catheterization or as a consequence of embolization. Although many of our patients are quite elderly and, as such, may be confused in the intensive care unit, a simple neurologic examination as documented should rule out any gross pathology. Nevertheless, because cardiopulmonary bypass can result in perioperative stroke, any neurologic change should be assessed by the surgeon before proceeding to surgery.

Fortunately for Mr. XY, we have gotten through the preoperative phase very well. He has had no other disease to speak of, not yet anyway, and he has contained his nervousness so that he is, in fact,

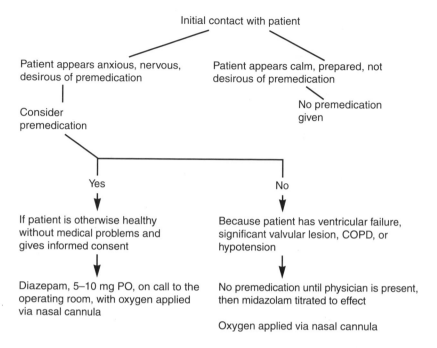

Should patients have a history of ethanolism or other substance abuse, cross tolerance will require higher premedication and anesthetic requirements. Should the patient initially not appearing to require sedation suddenly decompensate, intravenous midazolam can be administered after first being certain that any change in mental status is not the result of ventricular dysfunction, arrhythmia, stroke, or other acute pathology.

Figure 2-1. *Patient contact. (COPD = chronic obstructive pulmonary disease.)*

rather pleasant to work with. Indeed, we collectively do not believe that he is in need of premedication at all, so he comes to the operating room with a clear head and relatively strong heart as he proceeds for revascularization.

3

Here We Are in the Operating Room

Successful conveyance of Mr. XY and those like him to the surgery suite should be uneventful. Nevertheless, there are a few things to note. Remember to observe carefully how the patient's head is positioned on the stretcher. This is a good time to note if the patient suffers from any restriction of neck movement as mentioned previously, especially if this has been overlooked during the preoperative visit. Indeed, if this is same-day surgery, this may well be the first opportunity that the anesthesiologist has to visit with the patient. The immediate preoperative period may be the first time that the anesthesiologist is able to assess the patient and the family to obtain some sense of their level of expectations and understanding. We always emphasize that the patient is about to have cardiac surgery, which, of course, has implicit risks. Although patients and their families generally do not want to know the risks, they will most surely claim that they were not informed of them when they complain about their loved one's chipped tooth, injured throat, stroke, or death. Informed consent is the law, and we must be certain that the patient and family understand the risks of anesthesia. Should patients express reservations about surgery, we do not consider it our role to dissuade them. Rather, we inform the surgeon and cardiologist and allow them to talk to the patient about the appropriate course of action.

If the Patient Does Not Cancel Surgery, What Do We Need To Know So We Can?

An odd approach, you might think; after all, we are in the business of providing anesthesia, not looking for ways to deny care—well, not yet anyway. Still, this question is helpful because it forces us to look at the patient closely to identify those situations in which it would benefit the patient to have surgery delayed.

Attitude

As mentioned previously, we never force anyone to have surgery. If a patient expresses any doubt, we simply do not administer additional sedation so that we do not have to deal with the patient's reluctance. After all, we never regret the case that we do not manage. In essence, should a patient desire to cancel, we leave it to the patient and primary doctors to come to a decision. As anesthesiologists, our role is that of consultants, who need not be involved in encouraging or discouraging a patient from surgery. We believe it is the patient's choice.

Physical Condition and Laboratory Review

Ideally, we have gone over most of the patient's physical examination and laboratory data in the preoperative assessment. If this is the first contact with the patient, we should follow guidelines as previously described. If we are seeing the patient again, a quick reassessment is warranted (Table 3-1). Obviously, if renal insufficiency, infectious disease, or a new onset of myocardial infarction has just presented, those risk factors need to be addressed with the surgeon before proceeding with anesthesia.

Neurologic Condition
The possibility of preoperative strokes secondary to embolization as a consequence of catheterization was previously mentioned. Again, in the immediate preoperative period the patient is examined for changes in neurologic function.

Ventricular Performance
Barring any new onset of myocardial infarction, ventricular performance will not in and of itself move us to cancel the case. Rather, if ven-

Table 3-1. Guide to Patient Reassessment Immediately Preoperatively

---

Vital signs: Hypotension, tachycardia, and tachypnea may indicate new ischemia, infarction, ventricular failure, or an infectious process. Hyperthermia may indicate the presence of infection.

Auscultation: New murmur, rales, and wheezes may suggest ventricular failure, myocardial infarction, or the development of pulmonary pathology.

Laboratory review: Hyperglycemia or hypoglycemia may indicate inadequate diabetes management preoperatively. Anemia may signify continued bleeding as a consequence of anticoagulation. Elevated blood urea nitrogen, creatinine, and potassium levels may signify renal dysfunction secondary to contrast dye administration at the time of catheterization.

---

tricular performance is impaired as measured by tests of cardiac function or physiologic signs (edema, tachypnea, dyspnea, orthopnea, tachycardia), we may be prepared for increased difficulty in perioperative management as compared with that of the average patient. It is important that we note these findings in the immediate perioperative period, especially for individuals who are relatively new to cardiac anesthesia practice. If patients present in the operating room with impaired ventricular function, such cases are best initially managed by a more experienced cardiac anesthesiologist.

Okay, We Are Going To Manage the Case—Now What?

Now we have exhausted every possible reason not to manage the case (remember this is not because we don't want to bring the patient to surgery—it is a safety issue). If there are good reasons not to manage a case, we do not do it, and, in fact, generally our surgical colleagues do not want us to take any chances either. Therefore, with joint concern and with good communication we decide together first and foremost what is best for our patient, even if that does involve cancellation of a procedure.

Intravenous Access

What can we say at this stage about starting an intravenous (IV) line? It is hoped that, if you are considering providing cardiac anesthesia, this should not be an issue. Actually, for routine cases, an 18-gauge peripheral IV is all that is required for induction of anesthesia, assuming that large additional IVs (gauge 14 or 16) are started after induction is completed. No one ever regrets placement of as large a peripheral IV as possible. On the other hand, all cardiac patients do require central access. Therefore, we see no need to excessively poke and probe the patient in search of a 14-gauge IV site peripherally when all that is readily apparent are 18- to 20-gauge veins. In those patients in whom peripheral access is limited, and there are many, we advise obtaining as large an IV catheter as possible to facilitate induction of anesthesia and then provide either larger peripheral IV access or appropriate central venous access after induction of anesthesia. In fact, vasodilation after induction often reveals veins that seemed hidden, transforming the 20-gauge vein into one that can accommodate a 14-gauge cannula.

Arterial Cannulation

Having secured IV access, applied pulse oximeters, 5-channel electrocardiographic (ECG) leads, and supplemental oxygen via a nasal cannula, we quickly proceed to arterial line placement. As with IV placement or any particular technical skill, there is no magic that can be conveyed in a text or video that can give the anesthesiologist the feel or praxis understanding by which he or she may accomplish the task. Obviously within the boundaries of acceptable practice there may be as many techniques for arterial line placement as there are practitioners. We can only offer a few suggestions to aid in arterial cannulation. Of course, the real teachers for arterial cannulation are our many patients. Although unwilling instructors to be sure, they are by far more helpful than the many so-called teachers of the practice, ourselves included.

Generally, we prefer the left radial arterial pulse as a site for cannulation, assuming we have confirmed equivalency of bilateral radial arterial pulses. Subclavian stenosis and previous brachial arterial catheterization may result in a diminished radial artery pulse ipsilaterally. As such, the contralateral pulse may be preferable. Blood pressure (BP) determinations should be made in both arms during the history taking and physical examination by the surgical team. It is usual to check to be sure the left radial pulse is not in some way diminished compared with the right. In general, since the surgeon stands on the right side of the patient and frequently leans into the right arm, there may be a tendency to compress the right radial artery, resulting in diminished pressure tracing. Therefore, the left radial artery is the preferred cannulation site.

Other sites include the brachial, femoral, and axillary arteries. All of these sites may be employed for cannulation as necessary. In general, we prefer to have our surgical colleagues cannulate the femoral artery if radial cannulation is not possible because lower extremity vascular compromise may occur. Having the surgeon involved from the start with line placement gives them a sense of participation in the management of any problem that may result as a consequence of femoral arterial cannulation. Should radial artery grafts be planned, the radial arterial line and IV access need to be in the contralateral arm (generally the nondominant artery is taken as a bypass conduit).

As for techniques of arterial line placement, the best advice most assuredly is to "keep it simple, stupid." We do not perform the Allen's test, which is the occlusion of the radial and ulnar arteries followed by release of ulnar compression and inspection for rapid return of pinkish color to the ischemic hand. Because there are many false-positive and false-negative results with the test, our surgical team considers it essentially useless. As to technical placement, see Figures 3-1 to 3-3 for arterial line placement.

Once the arterial line is secured, the patient's arms are tucked along side the body. Be certain that the waveform remains distinct and that the arterial line is aspirated so that blood samples can be easily accessed after patient positioning.

Although arterial cannulation can result in infection of the cannulation site, arterial air emboli, and vascular occlusion, these are rare occurrences. In general, should ischemia or infection be noticed at the cannulation site, the arterial line needs to be removed and arterial access obtained at another location.

In interpreting waveforms obtained for arterial cannulas, it is important to note that central arterial pressure may differ significantly from radial or other peripheral arterial pressure measurements. The arterial pressure waveform changes depending on the cannulation site. The more distal to the aorta, the greater the systolic pressure. Mean and diastolic BP determination is less affected by catheter location. Figure 3-4 provides a sense of how pressure measurements may be altered by cannulation site.

At the time of weaning from cardiopulmonary bypass (CPB), the radial arterial pressure trace may be diminished and an accurate central aortic pressure may be needed. Fortunately, once bypass flow is discontinued, central aortic pressure can be measured from the aortic perfusion cannula. That pressure, although artificially elevated while the patient is on CPB, becomes an acceptable measure of central aortic pressure after the discontinuation of bypass flow.

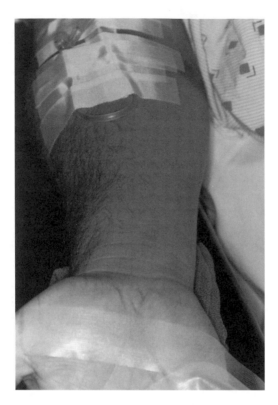

Figure 3-1. *Arm position and arm board.*

Last, a word of encouragement considering arterial cannulation: Every now and then we occasionally cannot get the arterial line. For whatever reason, the artery is just not where we think it is. Here is a suggestion that might help: Allow a colleague to attempt placement. Generally, anesthesiologists try to work with one another in a supportive way to permit this kind of assistance. Unfortunately, all too often, other anesthesiologists burst onto the scene acting like an incarnation of Mighty Mouse attempting to save the day and the patient from our inability to provide arterial cannulation. Such individuals have no sense of collegiality and it is hoped will whither under the teamwork approach demanded by health care reform. Of course, Mighty Mouse anesthesiologist often does get the arterial line. Why? Is it that Mighty Mouse really is more skilled than our frustrated clinical anesthesiologist? Of course not. Rather, Mighty Mouse anesthesiologist has two advantages: (1) Mighty Mouse is not frustrated having been unable to achieve arte-

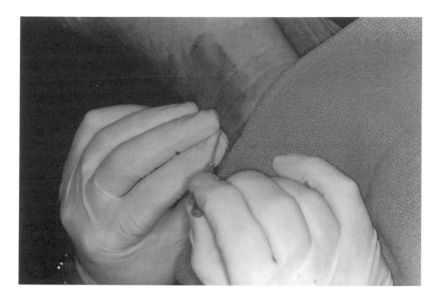

Figure 3-2. *A 20-gauge arterial line catheter at an approximately 30-degree angle.*

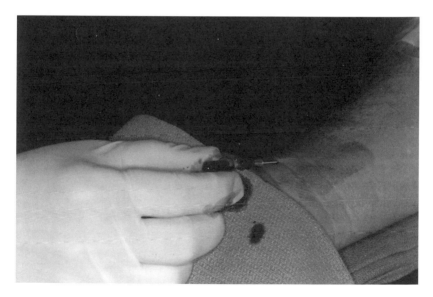

Figure 3-3. *Penetration of artery with blood flow.*

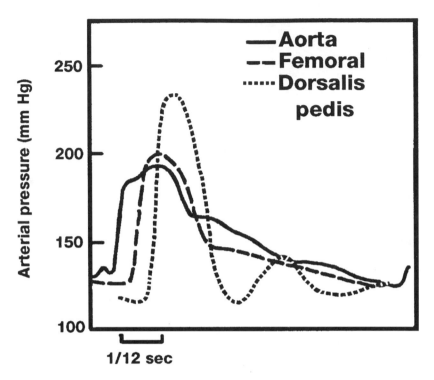

Figure 3-4. *Arterial pressure tracings. In comparison with central blood pressure pulses, peripheral pulses are narrower, with generally higher systolic pressures and dicrotic notches occurring later in the pulse. Peripheral pulse diastolic and mean pressures are approximately equal to or slightly lower than measurements. (Modified from WJ Hoffman, JD Wasnick [eds]. Postoperative Critical Care of The Massachusetts General Hospital. Boston: Little, Brown, 1992;102.)*

rial access in the first place; and (2) Mighty Mouse anesthesiologist knows that the artery is not where the frustrated anesthesiologist thinks it is. Mighty Mouse anesthesiologist generally attempts placement either more laterally or more medially than the frustrated anesthesiologist's previous attempts. Often this proves to be successful.

We hope you work together as do we (occasionally) when confronted with this issue and that you are not burdened by too many Mighty Mouse anesthesiologists in your practice. Of course, we can learn one thing from Mighty Mouse anesthesiologist, and that is go elsewhere. If arterial placement is frustrated by our own perceptions of where the artery might be, perhaps we can be Mighty Mouse ourselves by simply changing the site of where we believe successful cannulation will occur. In fact, we may well find that we achieve arterial cannulation just like Mighty Mouse. So do not despair, you too, can be a Mighty Mouse anesthesiologist. But let's be frank, shall we—aren't there enough of them already?

Central Venous Access

When we considered peripheral venous cannulation previously, we noted that we need not worry too greatly about our inability to provide large peripheral access. We mentioned that we had plenty of opportunities to secure adequate central access. Of course, we must achieve central access to effectively manage the cardiac surgical patient. That said, we should note that if we have adequate peripheral venous access for safe induction of anesthesia, we generally can proceed with central access after induction. This way, we do not force the awake or sedated patient to be placed head down under the drapes while we stick the neck looking for venous access and performing pulmonary arterial cannulation. Although some may argue that securing pulmonary artery (PA) monitoring before induction of anesthesia assists in guiding patient management after induction, we believe this argument is limited. As a monitor of ischemia, PA pressures are useful only when significant ventricular dysfunction has occurred. As to peri-induction hypotension, the ECG readily rules out dysrhythmic and ischemic causes, and we generally conclude that most peri-induction hypotension is a consequence of vasodilation unless proven otherwise. This, of course, is readily correctable, as described later in this chapter. In any event, should the patient deteriorate with induction, we believe that PA pressure monitoring will not provide any significant information that will alter therapy to the degree that would justify awake or sedated central line placement.

Additionally, the rapid availability of transesophageal echocardiography (TEE) allows us to assess ventricular function and monitor for signs of ischemia as manifested by wall motion abnormalities. Thus, we may rule out ischemia not detected by ECG. Should a patient deteriorate on induction, we can provide central access quickly so that central pressure monitoring may be employed to assist in guiding therapy. Although some argue that these pressure measurements provide valuable information in guiding the anesthetic induction, particularly if the patient deteriorates ("crashes" in the peri-induction period), this information simply does not prove valuable from a praxis understanding. Of course, the information that a patient is hypotensive in the setting of elevated PA pressures with a low cardiac output (CO) is helpful. However, as central access and PA pressure monitoring are readily achieved and as ischemia and dysrhythmia monitoring are easily detected by ECG and TEE, it is reasonable to assume that hypovolemia or vasodilation is the principal cause of peri-induction hypotension once other causes are ruled out. Rapid assessment by TEE can eliminate significant ventricular dysfunction as being responsible for deterioration on induction. Of course, vasodilation on induction can lead to ischemia and the development of decreased coronary perfusion, resulting in ventricular dysfunction. Nevertheless, our initial treatments are generally aimed at restoration of BP, and it seems unlikely that the information provided by PA monitoring would be of any great additional help for those patients who experience acute deterioration in the peri-induction period. Therefore, as a rule, we do not provide awake PA monitoring for every patient prior to induction.

Although a truly theoretical approach might dictate awake PA catheterization to provide complete information for each and every patient, a praxis understanding permits catheterization after induction. Indeed, the ready availability of TEE and close ECG monitoring provides more than acceptable surveillance for ventricular dysfunction, arrhythmia, and myocardial ischemia.

As to the technique of line placement, it is difficult for any text, video, or personal instructor to convey an approach for successful placement. The patients remain our greatest teachers. Regarding central access, we prefer a 9.0 French central venous introducer sheath placed via the right internal jugular vein. Additionally, we place a double-lumen central venous line via the right subclavian vein. Although this second line is not essential for intraoperative management, it is useful to the intensive care unit staff and patient postoperatively. Not only does this provide additional central access for vasoactive infusions, but it also frees the patient from both peripheral IVs and having to maintain jugular vein cannulation once PA pressure monitoring is no longer considered essential. This freedom permits additional movement of the patient while retaining good central venous access throughout the recovery period.

Of course, only one central venous access is essential, and this we reserve for the Swan-Ganz introducer sheath. Thus, we always place the Swan-Ganz introducer sheath first and any additional central access subsequently. Generally, we prefer to cannulate the right internal jugular vein with our sheath introducer. Figure 3-5 demonstrates an approach to internal jugular vein cannulation. Figures 3-6 to 3-11 provide a pictorial walkthrough of the anterior approach to internal jugular vein placement.

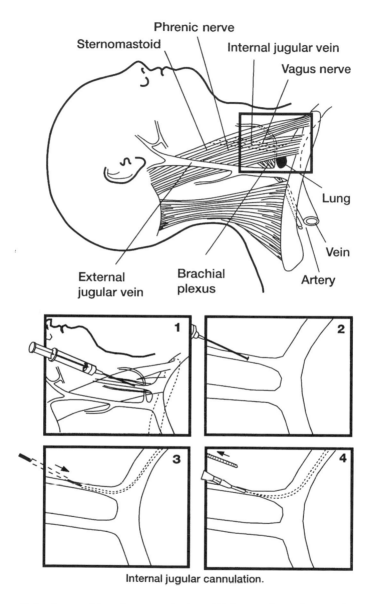

Internal jugular cannulation.

Figure 3-5. *Internal jugular cannulation. (1) Internal jugular vein located. (2) Thin wall needle passed into internal jugular vein. (3) Wire passed into internal jugular vein. (4) Catheter placed. (Modified from N Soni Practical Procedures in Anaesthesia and Intensive Care. Boston: Butterworth–Heinemann, 1994;34.)*

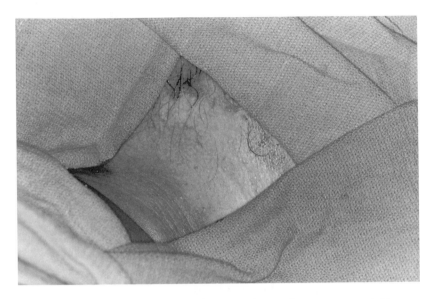

Figure 3-6. *Preparation and identification of carotid artery, sternocleido-mastoid muscle, and other landmarks.*

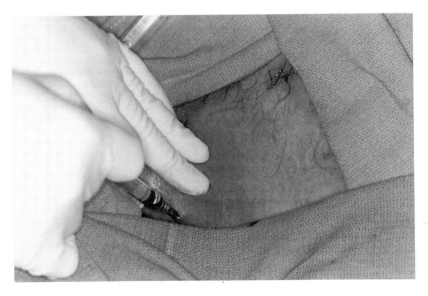

Figure 3-7. *Location of the internal jugular vein with a finder needle.*

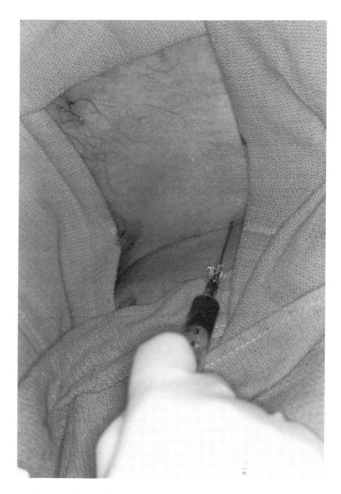

Figure 3-8. *Thin wall needle introduced into internal jugular vein.*

The potential complications from internal jugular vein cannulation include pneumothorax, carotid puncture, and brachial plexus injury. Of these three, carotid puncture is perhaps of greatest concern. As carotid puncture and even cannulation of the carotid artery can occur, it is important to always check for pulsatile flow and blood color when placing the finder and thin wall needle to ensure venous entry. Even so, carotid puncture and cannulation can and do occur. Should this happen, the introducer needle is withdrawn and pressure applied. Neck exploration may be

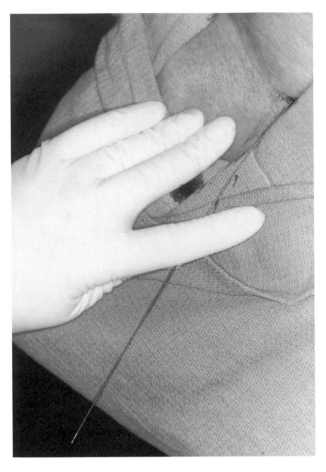

Figure 3-9. *Passage of wire via Seldinger's technique.*

required if cannulation of the carotid has occurred. Obviously, neurologic injury is a recognized risk both from embolization following penetration and palpitation of the carotid artery. Should hematoma develop, we must be cognizant of the possibility of airway compromise. Because cannulation generally occurs after the induction of anesthesia, the airway should already be secured. Nevertheless, should hematoma develop in patients undergoing awake central line placement, we must be prepared for rapid endotracheal intubation, evacuation of the expanding neck hematoma by our surgical colleagues, or both.

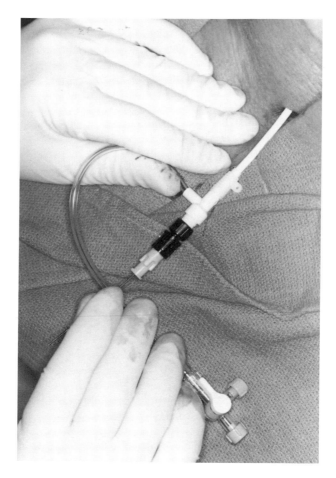

Figure 3-10. *Passage of introducer.*

Although we prefer the anterior approach to internal jugular vein cannulation, we proceed with either the middle or posterior approaches if necessary. In some patients, the triangle formed by the sternal and clavicular heads of the sternocleidomastoid muscle is so prominent that the middle approach (needle at apex of the triangle directed toward the ipsilateral nipple) is so inviting that it is an obvious choice. The posterior approach (where we aim toward the sternal notch by passing the needle posterior to the sternocleidomastoid) is less attractive. Because we are trying to avoid the carotid artery and other structures, we infrequently use the posterior approach.

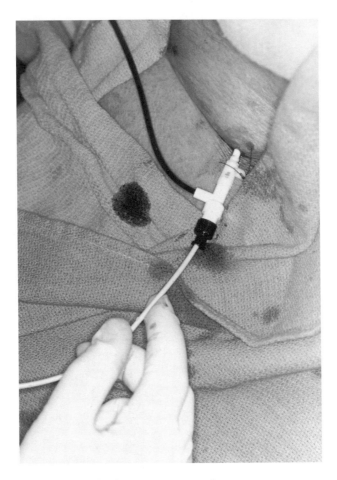

Figure 3-11. *Passage of pulmonary artery catheter.*

Generally, after a few attempts at internal jugular vein cannulation, we proceed to subclavian vein cannulation for the sheath introducer. If we have successfully placed the internal jugular vein catheter, we then place additional access via the right subclavian vein. Figure 3-12 presents central line cannulation via the right subclavian vein.

As with any technical procedure, Mighty Mouse anesthesiologists are always available to "help" you should you have difficulty securing central access (Figure 3-13). Beware, however, because Mighty Mouse generally does not have the same interest that you do should carotid

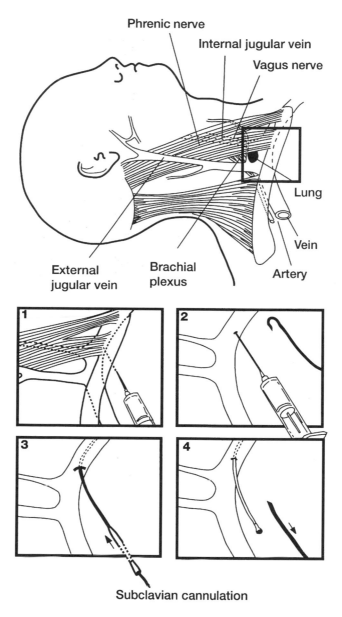

Figure 3-12. *Right subclavian vein cannulation. (1) Subclavian vein identified. (2) Thin wall needle placed. (3) Wire passed. (4) Catheter placed. (Reprinted with permission from N Soni. Practical Procedures in Anaesthesia and Intensive Care. Boston: Butterworth–Heinemann, 1994;25.)*

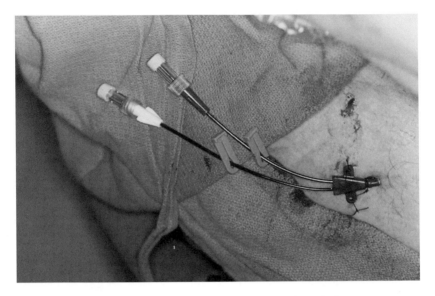

Figure 3-13. *Passage of double-lumen catheter into the subclavian vein.*

puncture or pneumothorax occur. As such, it is always prudent to choose your help wisely. Although pneumothorax is a constant risk whenever central access is planned via the internal jugular and subclavian veins, it is readily managed in the cardiac surgical patient because the chest will be quickly opened and any air easily evacuated. Additionally, because the patients require chest tubes of one variety or another, the impact of pneumothorax in this setting is hardly as significant a complication as in other situations requiring central line placement. Last, it is important to note that not every pneumothorax that occurs in the cardiac surgical patient is the result of line placement. Surgical manipulations can result in pneumothorax. Of course, surgeons will not often admit that.

Pulmonary Artery Catheterization

In these times of increased managed care and cost containment, there is a tendency to call into question the need for PA catheterization in each and every patient undergoing bypass surgery. Although it is true that many patients with relatively good ventricular function can adequately be managed perioperatively with only central venous pressure monitoring, individual patient performance is too variable to deny PA monitoring simply because of cost restraints. It may be argued that with right atrial pressure monitoring and green dye dilution CO measurement that the essential information provided by PA catheterization may be obtained. Nevertheless, old methods such as this hardly provide for the ease in obtaining the continuous supply of information that the PA line provides. More recent questions into PA catheter use in the intensive care setting many retard Swan-Ganz catheter placement for cardiac surgery as well. For now, PA catheter placement is routine. New prospective trials will probably be forthcoming to determine the use of PA catheterization in the coronary artery bypass population.

So what then does a PA catheter tell us and why do we consider it useful for patient management?

Pulmonary Artery Pressure and Pulmonary Capillary Occlusion Pressure

When the balloon of the PA catheter is inflated, a small PA is occluded, and a continuous channel is made between the left atrium and the occluded PA. Thus, the pulmonary capillary occlusion pressure reflects the left atrial pressure, which approximates the left ventricular end-diastolic pressure (LVEDP), which roughly approximates the left ventricular end-diastolic volume (LVEDV). Therefore, the pulmonary capillary occlusion pressure approximates the volume loading conditions of the left ventricle. Naturally, this is just an approximation because a poorly compliant left ventricle requires a relatively lower volume load to produce elevated left ventricular end-diastolic, left atrial, and pulmonary capillary occlusion pressures.

Mitral valvular disease similarly makes the correlation between the LVEDP and the left atrial pressure uncertain. Pulmonary arterial diastolic pressure is a further approximation of pulmonary capillary occlusion pressure. However, alterations in pulmonary vascular resistance (as occur in hypoxemia or primary pulmonary hypertension) may result in an elevated pulmonary arterial diastolic pressure that does not reflect the pulmonary capillary occlusion pressure. As an estimate of volume and pressure loading to the left ventricle, the pulmonary capillary occlusion pressure is helpful in patient management, particularly when determining appropriate volume loading to and compliance of the left ventricle when separating from CPB (as described in Chapter 6). Additionally, the pulmonary capillary occlusion pressure is helpful in assessing the effects of vasodilator and inotropic therapy in the treatment of ventricular dysfunction (see Chapter 8).

Cardiac Output

The thermistor-tipped PA catheter provides a relatively easy way to measure CO. Employing the Fick thermodilution technique, we can assess global ventricular function. As shall be seen later in this chapter, we may use both pulmonary capillary occlusion pressure and CO determinations to provide a simple scheme by which we may respond to hemodynamic instability.

Mixed Venous Oxygen Saturation

Mixed venous oxygen saturation (SVO_2) measurements (normal mixed venous oxygen tension [pVO_2] approximately 40 mm Hg; SVO_2 approximately 75%) may be measured fiberoptically from certain PA catheters. The SVO_2 represents hemoglobin oxygen saturation in the pulmonary vasculature after the mixing of venous return from the heart and from both the superior and inferior vena cava. Although a decrease in SVO_2 may herald reduced cardiac function and therefore increased oxygen extraction, other factors such as anemias and decreased arterial oxygen saturation may likewise reduce SVO_2. Hemoglobinopathies and arterial venous shunting may similarly increase SVO_2. Reduced SVO_2 may serve to some degree as a warning of impending cardiovascular collapse. Nevertheless, its usefulness is hardly essential, and certainly SVO_2 monitoring is not indicated for every patient.

Similarly, certain PA occlusion catheters have the ability to assess right ventricular ejection fraction, which may prove useful with right ventricular dysfunction. Such information generally supplements the assessment of right ventricular function as provided by TEE. Last, PA catheters have the ability to provide a pacing capability that we frequently employ in patients undergoing minimally invasive coronary artery bypass surgery (see Chapter 19) and in those procedures where direct access to the heart is limited and a pacing capability is required. Both pacing Swan-Ganz catheters and pace port catheters may be used depending on individual preference. Pacing capability achieved via a Swan-Ganz catheter is subject to catheter mobility and is less reliable than epicardial pacing.

Thus, the PA catheter provides a number of options and functions that assist in patient management, especially at the time of weaning from CPB. Although we do not consider it essential that all patients have PA catheter placement before induction, our team believes the information generated is valuable in the patient's intraoperative and postoperative management and therefore recommend that all patients undergo PA catheterization after anesthetic induction when bypass surgery is contemplated. Further studies are awaited to determine if this approach needs to be altered in the future.

Insertion of the Pulmonary Artery Catheter

Once the PA catheter introducer has been secured, we immediately pass the PA catheter. Because the PA line is relatively long, we are careful to avoid contamination and thus increase the risk of infection.

With the catheter sheath in place, the catheter is advanced with the balloon deflated until the 20-cm mark is reached. The balloon is inflated, and the catheter is passed through the right atrium, right ventricle, PA, and finally into occlusion position. Figure 3-14 presents a graphic of pressure changes associated with the various chambers of the heart as the PA line is passed.

There are many frustrating moments that the clinical anesthesiologist experiences attempting to float the catheter into the PA. A few clues are provided should we find the PA catheter does not go where we desire it to. Is the distal PA port lumen actually being measured by the designated PA transducer? That is to say, with the many IV lines, other lines, and cables, often the distal port is in fact attached to the central venous monitor rather than to the PA pressure transducer. Thus, the catheter routinely is placed into the PA, but because it is not attached to the appropriate transducer, it is not possible to confirm correct placement. Often, the only sign of this is the appearance of a right ventricular pressure trace once you have already passed the catheter far into the PA appearing on the PA transducer attached to the central venous pressure port.

Sometimes, the PA line coils in the right ventricle, never passing into the PA. Often this occurs when the PA catheter is passed well beyond 60 cm, with only a right ventricular tracing appearing. Should this happen, it is wise to pull the PA catheter back into the right atrium so to prevent the possibility of coiling the PA line and potentially knotting the line in the right ventricle. If the heart rate (HR) is relatively slow, a relatively slow advancement through the right ventricle increases the possibility of advancing into the PA. It is always important to be watchful for the increase in diastolic pressure that occurs when successful entry into a PA has been achieved.

Last, arrhythmias frequently occur as the PA line passes through the pulmonary outflow tract. Advancing into the pulmonary circulation

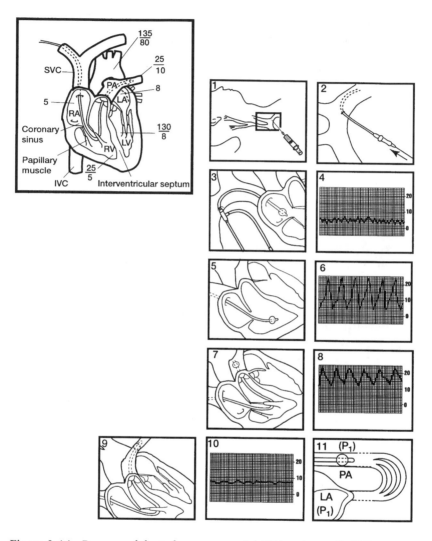

Figure 3-14. *Passage of the pulmonary arterial (PA) catheter. (1–2) Passage of the introducer. (3–4) PA catheter with central venous pressure tracing. (5–6) Catheter tip in the right ventricle and right ventricle tracing. (7–8) Catheter in PA and pressure tracing. (9–10) Wedge position and tracing. (11) Direct communication between the distal end of the catheter (sealed off by the balloon) and the left atrium. (SVC = superior vena cava; PA = pulmonary artery; LA = left atrium; RA = right atrium; LV = left ventricle; RV = right ventricle; IVC = inferior vena cava.) (Reprinted with permission from N Soni. Practical Procedures in Anaesthesia and Intensive Care. Boston: Butterworth–Heinemann, 1994;43.)*

generally corrects the rhythm disturbance. Reappearance of arrhythmias generally requires a quick check of the PA line pressure waveform to confirm that the distal tip is in a PA and has not floated back into the right ventricle, producing dysrhythmias. PA catheterization can be associated with infection as with any other catheter. Other serious complications include PA rupture. To avoid the risk of pulmonary rupture, we are certain that the distal tip is not occluded in the PA wedged position. Additionally, we are certain to withdraw the pulmonary catheter slightly before institution of CPB. We do not encourage nursing staff to frequently inflate the catheter balloon. Chapter 8 discusses the hemodynamic measurements obtained from these monitors and how we may use them to help our patients, particularly Mr. XY.

As it happens, Mr. XY will be fortunate enough to have uneventful line placement. Not all patients, of course, are as fortunate. Generally, pneumothorax, as we have mentioned, is not of too great a concern, because the chest is readily open and air can be seen lying beneath the pleura. The surgeon opens the pleura and evacuates the air. Carotid puncture is a more serious concern; however, the application of pressure should prevent any significant hematoma formation.

Electrocardiographic Monitoring

ECG monitoring is an essential part of anesthetic management. Monitoring of the five-lead ECG at leads II and V5 provides effective surveillance for myocardial ischemia and for dysrhythmia detection. It is important to secure the leads in such a way that they provide an appropriate ECG distribution without interfering with the surgical field. Placement of an occlusive dressing over the ECG leads may be essential to prevent them from becoming wet as a consequence of preparation solution or other irrigation.

Positioning

Once lines are secured, it is important to be sure that they are functioning in the position in which the patient will be during the course of the procedure. Arms and elbows must be padded and tucked along side the patient. The eyes should be taped shut to avoid corneal abrasions, and the head should be placed in a neutral position to prevent any flexion-extension injury. From an anesthesiologist's perspective, an effective anesthetic can be adversely affected by the development of a neuropathy or corneal abrasion. Thus, we pay great attention to routine anesthesia care in addition to concentrating on specific cardiac factors. As always, we remember it is just anesthesia.

Anesthetic Induction: Why It Really Does Not Matter What You Use

So much has been published on this subject that it is difficult to even begin to distill a few clinically relevant maxims from the great body of accumulated literature. To be sure, many an academic career has been secured by measuring the ability of this or that anesthetic to produce depression of myocardial function, coronary steal, vasodilation, reflex tachycardias, and, of course, hypotension. It is noteworthy from a praxis perspective to understand that the literature is replete with so many possible confounding factors that may lead to perioperative myocardial ischemia and ventricular failure that at times we may think all of our choices lead to patient jeopardy. Thus, before proceeding to analyze which potentially undesirable effects we are to cause as a consequence of our pharmacologic manipulations, we need to be clear what we are in fact trying to do and trying to avoid. Well that's easy. To paraphrase from the world of political sound bytes, "we're putting them to sleep, stupid." Okay, so it is just anesthesia, as we have maintained throughout this text so far. So then what else do we need to consider? Obviously, this great subspecialty would not have developed if it were that simple. Or would it? In fact, providing anesthesia for the cardiac patient may indeed be that simple after all, once we consider one or two provisions.

We have previously mentioned that myocardial ischemia is the consequence of an imbalance between myocardial oxygen supply and demand. There is obviously nothing revelatory here. What we must now take into account is how anesthetic agents and their effects, both desired and undesired, alter that balance. The effects of anesthesia are not all that bad, although we may be led to believe so. By providing anesthesia, we are not going to automatically provide conditions leading to myocardial ischemia. Rather, anesthesia may in fact have beneficial effects. Indeed, by slowing the HR and providing vasodilation (with a subsequent reduction of LVEDV and LVEDP), we may in fact contribute to improved myocardial oxygen balance. Conversely, tachycardia, hypotension, and myocardial depression may result in a tilting of that balance, leading to ischemia and potential cardiovascular collapse. Inadequate anesthesia resulting in hypertension and tachycardia can give the patient a stress test right before our eyes, leading to ischemia and ventricular dysfunction.

If we provide too little anesthesia we find ourselves running an intraoperative stress test that we know the patient is going to fail; after all, that's why the patient is in surgery. Too much anesthesia, and again, we are running a chemically induced stress test as a consequence of hypotension and vasodilation. Still, with the right administration of anesthesia, maybe, just maybe, not only will we put our patient to sleep, but also sleep with the best possible balance between myocardial oxygen supply and demand. This, of course, would definitely be in the patient's favor. And, after all, what is good for the patient is always good for us.

But here is the problem. We have our favorite patient, Mr. XY, whom we must now anesthetize. What are we going to use? How will we both induce and maintain anesthesia and preserve his myocardial oxygen supply-and-demand ratio? What magic have we? Well, in spite of the fact that cardiac anesthesiologists for years have been running about with syringes replete with large doses of synthetic narcotics, these confer no special magic or guarantee. Indeed, the pharmacologic approaches to anesthetic maintenance may vary greatly from physician to physician and institution to institution. Often for an institution, a given combination of a narcotic, an amnestic, and a muscle relaxant becomes anointed as having special utility in providing anesthesia for the coronary artery bypass patient. Of course, collectively we know that such lore is of what myths are made. Remember that Mr. XY has simple stable angina with preserved ventricular function. In fact, we have for the most part the entire anesthetic armamentarium to choose from. (We discuss management of the patient with poor ventricular function in Chapter 8.) As such, it is not the drugs per se that will keep Mr. XY free from ischemia perioperatively, but how the anesthesiologist employs those agents.

This is a critical point to make to surgeons and other interested parties. Too often anesthesia proceeds so smoothly that the anesthesiologist is seen by other physician colleagues as simply following a set formula without any specific thought process. Following rigid protocols further establishes that only certain regimens can mythically provide safe anesthesia. Indeed, the drug regimen or protocol soon comes to be the cherished guarantor of intraoperative patient safety, rather than the anesthesiologist. Naturally, this kind of thought reinforces the view that anesthesiologists are somewhat less worthy of compensation than perhaps other members of the care team. As we see managed care now bundling reimbursement for all physicians, there is hardly a desire to overly reward someone if they are merely perceived as doing little more than following a set protocol. As such, we encourage all to emphasize not that the pharmacology provides safe anesthesia, but rather it is the skill of the anesthesiologist using the anesthetics that insures patient safety. Although self-promotion is generally distasteful— and no doubt we all have known many, many masters of this dubious art—this may be the time for anesthesiologists again to remind the operating room community of the thought processes we follow as we anesthetize the heart patient. So then, let us not think about miracle drugs, but miracle-working anesthesiologists who employ those drugs.

If our miracle anesthesiologist is, in fact, to provide outstanding care, he or she will have the opportunity to demonstrate his or her abilities rapidly at the time of anesthetic induction. To begin with, the anesthesiologist needs to assess the patient immediately preinduction. Obviously, if a patient is ischemic before induction (as noted by ECG changes, chest pain, and so forth), it is likely that he or she will be so after induction. Unless, of course, the patient is ischemic as a consequence of tachycardia resulting from inadequate anxiolysis or failure to continue the anti-ischemic regimen perioperatively. Thus, if the patient is acutely ischemic, this needs to be corrected. Nitrates and beta blockers (i.e., esmolol) may readily correct myocardial ischemia in the patient with preserved ventricular function before induction of anesthesia. Additional premedication with midazolam (as described in Chapter 2) may also relieve any anxiety contributing to that ischemia. It is hoped, however, we will have avoided overt ischemia as we prepare the patient for induction. Of course, silent ischemia may nonetheless be present.

Having corrected any preinduction angina, we proceed with anesthesia. A wide assortment of IV and inhalational agents is available. Tables 3-2 to 3-4 present several commonly used drugs and their hemodynamic effects.

Although these tables summarize the hemodynamic effects of various agents, it is quite clear that no one drug alone is adequate for total cardiac anesthesia care. Thus, we are not simply going to use just isoflurane or just sufentanil or just midazolam in providing anesthetic management. The actual importance of Tables 3-2 to 3-4 is questionable at best. Of course, for those preparing for written examination, these tables are of critical importance, considering the limited format of our

Table 3-2. Hemodynamic Effects of Inhalational Agents

Agent	Myocardial Contractility	Blood Pressure	Heart Rate	Vaso-dilator	Other
Isoflurane	Decreased	Decreased	Increased	Yes	May produce coronary steal
Desflurane	Decreased	Decreased	Increased	Yes	—
Enflurane[a]	Decreased	Decreased	Increased	Yes	Fluoride ion production
Halothane[b]	Extremely decreased	Decreased	Decreased	Yes	Hepatic toxicity

[a]Enflurane is associated with fluoride ion production and potential renal injury.
[b]Halothane is included for historical purposes. Coronary steal occurs when vasodilation of normal coronary vessels steals blood away from ischemic areas of the heart.

Table 3-3. Hemodynamic Effects of Selected Narcotics

Agent	Myocardial Contractility	Blood Pressure	Heart Rate	Vasodilator
Sufentanil	—	Decreased	Extremely decreased	Yes
Fentanyl	—	Decreased	Decreased	Yes
Morphine*	—	Decreased	Decreased	Yes

*Morphine is associated with histamine release and slow onset, and is mentioned primarily for historical purposes. Decreased sympathetic outflow can lead to vasodilation.

Table 3-4. Hemodynamic Effects of Selected Intravenous Anesthetics

Agent	Myocardial Contractility	Blood Pressure	Heart Rate
Thiopental (Pentothal)	Decreased	Decreased	Increased
Propofol	Decreased	Decreased	± Increased
Ketamine	Increased through catecholamine release	Increased	Increased
Midazolam	± Decreased	Decreased	± Increased

multiple choice test. Yet, for those who have already transcended the need to prepare for written examination (at least those certified before the millennium) much greater questions need to be addressed. Namely, with so many hemodynamic data available, how do we construct an appropriate anesthetic plan? Obviously, all of these agents can produce potential myocardial ischemia as a consequence of tachycardia, hypotension, and ventricular depression to a greater or lesser degree. Other agents, by reducing myocardial contractility or producing brady-cardia and vasodilation, may likewise relieve myocardial ischemia. Whether anesthesia contributes to the development of ischemia and ventricular dysfunction, relieves ischemia and improves ventricular function, or, in fact, does not affect the ventricle at all, is the result of the interplay between the patient and the anesthesiologist as they both react to changes brought about by the combination of these drugs, rather than from the effects of any one agent, per se.

Although we resist stating that there is any particular regimen appropriate for anesthesia induction and maintenance, in general we proceed with an induction using a combination of sufentanil (10–20 µg per kg) and midazolam (7–10 mg) supplemented with isoflurane. This approach is relatively easy to follow and additional sufentanil and midazolam can be titrated as needed. Obviously, other agents may be substituted. Fentanyl, 50–100 µg per kg, has long been employed by cardiac anesthesiologists. We have chosen sufentanil simply because of the smaller volume and relative ease in administration. (In other words, we do not like drawing up the big syringe.) But, it hardly matters whether one uses fentanyl or sufentanil as a narcotic, provided that one focuses on the balance between oxygen supply and demand. Morphine sulfate, because of its slow onset and histamine release, is included simply for historical purposes and is unlikely to find its way into current high-dose narcotic anesthetic practice. Additionally, we have used varying amounts of thiopental (Pentothal), propofol, and etomidate to supplement anesthesia induction, especially in patients with significant cross tolerance from ethanol or other substance abuse. Propofol is particularly useful as a continuous infusion to maintain sedation through to the intensive care unit. When the patient is stable, propofol is discontinued, leading to quick emergence and extubation.

At all times, we are primarily concerned with preventing, detecting, and responding to myocardial ischemia and ventricular dysfunction during the period of anesthetic management.

Last, we briefly consider the question of muscle relaxants. Muscle relaxants are essential to facilitate intubation and provide for immobility during cardiac surgery. Although anesthetic agents alone should render the patient immobile, the possibility of movement during this type of procedure would be totally unwelcome and potentially dangerous. Additionally, the temperature changes that occur during cardiac pulmonary bypass could lead to shivering and to increased myocardial oxygen consumption. As such, paralysis is essential to effective management of the bypass patient. Muscle relaxant selection is of concern to the anesthesiologist again based on how drug use affects the balance between myocardial oxygen consumption and demand.

Indeed, in cardiac anesthesia practice, muscle relaxants have often been chosen principally based on their side effects, or lack thereof, as they relate to hemodynamic stability. Indeed, gallamine at one time was administered more for its effect on HR than for its usefulness as a muscle relaxant. Pancuronium (0.1 mg per kg) has frequently been used to prevent bradycardia that may result from a combination of a benzodiazepine and sufentanil. On the other hand, pancuronium is associated with vagolysis and the development of tachycardia, which, as we have previously discussed, can result in ischemia. Vecuronium may similarly be employed in routine cardiac care, but it lacks the vagolytic effects of pancuronium. It does not offset the potential bradycardia that occurs with the coupling of a benzodiazepine and narcotics during anesthetic induction.

Histamine-releasing agents may be considered less desirous in cardiac anesthesia practice as a consequence of histamine-induced hypotension that leads to ischemia and ventricular dysfunction. New muscle relaxants appear to come to the market daily accompanied by scores of papers purporting their particular advantages or disadvantages, cardiac effects, and durations of action. Although newer agents such as rocuronium appear to facilitate rapid intubation, pipecuronium and doxacurium simply are long-acting muscle relaxants relatively free of significant hemodynamic effects. Which of these muscle relaxants is chosen appears to have little effect per se as long as the overall balance between the oxygen supply and demand is maintained throughout their use.

Should tachycardia or bradycardia develop as a consequence of muscle relaxant choice, no doubt these developments will be readily corrected. Certainly, we are not going to permit tachycardia and bradycardia to go untreated. Even if a muscle relaxant contributes to a particular rhythm disturbance or hypotension, this hardly leads our patient to disaster as a consequence of muscle relaxant choice. Any given side effect will be readily corrected.

In general, we provide relaxation using pancuronium for a sufentanil and midazolam induction. We do not routinely experience either profound tachycardia or bradycardia. We do not employ atropine or scopolamine premedication, thereby eliminating the combination of a muscarinic antagonist coupled with pancuronium. Even before considering the hemodynamic effects in choosing an anesthetic plan and muscle relaxants, we first remember basic anesthesia practice. If securing the airway seems problematic, the administration of long-acting narcotics and muscle relaxants for induction may not be prudent. Although this is explained in greater detail later in this chapter, we should remember that in those patients in whom mask ventilation and intubation appear difficult (but not so difficult as to warrant awake intubation), prudence might well dictate induction with a short-acting agent (i.e., propofol or etomidate) and succinylcholine. Small amounts of fentanyl may be used to blunt the hemodynamic effects of laryngoscopy. Additionally, should the depth of anesthesia be relatively light, we may control tachycardia and ischemia by the administration of small amounts of esmolol in those patients with good ventricular function. Such a plan may permit the patient to be intubated asleep without having to pursue the option of awake intubation.

Before we consider those things that specifically relate to cardiac surgery, we should be mindful of general anesthesia principles. Difficulty with airway management, no matter how much attention is given to the hemodynamic concerns can lead to disaster quickly.

What Really Matters in Induction: Remember, It Is Just Anesthesia

To what degree you have been convinced that anesthetic drug selection is relatively unimportant is, of course, moving us toward a demythologized understanding of cardiac anesthesia practice. If you are mindful of the effects of these agents alone and in combination, you should be able to design a regimen that secures hemodynamic stability, anesthetic induction, and most importantly, patient safety. The actual combination of drugs you employ is less important than your certainty that you are applying them well.

What is meant by applying the drugs well? Namely, we are the ultimate agent for anesthetic delivery. We continually interact with the patient. In essence, the skilled cardiac anesthesiologist, like all anesthesiologists, is both active and reactive. We are active in that we are cognizant of the effects that our actions have, and we are ever mindful to ensure that they do not lead to airway compromise, ventilatory embarrassment, myocardial ischemia, and ventricular failure. We are reactive in that when such events occur, we take action to immediately correct those events that threaten the patient's well-being. In this section, we take our patient, Mr. XY, through the many difficulties that can occur during anesthesia induction and maintenance up to placing the patient on CPB.

Preventing and responding to the unexpected is the essence of being both an active and reactive anesthesiologist. Thus, what really matters in cardiac anesthesia is not drugs, protocols, or monitors, but a physician who is part seer (i.e., knows what is likely to happen) and part damage control officer (i.e., corrects those things that go awry before the patient is threatened).

Securing the Airway

No matter how carefully we plan for hemodynamic stability, inability to ventilate and oxygenate will surely result in the greatest of anesthesia horrors—an airway catastrophe. Just because we are in the cardiac operating room provides no special protection against the difficult airway. So we must ask the question why does it appear that there are fewer airway crises in the heart operating room? This is because the heart team may encounter only one to two patients per day. As such, the risk of meeting the impossible airway declines as compared with a room with a rapid turnover. Therefore, the cardiac anesthesiologist may encounter fewer difficult airways simply because the number of patient contacts is reduced.

Before entering the room we must have a plan to manage airway difficulties. Again, this should not be a generic plan, but one that is based on careful patient evaluation. We should always be focused on a realistic assessment of our ability to secure effective oxygenation, ventilation, and then intubation. We must be especially careful if we plan to use drugs that promote hemodynamic stability and commit us to long periods of anesthesia. We must therefore be prepared to provide for airway management and controlled ventilation for some time if long-acting induction drugs are to be employed.

We have previously discussed those identifying features that could mark a particular patient as one who might have an airway difficulty. Should we find any of those conditions present, we must decide on our management plan for the expected difficult airway.

When we identify either by history or physical examination a patient obviously at risk for postinduction airway compromise, we have two choices. Namely, we can proceed with an awake intubation, being cognizant of potential hemodynamic ramifications that could lead to myocardial ischemia or we can proceed with induction of anesthesia after taking a few precautions and making appropriate preparations.

Awake Intubation for the Expected Difficult Airway

Patients with airway anatomy that puts them at risk for intubation difficulty have been previously described. Generally, if the case is elective, we frequently arrange for ear, nose, and throat evaluation with a flexible fiberoptic laryngoscope. This permits us to see if we may proceed with induction of anesthesia and asleep intubation. On the other hand, if the ear, nose, and throat physician informs us that the larynx is too anterior, we may make plans for alternative approaches.

Often, however, we do not have the luxury of obtaining such an evaluation and thus must rely on our own examination and experience to dictate whether any particular constellation of airway anatomy constitutes a particular difficulty. Thus, deciding whether to proceed with an awake or asleep intubation depends on our particular comfort level with a given patient. There are few stark anatomic features that in and of themselves will lead us to proceed with awake intubation. Inability to open the mouth and exceptionally morbid obesity are two situations in which we would favor awake intubation in the cardiac patient. Otherwise, physical clues to intubation difficulty are often not that alarming (i.e., prominent dentition, recessed chin). In fact, we may view such findings as being easily dealt with by taking appropriate precautions. More important perhaps than any physical signs is the patient who appears relatively normal except for a particular anesthesia history. Fortunately, many of these patients have had anesthesia in the past, and frequently they have been told by previous anesthesiologists that they possess an airway problem. We never ignore this information once we are told of a past airway difficulty. Only an arrogant anesthesiologist will ignore such a warning given to a patient by a previous doctor. If we are told of previous intubation failure, we attempt to acquire old records to see what the problem may have been. Those patients who present with a history of difficult intubation undergo awake intubation. Table 3-5 provides a guide to awake fiberoptic intubation in the cardiac patient.

Although it is not our purpose to provide a complete guide to basic anesthesia skills, such as awake intubation, we do need to address the

Table 3-5. A Guide to Awake Intubation in the Cardiac Patient

1. Apply full preinduction monitoring, including arterial line.

2. Sedate the patient with midazolam, fentanyl, and droperidol as indicated by history and physical condition. Our goal is a sedate patient breathing spontaneously.

3. Topically anesthetize the airway with 4% lidocaine spray. Additionally, superior laryngeal blocks or transtracheal blocks may be applied.

4. Cocaine 4% or phenylephrine lidocaine is applied to the nasal mucosa if a nasal intubation is planned.

5. Proceed as follows with intubation attempts:

    a. Attempt direct laryngoscopy: If cords are visible easily, proceed with induction of anesthesia.

    b. Attempt direct laryngoscopy: cords potentially visible; attempt tube placement; if successful, induce anesthesia.

    c. If unsuccessful at intubation, attempt oral or nasal fiberoptic intubation or other intubation techniques.

    d. If unsuccessful at intubation, consider awake tracheostomy in consultation with surgical team.

6. Always react to maintain hemodynamic stability.

7. If available, a second anesthesiologist should monitor the patient and treat hemodynamic changes during the intubation attempt.

cardiac ramifications of undertaking this type of approach. Obviously, awake intubation of any kind is going to cause hemodynamic stress. The hemodynamic responses to airway manipulation are tachycardia and hypertension. These can contribute to arrhythmias, ischemia, and ventricular dysfunction. As such, the decision to proceed with awake intubation should not be made lightly. Nevertheless, a secure airway is essential to anesthesia safety. If any doubt exists about the ability to ventilate and oxygenate a patient either by mask or laryngeal mask airway, clearly we must accept the risk of hemodynamic instability and attempt to secure the airway. After all, it is just anesthesia, which means focus on the airway, airway, airway, doesn't it?

During awake intubation, it is often helpful to plan to have two anesthesiologists present. One can perform the airway manipulation while the other concentrates on monitoring the patient. Adequacy of ventilation and oxygenation during intubation attempts and close attention to the signs of arrhythmias and ischemia are essential. Reacting to hemodynamic changes that occur is necessary to safely complete awake intubation. Intravenous lidocaine, atropine, esmolol, and nitroglycerin should be available instantly to correct any arrhythmias or ischemia that might develop as a consequence of tachycardia and hypertension. As always, maintaining the balance between myocardial oxygen supply and demand is essential if awake intubation is anticipated.

Occasionally, nasal intubation appears particularly inviting as a method for awake intubation. Because many patients arrive in the cardiac operating room having already been anticoagulated, this approach may lead to significant hemorrhage. Additionally, anticoagulation for CPB may similarly lead to significant hemorrhage well after successful placement of the endotracheal tube. Although we do not preclude this approach by any means, we are cognizant that nasopharyngeal bleeding may both obscure the view of the larynx and lead to significant aspiration of blood. Blood aspiration may lead to potential hypoxemia secondary to ventilation perfusion mismatch.

In many cases, we may not consider the patient's history and airway examination significant enough to warrant subjecting the patient to the stress of awake intubation. Such patients would include those who have a slightly recessed chin, profound dentition, or are somewhat obese but not overwhelmingly so. In these individuals, we suspect airway difficulty, but more than likely do not believe it is necessary to apply topical anesthesia to the larynx to perform awake laryngoscopy. Induction of anesthesia with relatively short-acting agents may be considered. Recognizing that because we consider the patient likely to be adequately ventilated either by mask or laryngeal mask airway, we can induce anesthesia and then awaken the patient if unsuccessful.

The exact agents for induction of anesthesia in this setting are, of course, subject to individual choice. Propofol, etomidate, pentothal, along with succinylcholine or short-acting nondepolarizing muscle relaxants may be employed. Inhalational anesthetics may be added to blunt the hemodynamic response to intubation. As always, which combination of anesthetics employed is less significant than being certain that the anesthesiologist reacts to changes in BP, rate, and rhythm that could lead to an unfavorable balance between the myocardial oxygen supply and demand. Phenylephrine, ephedrine, nitroglycerin, esmolol, lidocaine, and atropine should be available instantly to correct any change in hemodynamic behavior that might lead to ischemia, hypertension, and arrhythmias.

After induction with short-acting agents, direct laryngoscopy is performed. If the patient is readily intubated, then longer-acting narcotics,

Table 3-6. Approach to the Unexpectedly Difficult Intubation

1. Mask ventilate; obtain laryngeal mask airway.
2. Place laryngeal mask airway.
3. Ventilate via laryngeal mask airway and attend to hemodynamic stability.
4. Take no. 6.0 uncuffed endotracheal tube and place over fiberoptic laryngoscope.
5. Complete fiberoptic laryngoscopy via the laryngeal mask airway.
6. Advance no. 6.0 uncuffed endotracheal tube through the laryngeal mask airway guided by the fiberoptic laryngoscope.
7. Using two clamps and an assistant, push the no. 6.0 endotracheal tube through the laryngeal mask airway at the same time as withdrawing the laryngeal mask airway.
8. Using a flexible endotracheal tube changer, replace the no. 6.0 uncuffed tube with an appropriately sized cuffed endotracheal tube.
9. Have an assistant monitor the patient during these manipulations, reacting to hemodynamic changes as necessary.

amnestics, and muscle relaxants are given to provide anesthetic management through the procedure.

If direct laryngoscopy proves unsuccessful and ventilation is easily maintained via a mask airway, we may proceed with intubation attempts as described in the following section for the unexpected difficult airway. Should ventilation be marginal, even with the use of a laryngeal mask airway, the patient may be awakened; if that proves not to be an option, tracheostomy can be performed.

Unexpected Difficult Intubation of a Cardiac Patient

Of course, it is rarely the patient we think will be difficult to intubate who actually is difficult. In this setting, we may assume two things: (1) that we have established that we can adequately ventilate the patient and (2) that we have already given fairly long-acting drugs and muscle relaxants. In essence, we are more or less committed to proceeding with intubation and surgery.

Table 3-6 describes an approach for the management of the unexpected difficult airway. Although we prefer to use the laryngeal mask airway to guide fiberoptic intubation, there are many approaches that could prove acceptable. Various guides to intubation are available, including lighted stylets, and other intubation aides. Which approach

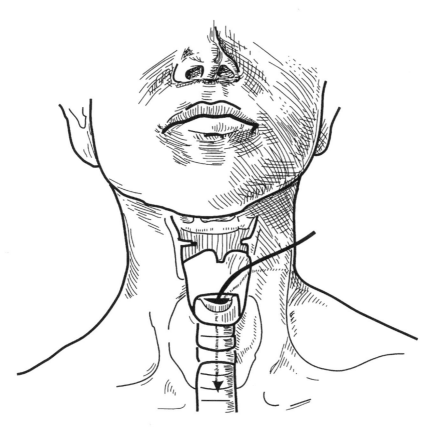

Figure 3-15. *The cricothyroid membrane is the entry point of an artificial airway during cricothyrotomy. (Reprinted with permission from WJ Hoffman, JD Wasnick [eds]. Postoperative Critical Care of The Massachusetts General Hospital. Boston: Little, Brown, 1992;13.)*

a given physician may employ is subject to individual preference. Nonetheless, the laryngeal mask airway approach has been, for the cardiac group at North Texas Anesthesia Consultants, very useful in this setting.

No matter how skillful we may be, there are times when we simply are not successful in securing the airway. Although we hope these times are rare, we must be prepared to take significant measures when we find ourselves in difficulty. The cricothyroid membrane serves as a ready site for placement of a 14-gauge catheter attached to an oxygen source should oxygenation be impaired (Figure 3-15). We must remember that such an approach fails to provide generally for adequate ventilation. Catheter oxygenation can secure oxygen delivery while we mobilize the surgical team for tracheostomy. It is important that we remember that we are, in fact, working with cardiac surgeons who should be able to perform tracheostomy and cricothyroidotomy relatively quickly. Surgeons should be engaged early on if we conclude we are unable to adequately oxygenate the patient. Indeed, even if we provide adequate ventilation and oxygenation, some patients may simply require a tracheostomy to facilitate surgery. Our thoracic surgeon should be of some use in this situation. Of course, we use the word *should* because nothing is ever guaranteed.

Last, a word about our friend Mighty Mouse anesthesiologist and the "let me have a try" attitude. Whenever there are intubation difficulties, a parade of mighty mice frequently appear uninvited in the operating room. Although it is wise to have assistance, one needs to choose assistance wisely. Many Mighty Mouse anesthesiologists have a no-lose attitude at times of intubation difficulty. If they successfully arrive in the operating room and place the endotracheal tube, they are, of course, the hero of the day and you become a slug. On the other hand, if they fail, there is no loss for them because it has already been shown that it is difficult and now that they have been unsuccessful, it must be really difficult to do. So there is no loss for an assistant to attempt an intubation. Indeed, this is particularly so because you as the physician of record are principally responsible when the teeth are dislodged or tissues perforated. You are the one who must take responsibility. Therefore, it is wise to limit Mighty Mouse assistance. Generally, one additional attempt at laryngoscopy by another individual seems appropriate. If you are experienced, it is foolish to allow a parade of anesthesiologists to attempt intubation. It is unlikely Mighty Mouse is any more skilled than anyone else in the operating room suite. Rather, he or she has no vested interest in how the case turns out. Unfortunately, in the politicized atmosphere of many operating room suites, many misguided anesthesiologists frequently enjoy seeing their colleagues suffer clinical difficulties. It is regrettable that such behavior remains a part of anesthesia practice. Ideally, when a difficult intubation is encountered, the appropriate response from a praxis perspective is to ask the physician in charge of the case one simple question: "How may I help you?" and then the assistant should act at the direction of the physician of record to assist him or her in facilitating intubation. It is not appropriate for the physician assistant to usurp authority for management of a case when it is not his or her responsibility or duty so to do.

Okay, Now the Tube Is In, But the Blood Pressure Is All Wrong

Now that we have successfully intubated our patient Mr. XY, he should be sailing happily along his anesthesia course. Because this is anesthesia, any number of hemodynamic changes may occur in the immediate postintubation period. Fortunately, none of these is as frustrating or lethal as failure to ventilate and oxygenate. Always remember that no matter how desperate a hemodynamic situation may be, sitting in the corner of the room is a perfusionist with a fully primed bypass machine. Although "crashing" onto bypass is highly undesirable, CPB is available as a readily accessible escape when hemodynamic catastrophe strikes. This is one distinct advantage of the cardiac operating room over the general surgical suite. Even though establishing CPB in the acute setting may be difficult, CPB is an escape mechanism that must not be forgotten. We discuss bypass management in greater detail elsewhere in this chapter and in Chapter 10. CPB is mentioned now only as a reminder that no matter how we may fail to correct or to prevent hemodynamic instability perioperatively, we always have this escape available to us.

Hypertension or hypotension may be frequently encountered in the immediate postinduction and peri-intubation period. Reviewing hemodynamics 101, we remember that

$$BP = CO \times \text{systemic vascular resistance (SVR)}$$

$$CO = \text{Stroke volume (SV)} \times HR$$

$$SV = LVEDV - \text{left ventricular end-systolic volume (LVESV)}$$
(Normal SV is approximately 70 ml per beat.)

$$SVR = \frac{\text{Mean arterial pressure (MAP)} - \text{central venous pressure (CVP)}}{CO} \times 80$$
(Normal SVR is approximately 800 and 1,200 dyne per second per cm^{-5}.)

From these basic formulas, we see that, in fact, elevated or reduced systemic BP can only result from changes in vascular tone, CO, or both. Of course, during the peri-induction period, we may well be affecting both of these variables. That is the bad news. The good news is that we need to correct only one or two variables for restoration of the "railroad track" hemodynamics that we all desire.

Postinduction Hypertension

Applying these formulas to postinduction hypertension is relatively straightforward, and hypertension is generally more easily treated than profound hypotension. Of course, hypertension and tachycardia can lead to ischemia and resulting ventricular failure. Still, the cause of perioperative hypertension is generally too little anesthesia and therefore is readily corrected. Unfortunately, we often overcorrect hypertension, resulting in the development of hypotension, which starts the patient on a hemodynamic roller coaster. Before we do that, however, we need to focus on an approach to the treatment of postinduction hypertension. Obviously, we should be aware of our patient's preinduction BP and what history he or she may have regarding antihypertension therapy. As previously mentioned, all antihypertensive drugs should be continued through the preoperative period to preclude withdrawal hypertension and tachycardia (e.g., secondary to clonidine or beta-blockade withdrawal).

Even though a patient may be hypertensive preoperatively, that does not imply that he or she will be so after anesthesia induction. Indeed, many patients who are hypertensive frequently become profoundly hypotensive once sympathetic outflow is reduced by the anesthetic state. Such patients must be closely monitored for development of significant hypotension after induction. Hypotension in this population is especially worrisome because autoregulation of blood flow may be significantly impaired, no longer ensuring adequate blood flow to vital organs at pressures significantly reduced from the patient's baseline.

Nonetheless, if a patient becomes hypertensive to the degree that it is necessary to treat the patient (as with so many things, absolutes rarely exist in anesthesia), we can employ our hemodynamic formula. If systolic BP is in excess of 200 mm Hg and 100 mm Hg diastolic, we advocate treatment in the peri-induction period. Even if these pressures are within the patient's BP range, the surgeon generally insists on lower pressures at the time of aortic cannulation prior to institution of CPB. Ideally, we aim to have the patient's BP at the lower end of their normal BP range. If the surgeon desires even lower pressures for aortic cannulation, we can quickly provide this and then permit the systolic pressure to return to the patient's lower normal baseline value.

Elevated BP can occur because of increased CO, increased peripheral vascular resistance, or both. CO may be increased either by an increase in SV, increase in HR, or both. SV increases because of either increased volume delivery to the heart, increased myocardial contractility, or both. HR can increase for many reasons (i.e., drug effects secondary to muscle relaxants [pancuronium], reflex response to vasodilation, increased catecholamine release). Certainly the release of catecholamines secondary to inadequate anesthesia can be a significant contributor to postinduction hypertension.

Elevated vascular tone and tachycardia are common responses to catecholamine production secondary to inadequate anesthesia. Of course, should the patient become significantly hypertensive, we must always consider error in administering vasoactive pressor drugs during the course of anesthetic induction.

Knowing the possible fundamental causes of hypertension (i.e., increased CO, increased vascular tone, or both), we can determine an effective response. Obviously, if HR and BP are elevated at the time of intubation, we readily conclude that most likely the patient has been inadequately anesthetized and may need supplemental narcotics, amnestics, or inhalational agents as appropriate to facilitate the overall management plan.

In the setting of a relative bradycardia and increased systemic pressure, we might conclude that peripheral resistance is elevated with a concomitant reflex decrease in HR. Again, inadequate anesthesia may be manifesting itself, but we must also consider that perhaps phenylephrine or other agents may have been given in error. Anesthetic agents or vasodilators may be given at this time, with due care as a response to periinduction hypertension.

If vasodilators are to be employed, it is prudent to use short-acting IV agents. Generally, IV nitroglycerin is our preferred vasodilator because of its beneficial effects in reducing ventricular volumes and myocardial wall tension, as well as its role as a coronary vasodilator. The pharmacology of IV nitroglycerin is reviewed later in this chapter. Other antihypertensive agents may be employed depending on circumstances. Labetalol has alpha-adrenergic blocking abilities in addition to nonspecific beta blockade. Of course, in a patient with compromised ventricular function, beta blockers could lead to cardiovascular collapse. As with all nonspecific beta blockers, labetalol may also produce bronchospasms. Five to 10 mg IV is given as necessary.

Hydralazine is an arterial vasodilator that may produce a reflex tachycardia, making it potentially undesirable in the cardiac patient. Five to 10 mg IV is given as a single bolus. The availability of hydralazine varies from institution to institution.

Nicardipine is a calcium antagonist. Nicardipine is a vasodilator that can produce a reflex increase in HR.

Nitroprusside is a direct-acting vasodilator of both arterial and venous vessels. As a consequence of vasodilator administration, tachycardia may occur, leading to ischemia. Coronary steal may likewise present as a consequence of coronary vasodilation leading blood flow away from ischemic tissues. Nitroprusside may result in increased cerebral blood flow, raising intracranial pressure, and like nitroglycerin, may impair hypoxic pulmonary vasoconstriction resulting in ventilation-perfusion mismatch and worsening any potential hypoxemia.

Cyanide toxicity is a concern with protracted use and in those with deficiency of the enzyme rhodanese. Cyanide toxicity is identified by an increasing mixed venous oxygen content in the setting of metabolic acidemia. Increased nitroprusside requirements and tachycardia may also indicate cyanide toxicity.

It is unlikely that sodium nitroprusside could be administered in the perioperative period to the degree necessary to develop cyanide or thiocyanate toxicity. However, as any anesthesia examinee will strangely remember, tobacco amblyopia patients as well as those with Leiber's optic atrophy are particularly at risk for nitroprusside-induced cyanide toxicity. Although it is conceivable in the peri-induction period to require nitroprusside to correct profound hypertension, this should be employed only after correction of any inadequate anesthesia that might be contributing to the patient's hypertension. Sodium nitroprusside is most frequently used postoperatively in intensive care units to correct hypertension.

Therefore, when we encounter peri-induction hypertension, we treat inadequate anesthesia by supplementing narcotics, amnestics, or inhalation agents as necessary. If BP remains elevated, the HR is elevated, and ventricular function is adequate, beta blockers or calcium antagonists along with nitroglycerin may be applied. Should elevated BP prove refractory to all interventions, sodium nitroprusside along with judicious beta blockade may be safely employed.

There is no magic formula to treating peri-induction hypertension. In the course of these interventions, you are likely to produce hypotension requiring treatment or perhaps even ischemia as a consequence of reflex tachycardia in the setting of a lower BP. Being both an actor and reactor should help to minimize any hemodynamic disturbance likely to cause significant patient injury.

Postinduction Hypotension

Even more than the threat of hypertension, nothing generates more anxiety among anesthesiologists, surgeons, and the operating room team than hypotension. By this we do not mean a relative hypotension compared with the patient's normal BP range. For Mr. XY, whose normal BP is 140/80, a pressure of 90/70 is a relative hypotension. Nonetheless, autoregulation of cerebral blood flow should compensate for this degree of relative BP decrease. On the other hand, a systolic BP of less than 60 mm Hg systolic is likely to precipitate great concern among all present. The interval in systolic BP between 90 mm Hg systolic in the patient who is generally normotensive and 60 mm Hg systolic remains a gray zone. It may not be considered worthy of treatment depending on the individual. Obviously, an elderly woman who generally maintains a significantly higher BP may not tolerate a systolic BP of less than 90 mm Hg adequately. Decreased urine output is but one manifestation of a systemic pressure too low to guarantee organ perfusion. What constitutes a pressure that is too low varies from individual to individual. Reduced systolic pressure much below 60 mm Hg systolic seems to warrant treatment in any instance.

Coronary perfusion pressure is equal to diastolic arterial pressure (DAP) minus LVEDP (CPP = DAP – LVEDP). Left coronary artery blood flow occurs for the most part during diastole. Therefore, systolic pressure is not in and of itself an adequate guide to ensure appropriate left coronary arterial perfusion pressure.

Mean BP may prove more helpful in assessing the pressure gradient established during coronary perfusion. This is hardly consistent with a praxis understanding of clinical cardiac anesthesia. No matter to what degree we may educate ourselves and the operating room community to the appropriateness of mean pressures, it is obvious that if the systolic pressure decreases too low, mean and diastolic pressure will likely decrease as well. In a patient at risk for myocardial ischemia, as systolic pressure decreases to the 70s and 60s, it is important that we both act and react to secure adequate perfusion pressure, but also to assure the surgeon and staff that the patient has not gotten out of our control. We must repeatedly demonstrate that we cannot only prevent wide hemodynamic swings through our careful management, but also correct them with little effort once they do occur. After all, it is just anesthesia.

Once again, we turn to hemodynamics 101 as our guide to peri-induction hypotension. Just as there were only two determinants of hypertension, so too there can only be two determinants of hypotension. You will recall that BP = CO × SVR. If we have a decreased BP, then the CO, vascular tone, or both have been reduced. How does anesthesia alter the equation? Assume we choose a relatively standard cardiac anesthetic, namely a synthetic narcotic, benzodiazepine, and nondepolarizing muscle relaxant. What effects can we expect? Of course anesthetic induction is likely to result in the decrease of sympathetic outflow, thereby reducing vascular tone. Vasodilation may subsequently lead to decrease in venous return to the heart, lowering CO. Additionally, HR reduction as a consequence of the vagotonic effects of drugs such as fentanyl may further reduce CO. Remember, CO = HR × SV. Therefore, induction of anesthesia can reduce both CO and vascular tone. No wonder our patient is hypotensive. It's the anesthesia, stupid! Well, naturally, nothing is ever quite as simple and straightforward as this simple assessment. Both a decreased HR and decreased venous return to the heart may contribute to a decreased CO. They are not the only possible sources of a decreased CO, however. Ventricular dysfunction either as a consequence of obstruction to blood flow such as in aortic stenosis or idiopathic hypertrophic subaortic stenosis or secondary to inadequate myocardial contractility may also reduce both CO and systemic BP.

Therefore, we have to be able to distinguish among those causes that contribute to peri-induction hypotension. Previously, we argued that preinduction placement of a PA catheter appeared unnecessary. Now you may be thinking, if that PA catheter is in place we could make some definitive diagnosis about why the patient is currently hypotensive (i.e., crashing). So how then, we must ask, would the PA catheter and the information obtained from it contribute to our management scheme? Recall that we identified the PA line as assisting us in two principal ways. First, we can measure the CO, and second, we are aware that the pulmonary catheter occlusion pressure approximates the LVEDP, which further approximates LVEDV depending on the overall compliance of the left ventricle. By including these values with our basic hemodynamic understanding, we may further refine our interventions (Figure 3-16).

As Figure 3-16 demonstrates, we may calculate the SV and obtain a measure of the pulmonary capillary occlusion pressure so that we can determine whether the cause of hypotension in the setting of decreased SV is principally a consequence of hypovolemia or secondary to ventricular dysfunction.

From this approach we might conclude that to effectively diagnose and treat perioperative hypotension, we must have already placed our pulmonary capillary occlusion catheter. However, as previously mentioned, awake or sedated placement of a PA catheter may lead to its own particular problems. Oversedation, decreased ventilation, and tachycardia secondary to anxiety are but a few concerns raised by

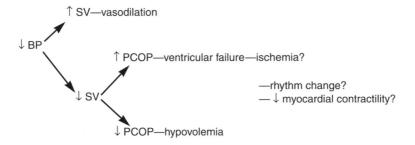

↓ systemic BP

Recall BP = CO × SVR

CO = SV × HR $SV = \dfrac{CO}{HR}$

SV = left ventricular end-diastolic volume − left ventricular end-systolic volume

NL = 60–80 ml/beat

↓ BP → ↑ SV—vasodilation

↓ SV → ↑ PCOP—ventricular failure—ischemia?

—rhythm change?
— ↓ myocardial contractility?

↓ PCOP—hypovolemia

If ↓ SV and ↑ PCOP, R/O ischemia, rhythm change;
administer inotropes/nitrates/mechanical assistance.

If ↓ SV and ↓ PCOP, correct hypovolemia.

If ↓ BP and ↑ SV, restore vascular tone.

Figure 3-16. *Diagnostic guide to peri-induction hypotension. (BP = blood pressure; CO = cardiac output; SVR = systemic vascular resistance; SV = stroke volume; HR = heart rate; NL = normal limits; PCOP = pulmonary capillary occlusion pressure; R/O = rule out.)*

placement of the PA line in the awake patient. Placement of the line can be readily done, and many institutions insist on awake catheter placement. In certain teaching institutions, surgeons are so concerned that the anesthesiologist will lacerate the carotid artery that they insist on line placement prior to induction so that the case may be canceled in the event of significant carotid arterial trauma or inadvertent cannulation. We believe this approach is of little benefit to the patient. In fact, safe induction of anesthesia and management of peri-induction hypotension can be readily achieved with PA cannulation after intubation. First, we must consider the time the PA line placement actually consumes. With some practice, both access to the central circulation and PA catheterization can be achieved in a few minutes. Thus, we place the PA line immediately after endotracheal intubation. Literally, this occurs within seconds after induction of anesthesia. Nonetheless, suppose that at the time of induction the blood pressure decreases to 60–70 mm Hg systolic—what then? Are we vasodilated? Hypovolemic? Ischemic? We have not yet placed our PA catheter, and we are in the situation where we need to treat the BP. So what are we to do? What do we know? The answer to what we know is as follows: (1) We have just administered an anesthetic capable of decreasing sympathetic outflow and reducing both HR and venous return to the heart. Additionally, we know that this vasodilation may result in hypotension. (2) We have in place a multi-lead ECG capable of looking for signs of ischemia or rhythm change. (3) We have a TEE probe and machine in the operating room. Again, with practice this can be easily placed after endotracheal intubation. TEE can provide a quick assessment of ventricular contractility. Although various volume-loading conditions may complicate the assessment for wall motion abnormalities, a quick examination of ventricular function by TEE should determine if myocardial function is indeed impaired. We must remember that all wall motion abnormalities are not a consequence of ischemia and infarction. Additionally, because the TEE probe is placed after induction, we will probably not have benefit of a pre-operative TEE result to compare as a baseline. Nonetheless, if the heart is not working, it will be clear on the TEE result. Indeed, with limited experience, it is quite possible to distinguish a poorly contracting ventricle from one that is unimpaired. Although such a level of skill no doubt falls short of a cardiologist for the purpose of TEE interpretation, this can nevertheless provide the anesthesiologist with a guide to therapy.

Therefore, if the BP is decreased without evidence on the ECG of ischemia or significant rhythm change, we must conclude that decreased sympathetic outflow as a consequence of induction is responsible for hypotension. This can be easily corrected by a combination of volume replacement and brief pressor support. Indeed, such quick bolus administrations of pressors are often necessary in the peri-induc-

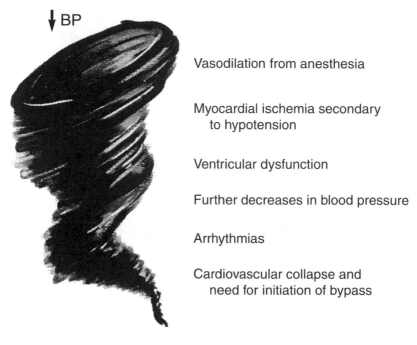

↓ BP

Vasodilation from anesthesia

Myocardial ischemia secondary
to hypotension

Ventricular dysfunction

Further decreases in blood pressure

Arrhythmias

Cardiovascular collapse and
need for initiation of bypass

Figure 3-17. *The hemodynamic spiral. (BP = blood pressure.)*

tion period. After all, even if the cause of hypotension is simply a consequence of vasodilation and decreased sympathetic outflow, if left untreated, the diseased heart may well become underperfused, leading to a downward hemodynamic spiral (Figure 3-17).

Thus, moderate hypotension can ultimately spiral out of control, producing an operating room crisis, recriminations, and of course, naturally a situation in which the anesthesiologist will be blamed for any misadventure encountered by the patient through the course of their entire admission. This spiral can be avoided through proactive, active, and reactive interventions.

Quick Pressor Support
This is not the elegant application of pharmacotherapy that many would like to project as the raison d'être of cardiac anesthesia. Rather, as we explained previously, barring obvious signs of ischemia by ECG or decreased ventricular function on TEE, generally peri-induction hypotension occurs as a consequence of anesthetic induction and

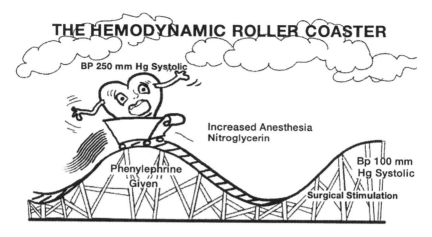

Figure 3-18. *The hemodynamic roller coaster. (BP = blood pressure.)*

decreased sympathetic outflow. In that setting, it becomes essential to avoid the hemodynamic spiral and restore sympathetic tone. Our surgical colleagues are going to help in that regard when they let loose with the sternal saw. Unfortunately, the preparation time in a cardiac case can seem intolerably long—that is, 20–30 minutes may pass between induction and the actual start of surgery. This is a long time to wait for sympathetic outflow to increase as a consequence of a patient encountering the reality of cold steel. Additionally, we are supposed to have been providing a stress-free anesthetic anyway. Thus, generally we do not want surgical stimulation to result in excessive tachycardia, hypertension, and increased sympathetic tone. So like it or not, we are at a point at which we must administer pressors to restore BP.

Small amounts of phenylephrine or ephedrine administered by IV bolus generally restores systemic pressure. We occasionally overshoot our mark. A hypotensive crisis that could lead to myocardial ischemia can readily be transformed into a hypertensive crisis that can lead to myocardial ischemia. Therefore, we should always start with a relatively small amount of phenylephrine or ephedrine and observe and react. Obviously, if the BP reaches 260 mm Hg systolic, we have overshot our mark and now must lower the BP. Such hemodynamic roller coasters are infrequent but can occur and complicate our peri-induction hemodynamic management (Figure 3-18). Avoiding the hemodynamic roller coaster can be difficult. Nevertheless, by the administration of small amounts of pressors given through bolus dosing we can restore BP with limited risk of overshooting our mark.

Phenylephrine Pharmacology

Phenylephrine is an alpha$_1$-receptor sympathetic agonist. It produces both arterial and venous vasoconstriction. It elevates PA pressures. CO may be decreased, along with decreases in renal blood flow. Phenylephrine may produce reflex bradycardia. Generally, 10–20 mg of phenylephrine may be mixed in a 250-ml bag of diluent. Administration is either by a bolus of 1–2 ml of 20 mg in 250-ml solution or by continuous infusion.

Phenylephrine restores BP, but there is a downside to its use as well. As mentioned previously, phenylephrine can decrease CO, decrease renal perfusion, and elevate PA pressures, potentially contributing to right ventricular dysfunction. If we take a purely theoretical look at phenylephrine, we might find it lacking as an appropriate response to peri-induction hypotension in the cardiac patient. Still, its benefits generally far outweigh its faults. If the patient remains hypotensive, we are in danger of starting down the hemodynamic spiral. We need to do something. By increasing BP without increasing HR, myocardial oxygen supply should improve, thereby reducing the likelihood of developing ventricular dysfunction. Of course, increased vascular tone could lead to increased myocardial wall tension and oxygen consumption.

Still, even if myocardial ischemia is the cause of hypotension, restoring systolic pressure should improve CPP, thereby correcting the oxygen imbalance. An infusion of nitroglycerin may simultaneously result in dilation of the coronary vasculature. Therefore, even as phenylephrine increases vascular tone, nitroglycerin may promote venous dilation to a degree. Additionally, nitroglycerin's ability as a vasodilator can reduce ventricular size even in the setting of increased arterial tone, thereby reducing ventricular wall tension and decreasing myocardial oxygen demand and ischemia. Thus, even if we conclude that ischemia is the true cause of hypotension, phenylephrine combined with nitroglycerin may effectively restore hemodynamic stability and relieve ischemia. On the other hand, if the heart is simply failing as a consequence of long-standing cardiomyopathy, administration of phenylephrine would not be the ideal choice to correct peri-induction hypotension. Although BP may be restored, increased vascular tone could simply lead to ventricular distention and hemodynamic collapse. In this instance, other inotropes might be indicated (i.e., dobutamine, dopamine, milrinone, or amrinone). These are discussed in Chapter 8.

Obviously, the patient's history will be of use to us in guiding the selection of vasoactive drugs. If patients are known to have a marginal ventricular function (i.e., ejection fraction of less than 30%), their ability to tolerate the effects of increased vascular tone may well be minimal. In this setting, we should titrate inotropes as necessary to restore BP. Obviously TEE can be of great value in assessing how our pharmacologic manipulations alter ventricular performance. In such a setting, the best move would be to titrate inotropes by infusion as necessary to improve CO and to increase BP. Nevertheless, such ventricular dysfunction should rarely surprise us if we have done an adequate preoperative assessment. The vast majority of our patients, such as Mr. XY, have more or less adequate ventricular function. Pressor support with phenylephrine with or without nitroglycerin may sufficiently stabilize the patient following induction should hypotension develop.

Ephedrine Pharmacology
At times you will want to provide a simple correction of hypotension in a patient with bradycardia (i.e., HR of less than 50 beats per minute). Decreased venous return to the heart, narcotics, and decreased sympathetic tone can often produce bradycardia and hypotension. Phenylephrine as an alpha$_1$-agonist can, through reflex mechanisms, contribute to additional reductions in HR. In this setting, small amounts of ephedrine may prove useful to restore HR and BP.

Ephedrine has both direct effects on alpha and beta receptors as well as stimulating the release of norepinephrine. Ephedrine increases HR and myocardial contractility and to a degree vascular tone. It is contraindicated in patients taking monamine oxidase inhibitors. Ephedrine can have an effect lasting several minutes. Ephedrine is administered in 5- to 10-mg bolus as needed.

Ephedrine increases both HR and myocardial contractility. Therefore, it can lead to increased myocardial oxygen consumption and potentially to ischemia. Nonetheless, it is useful when the HR is slow and BP reduced.

So what can be said about quick pressor support in the peri-induction period? Quick pressor support (1) restores BP; (2) can aggravate ischemia; (3) can correct ischemia; (4) may allow us to avoid the hemodynamic spiral; and (5) may start us along the hemodynamic roller coaster.

In essence, whenever we take an action, we hope that we achieve the stability that we desire. Of course, this does not always occur, and we are compelled to try something else. Only the foolish anesthetist continues with the same approach to therapy once it has been discerned that it does not achieve the goals. If a patient is hypotensive with ventricular dysfunction as discerned through TEE evaluation and direct vision, then by all means we need to improve myocardial contractility either pharmacologically with inotropes or mechanically with an intra-aortic balloon pump. Clearly, if the heart is failing, an additional dose of phenylephrine would be inappropriate. If one continues to administer phenylephrine, the heart fails and distends like a muscular balloon.

Try as we may, some patients simply deteriorate after induction to the degree we cannot correct their problems. The left main coronary artery may develop a thrombosis at any time during the induction, which can result in quick deterioration in spite of all of our efforts. A good reminder is to keep heparin anticoagulation therapy in place up until the time of surgery in those patients who are a risk for left main occlusion. In this instance, there is little the anesthesiologist can offer except to be prepared to provide for emergency institution of CPB.

It is no disgrace to have to have a patient go on bypass emergently. Surgeons should heed our recommendations and expeditiously place cannulas as needed on our instruction should we determine that the patient's hypotensive course is not salvageable through the administration of pharmacotherapy. Indeed, at times no matter which drugs we choose or how we employ them, bypass is the only mechanism to ensure an adequate systemic perfusion.

Peri-Induction Myocardial Ischemia

We have already discussed in some detail mechanisms and approaches to the treatment of myocardial ischemia. Ischemia that occurs after anesthesia induction is no different than myocardial ischemia produced at any other time. Inadequate myocardial oxygen supply unable to meet increased myocardial oxygen demand results in myocardial ischemia.

If patients become ischemic as a consequence of hypertension and tachycardia, additional narcotic, benzodiazepine, and inhalational agents may be administered to attempt to decrease myocardial oxygen demand. If ineffective, beta blockers (i.e., esmolol) or nitroglycerin can be given to improve the myocardial oxygen supply and demand balance.

Should hypotension be the precipitant of myocardial ischemia, as described previously, a combination of phenylephrine and nitroglycerin may be titrated to effect. In patients with refractory ischemia, intraoperative balloon counterpulsation may be initiated with the assistance of a surgical team or bypass initiated to reduce myocardial wall tension and myocardial oxygen demand.

In general, providing an adequate anesthetic depth produces an environment where hemodynamic perturbations are minimal. Still, the patient's ECG should be constantly monitored throughout the induction so that anti-ischemic interventions may be undertaken as quickly as possible.

Nitroglycerin vasodilates venous vessels as well as coronary arteries and arterioles. As such, venous return is decreased, reducing myocardial wall tension and thereby improving the balance between myocardial oxygen supply and demand. PA pressures are decreased. Nitroglycerin's ability to vasodilate pulmonary vasculature can impair hypoxic pulmonary vasoconstriction and with prolonged use may lead to tachyphylaxis and methemoglobinemia. Nitroglycerin is delivered by infusion and should be titrated to effect. As with other pharmacologic infusions, it is better to start with a relatively low dose and then titrate upward as needed. Like the pressor drugs, vasodilators too can put us on the hemodynamic roller coaster. Careful observation and acting and reacting can prevent iatrogenic hypotension leading to ischemia and yet another episode in which anesthesia and the anesthesiologist's actions are blamed for a patient's instability.

As a practical concern, we need to be cognizant that whenever a hemodynamic change occurs, even to the slightest degree, the surgeon is most likely going to ascribe any adverse outcome in the patient to that event. For example, if during induction the patient experiences a few moments of hypotension to say 60 mm Hg, if that patient subsequently develops renal failure, anesthesia will be blamed.

The patient may well have been on CPB for several hours or may have recently received a load of IV contrast dye or simply may have a history of renal or vascular disease. No matter what other factors may present, the surgeon tends to first and foremost be a spin doctor. The fact that a surgeon keeps a patient on bypass for an incredibly long time or embolizes material from the aortic cannulation site has little effect on these spin surgeons. It is important we collectively take every precaution to minimize hemodynamic embarrassment, not only to protect our patients, but also to prevent our surgical colleagues from having too easy a time spinning the case should complications develop.

Our team is privileged to work with surgeons who generally take responsibility for their own actions as we do for ours. Nevertheless, there are surgeons who in this era of constantly monitored morbidity and mortality attempt to ascribe blame for routine surgical complications on the anesthesiologist. Should an anesthesiologist have difficulty, he or she should seek surgical assistance whenever necessary. There is no embarrassment in working with a surgeon to secure the airway or in crashing on bypass if that will improve a patient's outcome.

Peri-Induction Dysrhythmia

Tachycardias
Having successfully managed to induce anesthesia without producing significant hypertension or hypotension generally implies that a normal sinus rhythm has been maintained. Of course, it is possible that the BP remains acceptable even with various rhythm disturbances. Nonetheless, it is important to correct arrhythmias because they can ultimately lead to an imbalance between myocardial oxygen supply and demand. Tachycardias can be particularly annoying to the cardiac anesthesiologist because they not only increase myocardial oxygen consumption, but also shorten diastolic time. Because much perfusion of the left ventricle occurs during diastole, tachycardias present a myocardial oxygen supply problem as well as one of increased demand. So obviously tachycardias need to be identified and corrected. In general, tachycardias may be classified as either primary or secondary. Primary tachycardias include atrial fibrillation or flutter, other supraventricular tachycardias, and ventricular tachycardias and fibrillation. These are briefly discussed with regard to treatment options in the cardiac operating room. Secondary tachycardias include those sinus tachycardias (i.e., HR of more than 100 beats per minute) that occur secondary to anemia, light anesthesia, pain, anxiety, fever, thyrotoxicosis, hypovolemia, hypercarbia, bladder distention, and vagolysis secondary to anesthesia.

Secondary Tachycardias
Secondary causes of sinus tachycardia need to be corrected before applying pharmacotherapy directed at decreasing the HR. A number of these secondary etiologies of sinus tachycardia are present in the cardiac operating room. Although it is unlikely that patients with significant anemia (i.e., hematocrit of less than 20) would be electively taken into surgery, it is possible that in certain emergency situations (e.g., chest trauma, reoperation for bleeding, emergencies from the cardiac catheterization laboratory), the patient may have developed significant anemia. Because hemodilution-associated CPB serves only to further decrease the hematocrit, anemias should be treated with packed red

blood cells as needed. Recall that anemia decreases the oxygen content of blood, which can lead to inadequate myocardial oxygen supply.

Inadequate anesthesia associated with hypertension and tachycardia is a relatively common occurrence and can generally be treated with additional narcotics, inhalational agents, or both. Of course, anesthetics themselves (i.e., desflurane, isoflurane) can be associated with reflex tachycardias secondary to vasodilation and vagolysis. Increasing the inspired inhalational concentration may further increase the HR. Of course, the beauty of inhalational anesthesia is the ease of administration. Should we determine that a patient is tachycardic because of light anesthesia and elect to increase the concentration of inhalational anesthesia, the patient's HR will decrease if this is the correct assumption. On the other hand, if an increase in the concentration of inhalational agents either does nothing or results in increased HR, then we know that we must try something else.

Bladder distension can be a problem in the cardiac surgical patient if a bladder catheter is not properly inserted or has become occluded. Patients should never be anuric. Even if they experience acute renal failure, small amounts of urine will be produced and collected into the drainage apparatus. If during surgery absolutely no urine is produced in the setting of hypertension and tachycardia, the bladder catheter must be checked to ensure that it is not obstructed, and the surgeon should palpate the abdomen for signs of bladder distension.

Having ruled out other precipitants of sinus tachycardia, if the patient remains tachycardic, small amounts of esmolol, 10–20 mg, may be administered to effect, assuming the patient is free of any contraindication to beta blockade. Esmolol is a $beta_1$-selective blocking agent with a relatively short half-life (i.e., $\tau 1/2 = 9$ minutes). Inactivated by red cell esterase, esmolol can be administered either by a small bolus (IV) to effect (i.e., 10–20 mg) or by continuous infusion. Should protracted beta blockade be desired, 0.5 mg per kg is given as a loading dose, followed by an infusion startup at 50 µg per kg per minute. The dose is then titrated to effect as needed to achieve the desired heart rate and blood pressure. Obviously, bronchospasm and congestive heart failure can be exacerbated by beta blockade. Fortunately, the dose needed to slow the heart is usually low, and esmolol's effects are short lived. (After the desired rate and rhythm are achieved the infusion of esmolol is reduced to a maintenance rate of approximately 20 µg per kg per minute. Therefore, if we wish to correct sinus tachycardia of uncertain etiology, esmolol may be relatively safely used.)

Table 3-7. Common Mechanical Sources of Intraoperative Arrhythmias

1. Ventricular tachycardias and premature ventricular complexes.
   a. Check Swan-Ganz catheter placement. Is a ventricular tracing present? If yes, advance catheter into pulmonary outflow track.
   b. Is the heart being manipulated out of the chest? Alert surgeon to stop.
2. Atrial fibrillation: Is the surgeon cannulating the right atrium? Arrhythmia often resolves following successful placement.

Nevertheless, if tachycardia is the compensation mechanism for a failing heart, beta blockade may well lead to cardiovascular collapse. As always, knowledge of the patient's preoperative condition will guide therapy.

Primary Tachycardias
Although the purpose of this section is not to provide a comprehensive review of arrhythmia management, we consider a few classic arrhythmias in general and their treatment in the cardiac surgery operating room. Before doing so, we must take account of the surgeon's actions. Many of the dysrhythmias encountered in surgery relate directly to surgical manipulation of the heart. Therefore, before panicking at the sight of ventricular tachycardia or rapid onset of atrial fibrillation, we must be aware of what the surgeon is doing (Table 3-7).

As Table 3-7 suggests, mechanical manipulation of the heart to achieve cannulation or release adhesions (especially for reoperative surgery) may be the source of numerous arrhythmias following sternotomy. Correction of the rhythm generally follows cessation of the precipitating cardiac manipulation. Nevertheless, occasionally an unacceptable rhythm presents requiring treatment. Still, if it is the surgeon who is causing a hemodynamically significant arrhythmia, it may be necessary to insist that the cannulas be placed to initiate CPB should further surgical manipulation of the heart be necessary.

Often arrhythmias that occur after induction are caused either by the PA catheter "tickling" the ventricle or as a consequence of surgical manipulation of the heart. These are by no means the only causes of such peri-induction dysrhythmias. Hypokalemia associated with hyperventilation, hypothermia, hypoxemia, hypercarbia, acid–base imbalance, and, of course, ischemia may contribute to the development of various abnormal rhythms. Many patients have a preoperative arrhythmia such as atrial fibrillation or suffer frequent premature ventricular contractions. Remember first and foremost that you are not a cardiologist. If the patient has made it to cardiac surgery, someone has already attempted to control the dysrhythmias. Therefore, it is unlikely that you will necessarily correct a previous arrhythmia in the peri-induction period. It is important, however, to continue anti-arrhythmia drugs preoperatively so that heightened sympathetic tone in the surgical suite does not lead to more malignant arrhythmias and patient deterioration. As such, antiarrhythmic as well as anti-ischemic agents must be continued perioperatively.

Anesthetic agents, as a consequence of their vagotonic and vagolytic effects, may also contribute to the development of various degrees of bradycardias and tachycardias. Accelerated nodal rhythms frequently accompany anesthesia in both the cardiac and noncardiac surgical patient. Thus, knowing that so many things may contribute to peri-induction arrhythmias, what actually do you need to do? If you are lucky, nothing. If arrhythmias appear related to some mechanical activity cessation, completion of the offending action should correct the problem. Problems related to electrolyte and acid–base disorders should not be a problem if we have carefully monitored our laboratory results preoperatively and adjusted our patient management accordingly. Similarly, continuing preoperative medical therapy should prevent any baseline arrhythmias from going out of control in the operating room. Last, we should choose anesthetics and doses in such a way that we do not provide unopposed vagotonia or vagolysis as a consequence of our drug selection. Of course, having done all of that, we still may end up with a patient who has significant arrhythmias after induction. Now what are we to do?

The particulars of rhythm identification can be found in any number of texts concerned with ECG interpretation. Obviously, once we determine that the rhythm is something other than sinus at an acceptable rate, we need to ask two questions: (1) What is the rhythm? (2) Does it matter? Question 1 is important as it will guide our therapy, and question 2 determines whether that therapy needs to be administered. What is the rhythm? Namely, is the arrhythmia of supraventricular or ventricular origin? This is crucial because treatment for most supraventricular rhythms differs from the treatment of ventricular arrhythmias. Does it matter? Well, if the rhythm causes no significant hemodynamic compromise, treatment may not be necessary. But we must be careful. Rapid HRs, as we have discussed previously, can lead to ischemia. Therefore, the decision not to treat an aberrant rhythm must be carefully considered. Additionally, most rhythm disturbances matter because they can herald underlying ischemia or some other problem.

Supraventricular dysrhythmias include atrial fibrillation, atrial flutter, and supraventricular tachycardia. Supraventricular dysrhythmias are characterized by generally well-preserved QRS complexes and by either an absent P wave, such as in atrial fibrillation, or a P wave lost among the QRS complex (i.e., supraventricular tachycardias). In the cardiac operating room with the chest open, electroversion paddles at hand, and a perfusionist standing by, quick synchronized cardioversion of new onset supraventricular arrhythmias (Figure 3-19) is preferred treatment if the ventricular response and hemodynamic effects appear to threaten the patient or lead to myocardial ischemia. Calcium antagonists and beta blockers may be employed to slow the ventricular response as necessary. Should a patient have a history of recurrent supraventricular tachycardia and accessory conduction bundle, therapy with digoxin, beta blockers, and calcium antagonists could lead to degeneration of the rhythm to ventricular fibrillation. Because the chest is opened and synchronized cardioversion is at hand, electroversion of supraventricular arrhythmias is easily achieved. Adenosine (6 mg) can be used for supraventricular rhythms. Rapidly metabolized, adenosine slows atrioventricular nodal conduction. If pharmacotherapy is planned for arrhythmias, cardioversion needs to be readily at hand. And since we are in the operating room with an open chest, most assuredly it is.

Digoxin is frequently used in the treatment of supraventricular dysrhythmias. In addition to increasing intramyocardial calcium concentration, digoxin slows conduction through the atrioventricular node. Therefore, it can slow the ventricular response to atrial fibrillation. Digoxin is eliminated via the kidneys; therefore, renal impairment can lead to a toxic dosage. In general, in the prebypass period, there is little reason to employ this drug for correction of supraventricular dysrhythmias. Occasionally, digoxin may be administered postoperatively for alleged prophylaxis against supraventricular tachycardia in the surgical patient. However, the success of this maneuver remains questionable. Obviously, care must be taken to ensure that hypokalemia is corrected to minimize the incidence of digitalis toxicity.

In treating supraventricular dysrhythmias in the prebypass, postinduction period, we aim to achieve hemodynamic stability as our guide to effective treatment. Because we have the benefit of an open chest and a perfusionist at our side to assist should our manipulation lead to ventricular tachycardia or fibrillation, we can readily escape from most complications of our antiarrhythmia management.

Ventricular Tachycardias
The development of ventricular tachycardia or ventricular fibrillation after induction of anesthesia in the coronary artery bypass patient will be

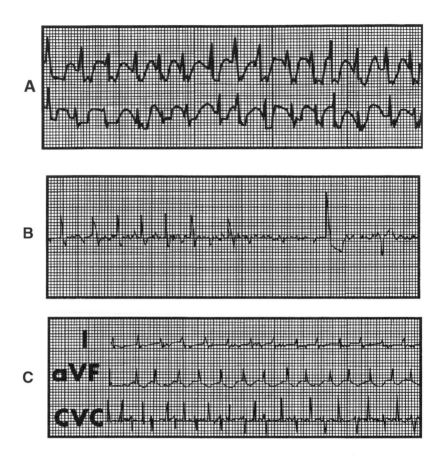

Figure 3-19. *Sample rhythm strips of supraventricular arrhythmias. (A) Atrial fibrillation with rapid ventricular response. Fibrillation waves are not obvious. QRS irregularity may be missed because ventricular rate is rapid. (B) Atrial flutter with 2 to 1 atrioventricular block. Carotid sinus massage increases the block and unmasks flutter waves. (C) Atrioventricular reentry tachycardias. No P waves are evident in surface leads (I, V$_F$). The atrial electrocardiogram form the central venous catheter (CVC) demonstrates atrial activity occurring some time after the QRS, suggesting that the rhythm is atrioventricular reentry tachycardia. (Reprinted with permission from TE Oh. Intensive Care Manual [4th ed]. Oxford: Butterworth–Heinemann, 1997.)*

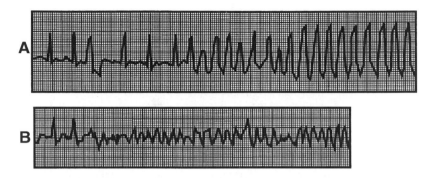

Figure 3-20. *Ventricular arrhythmias. (A) Ventricular tachycardia. (B) Ventricular fibrillation. (Reprinted with permission from TE Oh. Intensive Care Manual [4th ed]. Oxford: Butterworth–Heinemann, 1997.)*

of great concern. Generally, therapy is directed at immediate electrical conversion of the rhythm either with external or internal defibrillation paddles. As in cardiopulmonary resuscitation protocols, electrical conversion of the rhythm is essential. Unlike cardiopulmonary resuscitation in the intensive care unit or on the ward, a lethal rhythm can be survived as long as the surgical team is readily available to initiate CPB either through opening of the sternum in primary cases or through femoral bypass in patients undergoing re-do surgery. Ventricular fibrillation in the peri-induction period can be survived by open chest cardiac massage and the institution of CPB. What is essential in the treatment of ventricular fibrillation in the operating room is that definitive action be taken. Yes, the chest needs to be open. Yes, we must heparinize the patient. Yes, we must give epinephrine, lidocaine, and electrical shock as necessary. And, yes, we must do what is necessary to initiate effective resuscitative measures. Figure 3-20 demonstrates ventricular arrhythmias.

If the rhythm is corrected, one may safely proceed with surgery in a normal course. Intravenous lidocaine should be given and a lidocaine infusion begun. Alternatively, procainamide, bretylium, or both may be administered as necessary to secure sinus rhythm. Table 3-8 presents information regarding the use of lidocaine, procainamide, and bretylium in the cardiac surgical patient.

It is certainly not our purpose to review antiarrhythmic therapy in great detail. Suffice it to say, if you notice that Mr. XY is in ventricular fibrillation in the cardiac operating room, then you do, in fact, have a problem. Generally, you must first remember a few basic anesthesia

Table 3-8. Antiarrhythmics by Intravenous Infusion

Agent	Action	Dose	Adverse Effects
Lidocaine	Decreased automaticity; decreased conduction in injured myocardium	50–100 mg load 1–4 mg/min	Central nervous system toxicity; decreased myocardial contractility
Procainamide	Decreased conduction velocity; decreased automaticity	50 mg/min load to 600 mg maintenance 2–4 mg/min; watch QRS widening on electrocardiogram	Atrioventricular block; myocardial depression; torsades des pointes
Bretylium	Prolongs action potential; blocks adrenergic release	Load 5 mg/kg up to 30 mg/kg; infuse 1–2 mg/min	Initial hypertension, then hypotension

principles. Namely, is the PA line in some way irritating the ventricle? Also, less we forget the basics: acid–base and electrolyte balances and gas exchange, must be acceptable. Assuming we have corrected any obvious precipitants of ventricular dysrhythmias, we must conclude that the patient's primary disease process is responsible for the development of ventricular fibrillation or tachycardia. In general, should ventricular fibrillation present, the prompt application of electrical current is the appropriate therapy. If unsuccessful after a number of attempts, cardiopulmonary resuscitation should be instituted and epinephrine administered, following Advanced Cardiopulmonary Life Support routine. Of course, since we are not on a hospital floor unit, the chest can be quickly opened or the groins prepared so that CPB may be initiated. Rapid institution of bypass, along with cardiopulmonary resuscitation, can permit a patient who develops a life-threatening arrhythmia to survive to permit surgical revascularization and, it is hoped, successful resuscitation.

Peri-Induction Bradycardias
Bradycardias may also complicate the peri-induction period. Vagotonic agents such as sufentanil can result in the development of sinus brady-

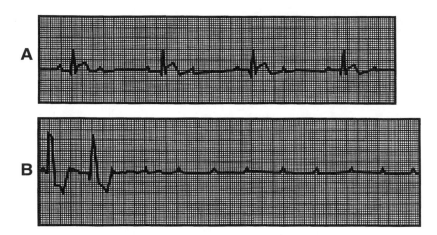

Figure 3-21. *Second-degree heart block. (A) Second-degree (2 to 1) atrioventricular block (atrial rate of 76/minute, ventricular rate of 38/minute). (B) Third-degree (complete) atrioventricular block and ventricular asystole. Failure of ventricular pacing is followed by complete heart block. Sinoatrial node discharge continues (P waves) but no ventricular escape pacemaker emerges. (Reprinted with permission from TE Oh. Intensive Care Manual [4th ed]. Oxford: Butterworth–Heinemann, 1997.)*

cardia. In and of itself, the HR is of little consequence except that such bradycardia may contribute to decreased CO and hypotension. Hypotension might then lead to the development of myocardial ischemia. Reflex bradycardias may also occur in the setting of hypertension. Often treatment of peri-induction hypotension with a small bolus dose of phenylephrine can produce a slowing of the HR.

Also, patients who are experiencing myocardial ischemia and infarction may develop any number of conduction defects. Second- and third-degree heart blocks that occur perioperatively should already have been treated by temporary pacing. On the other hand, if significant heart block develops in the postinduction period, temporary pacing should be initiated. Many PA flotation catheters are equipped with access for pacing wires or have pacing ability in themselves. Because the chest is open, the surgeon can place epicardial pacing wires if necessary. If varying degrees of heart block develop that lead to cardiovascular collapse in the postinduction period, signs of acute ischemia and decompensation should be sought and treated (Figure 3-21). In such instances, rapid institution of CPB corrects hemodynamic collapse and protects against patient injury as a consequence of hypoperfusion. Fortunately, bradycardia is often simply just a consequence of anesthesia induction. Therapy is therefore guided to increase the HR and restore BP. We previously described the usage of ephedrine in the peri-induction period. Small doses, 5 mg IV, may be given to increase HR and BP. Of course, there is always a danger in giving pressor agents that we may start the patient along a hemodynamic roller coaster. However, for the most part, ephedrine administration is very useful in this setting. Atropine, the muscarinic antagonist, increases HR. In addition to its antisialagogue and bronchodilator effects, atropine may produce central anticholinergic syndrome. Given as a 0.4- to 2.0-mg dose, atropine may lead to worrisome tachycardias that might exacerbate myocardial ischemia in the cardiac patient. Nonetheless, if the HR is really slow, a dose of atropine may well speed things up; however, you may need to subsequently slow things down. But as with so many things, we must face one problem at a time. Glycopyrrolate, 0.2 mg IV, may be similarly given as a response to significant sinus bradycardias. Vasoactive infusions of dobutamine, isoproterenol, and epinephrine likewise increase HR and BP. Starting infusions to correct sinus bradycardia at the time of induction may be overkill. Indeed, fluid administration and surgical stimulation often corrects BP and HR reductions. Small doses of ephedrine generally restore pressure if surgical stimuli are not immediately forthcoming. Although some may administer additional vagolytic muscle relaxants (i.e., pancuronium) to offset peri-induction bradycardia, we believe it is more prudent to treat bradycardias with ephedrine rather than to rely on the side effects of muscle relaxants. Transesophageal pacing and other pacing modalities may likewise be employed to correct peri-induction bradycardia if available.

So What Does a Good Induction Do Anyway?

Having presented a number of scenarios by which Mr. XY may end up riding the hemodynamic roller coaster, what is an ideal induction? First, we want the patient to be asleep. It is important that when providing a narcotic anesthetic we have not neglected to include amnestics. Whereas the large syringe of narcotics may well provide hemodynamic stability, it is important to remember that each patient is different. Alcoholics and other substance abusers may require significantly more anesthesia to achieve what we might consider to be a safe anesthetic depth. Likewise, it is always better if patients appear lightly anesthetized to assume that in fact they are lightly anesthetized and supplement additional narcotics, amnestics, and inhalational drugs as necessary. Second, we need to achieve some degree of hemodynamic stability if possible. This is not a static process. We simply cannot take one syringe of drugs, inject it, and sit back and expect the patient to maintain railroad track hemodynamics. Rather, we have to engage the patient actively with pressors and vasodilators to correct ischemia, hypertension, and hypotension as they are encountered. What is important is that when we see trends in hemodynamic behavior, we have to correct and respond to those trends. Rather than wait for the systolic pressure to become 50 mm Hg and the ST segments to drop, it is far better to correct a relative hypotension at 75 or 80 mm Hg systolic and prevent what we could consider an anesthesia-related crisis. It is also significant that as we secure hemodynamic stability that we do not forget our anesthesia basics. Simple things can truly make life miserable for both the patient and ourselves in this regard. Namely, we must remember how we positioned the arms. Are the eyes, ears, and nose free of any lines or wires that could produce pressure injuries over the course of protracted surgery?

Obviously, ensuring the adequacy of ventilation is always crucial. Many patients present for coronary artery bypass with significant chronic obstructive lung disease and can develop bronchospasms and ventilation-perfusion mismatch. Auscultation for wheezing and application of appropriate bronchodilator therapy should be done immediately after induction if necessary. A baseline blood gas measurement may be taken following induction; however, if end-tidal carbon dioxide and hemoglobin oxygen saturation monitors are acceptable, it is within the physician's discretion to delete this additional test. In medicine's new age, information should be obtained only as necessary. If we are confident in the adequacy of ventilation and oxygenation based on end-tidal carbon dioxide, arterial oxygen saturation, mixed venous oxygen saturation, and our clinical impressions, then additional laboratory studies are not needed.

Finally, a good induction should produce a calm environment in which to work. There are in this great medical world many individuals who will, no doubt, destroy a calm environment. Panicked surgeons in such great fear of appearing in the paper with less than stellar morbidity and mortality, frequently obsess to the point that they interfere with the responsibilities of other members of the team. Others become so insecure that they are unable to make a decision. Anesthesiologists are little better. So concerned with their image and decline in station, they respond by overemphasizing what they do to the point that operating room progress is slowed by anesthesiologists who simply cannot put the patient asleep. We reject both models of practice. The cardiac operating room should be a workplace where people are confident with those with whom they work. If we are not confident in the surgeon, we should not be working with him or her, and that should be true from the surgeon's perspective as well. The cardiac operating room should be a routine place. Even when the BP is 50 mm Hg systolic and the patient is about to "crash and burn," we need to remember that even this can be routine after a while. Yes, from time to time in spite of our best efforts, occasionally patients do not do well, so we must remember to stay calm.

4

Cruise Control: Anesthesia Maintenance in the Prebypass Period

Anesthesia Duties in the Prebypass Period

With the patient now prepared and draped and our calm induction completed, we have the opportunity to do some housekeeping and prepare the patient for initiation of cardiopulmonary bypass. Generally, this is a stable period for Mr. XY and patients like him, but it remains for us to be on guard for signs of ischemia. Most important, this is the time where we may get a feel for how the patient will behave. Generally, if we find the cardiac output decreased and blood pressure reduced, we can assume that the patient has impaired ventricular function, which might make weaning from cardiopulmonary bypass difficult later in the procedure. Specifically, we may attend to a few tasks during this lull in the action.

1. Make certain that antibiotic prophylaxis has been given. Generally, the surgeon asks us to administer antibiotics of some sort prior to incision. We do this after induction of the anesthesia but before central line placement. The period during which the patient is prepared and draped is the opportunity to ensure that antibiotics have been administered prior to incision. As always, antibiotic administration can be associated with allergic response or histamine release and may be associated with vasodilation and hypotension.

2.   Complete the transesophageal echocardiography study. This is discussed in greater length in Chapter 18. This is nonetheless a wonderful time to complete the examination. If a cardiologist is to assist or perform the examination, this is the time to allow him or her to complete the task.

3.   Organize lines and label items. As said before, it is just anesthesia, and what anesthesiologist does not want to organize lines and label things? Generally, a nitroglycerin infusion is available, as well as nitroprusside and phenylephrine. Other inotropes should be readily at hand.

4.   Recheck patient positioning. Often lines are draped over the ears, eyes, nose, and so forth of the patient. The elbows should be checked to assess padding. The patient's neck may have been extended to facilitate internal jugular cannulation. This should be checked so that the head and neck remain in a neutral position to prevent injury to cervical nerves.

5.   Obtain blood samples for activated clotting time baseline and other laboratory values. We discuss activated clotting time and other monitors of anticoagulation adequacy later in this chapter. Because many patients present to surgery having received several doses of heparin anticoagulation, a degree of heparin resistance may be anticipated. The baseline activated clotting time accompanied by heparin concentration analysis provides a guide to heparin administration prior to the institution of cardiopulmonary bypass.

Generally, if the patient's behavior remains otherwise normal, we can proceed without obtaining additional laboratory studies. We generally do not obtain a prebypass blood gas level if in our assessment the patient's performance, end-tidal carbon dioxide, and oxygen saturation monitors do not indicate any abnormality.

What Is the Surgeon Up To?

Unlike peripheral surgery, what the surgeon does influences what anesthesiologists must do in the cardiac operating room. Both the anesthesiologist and surgeon have the ability to interfere with one another greatly. Therefore, it is important to know what the surgeon is up to so that not only may we avoid difficulty for ourselves but perhaps help keep the surgeon out of trouble as well. After making the initial incision, the surgeon is ready to put the saw to the sternum. In addition to creating blood splatter, the sternal saw does have a potential to cut any number of vital structures. Generally, the patient is disconnected from the breathing apparatus prior to opening the sternum to minimize risk to any vital structure that the sternal saw might encounter. The command "lungs down" provides too little warning if unexpected. So it is important to anticipate this action. Additionally, it is wise to stand back from the surgical field to avoid blood splatter.

Sternal opening in reoperation, as discussed in Chapter 7, is associated with particular risks of injury to the patient as a consequence of adherence of bypass grafts and the right ventricle to the sternum. Sawing through the sternum in such cases may be complicated by rapid blood loss, ventricular failure, ischemia, tamponade, and the need for emergent resuscitation of the patient. At times, surgeons place a femoral cannula to initiate femoral bypass if sternal entry appears particularly problematic in a reoperative patient. Our vigilance in preparing for resuscitative efforts should be heightened in this setting.

While an assistant harvests saphenous vein, the surgeon proceeds to harvest the internal mammary artery. Generally, the left internal mammary artery is taken, but at times in younger patients, both mammary arteries are harvested. During mammary artery harvesting, a retractor lifts the ipsilateral hemithorax so as to expose the vessel. Occasionally, this action restricts flow through the ipsilateral subclavian artery, diminishing the arterial trace obtained via a radial artery line. Also, placement of the sternal retractor, which is attached to the operating room table, may put pressure on the left or right arm depending on which mammary artery is being harvested. Retractor placement is also associated with damaging intravenous lines and pressure lines that may run along the side of the operating bed. Fortunately, mammary artery harvesting generally should not take the surgeon long. However, some surgeons completely free the artery from surrounding tissues, adding considerable time prior to bypass. Other surgeons simply take down a pedicle of tissue about the mammary artery, which generally quickens the surgical procedure. During mammary artery manipulation, it is not uncommon for the vessel to go into a vasospasm. Papaverine is occasionally injected into the mammary artery to produce vasodilation. Although rarely seen, systemic vasodilation may occur as well. Radial arteries may likewise be taken to provide additional arterial conduits.

In general, this period should be relatively smooth from a hemodynamic perspective. Appropriate dosing of inhalational anesthetics, narcotics, muscle relaxants, and amnestics should be given to maintain relative normotension and to avoid tachycardia. Should hemodynamic instability present, the patient can be managed as previously described using the principles of hemodynamics 101 in Chapter 3. In essence, if the ventricle is relatively healthy, it is little trouble to provide additional anesthetic to offset the effects of surgical manipulation. On the other hand, the poor ventricle may need support with inotropes and vasodilators to provide suitable hemodynamic stability while bypass conduits are being harvested. In Chapter 5 we discuss in greater detail how we prepare the patient for bypass. Of course, even the patient with an otherwise healthy ventricle can become ischemic in the postinduction period. Supporting the blood pressure with phenylephrine and anti-ischemia therapy with nitrates can also correct or prevent the hemodynamic spiral associated with myocardial ischemia in the otherwise healthy ventricle. If the ventricle is well preserved and ischemic in the setting of tachycardia, esmolol may be judicially administered along with additional anesthetic agents in an effort to correct the myocardial oxygen supply and demand ratio.

The same basic hemodynamic management principles that guide induction are operative during the prebypass period as well. Of course, the autonomic stimulation resultant from surgical incision and manipulation can often complicate matters. Last, the unexpected can always happen during so-called lulls in the action. Arrhythmias, asystole, and ventricular fibrillation can appear without warning. It is wise to closely monitor the patient at all times.

5

Preparing for Cardiopulmonary Bypass

Okay, so we have successfully maintained Mr. XY through induction and the harvesting of the bypass conduits. The overwhelming majority of patients do just fine through these steps. Stable hemodynamics, easy intubations, and good gas exchange all are characteristic of the majority of cases whom we take to cardiac surgery. Of course, there are those few less fortunate types who become ischemic, hypertensive, fibrillate, bronchospastic, and are otherwise impossible to intubate. Nevertheless, with a little screening, we can identify some of our problem patients. The 5-ft tall, 350-lb individual who smokes two packs of cigarettes per day is not likely to be the best candidate for an uneventful anesthetic. In the future, managed care may simply prevent such individuals from coming to surgery. The morality of such decisions fortunately is not ours as anesthesiologists to address. Nevertheless, as we most likely will have to take such individuals to surgery for the time being, we certainly should not be surprised if they have a generalized failure to thrive in the surgical suite.

That being said, Mr. XY and those like him are now ready to "go on bypass." What does this really mean? For us, in fact, it means very little because the bypass period is a relatively easy one from an anesthesia standpoint. Except for administering the correct dose of heparin to secure proper anticoagulation, giving antifibrinolytics, and seeing that certain housekeeping functions are attended to, going on bypass is of little challenge to us. As we shall see, when problems with bypass occur, they are principally the responsibility of the surgeon and the perfusionist to correct. Anesthesiologists can be helpful observers and contribute as we can, but fortunately, we do not absolutely need to do anything more.

Heparin, Please

At some point the surgeon will request that the patient be anticoagulated with heparin. Failure to ensure adequate heparinization leads to the worst-case scenario—development of clots during cardiopulmonary bypass or, more likely, a consumptive coagulopathy resulting from inadequate heparinization. Making certain that the patient is fully heparinized with an acceptable activated clotting time (ACT) is an essential task that we must complete.

Timing

Heparin administration is requested generally after veins have been harvested and following mammary artery dissection. Before freeing the distal end of the mammary artery from the chest wall with vascular clips, the surgeon requests heparinization. If no mammary artery is being harvested, heparin is generally given prior to placement of aortic cannulation stitches. The adequacy of heparin anticoagulation must be confirmed and documented before the initiation of cardiopulmonary bypass in everything but the most extreme emergency.

Heparin Dosage

Generally, 3–4 mg of heparin per kg is administered via central access as a starting point in securing acceptable anticoagulation. The ACT and possibly a heparin concentration assay are performed after circulation of the heparin bolus. The ACT is obtained by mixing a small amount of blood with diatomaceous earth, which initiates coagulation. Normal ACTs are in the 110- to 120-second range. Acceptable anticoagulation for cardiopulmonary bypass is debated in the literature, but generally is considered to be greater than 400–480 seconds.

A measurement of heparin concentration may be completed. However, ACT does not always correlate with heparin concentration. It is also possible to achieve relatively high heparin concentrations and be less than adequately anticoagulated for the institution of cardiopulmonary bypass. Other assessments of the coagulation system focus on clot viscosity and elasticity. They have not found their way into routine practice. So we need to be certain that the ACT is greater than 400–480 seconds before starting bypass. If not, we must ask, "Why not?"

Why not can be answered briefly by reviewing the pharmacology of heparin. Heparin is a negatively charged mucopolysaccharide derived from bovine lung or pork intestine. Derived from various sources, heparin is a negatively charged molecule that bonds to antithrombin III. A complex of heparin and antithrombin III inactivates thrombin and clotting factor X, as well as other factors. Heparin is metabolized hepatically. Because heparin's anticoagulant effect is dependent on antithrombin III, reduced amounts of antithrombin III impair the ability of heparin to achieve anticoagulation acceptable for cardiopulmonary bypass.

Inability to achieve a suitable ACT for initiation of cardiopulmonary bypass is an occasional problem in the immediate prebypass period. Because many patients are anticoagulated after their initial presentation to the hospital for either unstable angina or myocardial infarction, it is not unusual for patients to have received heparin for some days prior to surgery. In such situations, antithrombin III concentrations may be reduced, thereby requiring a significant increase in heparin dose to achieve appropriate anticoagulation. Generally, enough heparin can be administered to achieve a safe level of anticoagulation. Antithrombin III can be administered through a fresh frozen plasma transfusion. Antithrombin III concentrates may well be readily available in your institution should additional antithrombin III be necessary. In the overwhelming number of instances, however, simply providing the patient additional heparin generally gets the ACT to an acceptable level. Obviously, it is critical that we are confident that the heparin has been correctly administered through a central line. Confirming ease of blood return should reassure us that the heparin has entered the central circulation.

Additional problems with heparin include occasional hypotension that occurs after administration, as well as an immune-mediated thrombocytopenia and thrombosis. This syndrome appears after a few days of heparin use and can lead to platelet consumption and significant end-organ damage. The history of a patient with heparin-related thrombocytopenia should be reviewed by a hematologist prior to taking the patient to the operating room so that appropriate corticosteroid or other therapies may be initiated. As to hypotension that occurs after administration, this is a consequence of vasodilation. Restoration of vascular tone should correct any transient decrease in blood pressure after heparin administration. Obviously, initiation of bypass can be commenced once the ACT is confirmed. If the patient is moribund for whatever reason, it may be necessary to initiate bypass after heparin is given but while the ACT is being determined. In this emergency setting, it is wise to administer a dose in excess of normal so to be as sure as possible that an acceptable level of anticoagulation is obtained. Patients taken to surgery in such distress are already likely to be significantly coagulopathic after cardiopulmonary bypass. As such, it is better not to include inadequate anticoagulation as yet another source of postbypass coagulopathy.

Prebypass Housekeeping, or What Obsessive-Compulsive Anesthesiologists Love to Do

Many would argue that it is a virtue to be obsessive and compulsive as an anesthesiologist. Throughout residency we are taught the virtue of a well-organized tray, a neat work space, and a legible record. Although all of these are worthy goals, unfortunately too many anesthesiologists can be incapacitated by obsessive compulsiveness. Surely organizational skills are helpful; but far less so than having an intrinsic feeling and understanding for what we are doing. So as we attend to the housekeeping before bypass, we should be ever mindful exactly what we are about and pay close attention first and foremost to the patient.

Intravenous Fluids

Generally, we use lactated Ringer's solution as our intravenous fluid in the prebypass period. Patients with renal failure require judicious amounts of normal saline as necessary. We try not to give patients such as Mr. XY exceedingly large amounts of intravenous crystalloid. Patients receive a large volume load at the time of institution of cardiopulmonary bypass, and there is little reason to add to this by excessive fluid administration in the prebypass period. Of course, crystalloid is given to facilitate administration of drugs and generally to compensate for the patient's NPO status and fluid loss associated with surgery. With uneventful surgery, this should generally amount to 1–2 liters of fluid before bypass is initiated. Fortunately, even if excess volume is administered, the perfusionist can hemoconcentrate the patient's blood volume during cardiopulmonary bypass. Still, we try to avoid volume overload in the patient, but remember that even if it occurs, we can always remove excessive volume during the bypass run. Before bypass is initiated, all intravenous lines are shut off.

Pulmonary Artery Catheter

With manipulation of the patient's heart and shifting volume status, it is possible for the pulmonary catheter to become wedged into a pulmonary artery during bypass. Obviously, we wish to avoid pulmonary artery rupture and therefore, we are certain the pulmonary artery line is withdrawn 1 or 2 cm prior to bypass. We are careful not to pull back too far, however, as the pulmonary artery catheter can then be placed in the right ventricle or pulmonary outflow tract in a position where it is more likely to generate ventricular dysrhythmias. As a handy rule, we rarely wedge the pulmonary artery line at the time of placement in any event. Thus, when placing the catheter, often it is helpful simply to advance the pulmonary artery line until a pulmonary arterial trace is obtained without advancing to a wedged position.

Confirmation of Patient Positioning

Occasionally, the transesophageal echocardiography probe, pulmonary artery catheters, or endotracheal tube may produce pressure on a patient's nose, lips, or eyes. Although some injuries will always occur, it is wise to check occasionally to be certain that the ears, nose, eyes, and face are free from any pressure-producing appliances. Unfortunately, the arms by this time are out of our reach and cannot be checked during the bypass run. A metal triangle is routinely placed over the patient's face to prevent members of the surgical team from leaning on the face during the bypass run. Attending to details such as these is important in providing quality care.

"Go On to Bypass"

Chapter 10 provides a guide to perfusion and myocardial protection from the perspective of a perfusionist—namely, someone who actually

Table 5-1. Going on Bypass

1. Aortic and venous cannulas are placed (see Figure 1A-10).
2. Anterograde and retrograde cardioplegia cannula are placed (see Figure 1A-11).
3. Final activated clotting time measurement is confirmed.
4. Surgeon releases clamp on venous cannula.
5. Venous return commences; bypass is initiated.
6. Central venous and pulmonary artery pressures decrease.
7. Heart empties; ventricular ejection decreases.
8. Ventilation is discontinued once full bypass flow is obtained, leaving circuit disconnected.
9. Surgeon and anesthesiologist inspect the heart.

is responsible for management of cardiopulmonary bypass. Generally, a coordinated effort between the surgical team and the perfusionist with the anesthesiologist as an interested observer is the best mechanism with which to work. In some institutions the bypass machine may, in fact, be operated by members of the anesthesia team. However, in actual cardiac practice, the anesthesiologist simply does not have a team. The anesthesiologist alone must manage the anesthesia, and so the perfusionist and the surgeon must coordinate difficulties with the bypass machine. That does not mean that we as anesthesiologists should be disinterested in what occurs. Remember, we still need to keep the patient asleep and paralyzed during the bypass run. Also, what happens during cardiopulmonary bypass affects our ability to separate the patient from bypass. Table 5-1 provides a guide to activities of the surgery-perfusion-anesthesia team as the patient is placed on cardiopulmonary bypass.

Inspection of the heart and close monitoring by the surgeon, perfusionist, and anesthesiologist are essential. The perfusionist confirms that adequate venous drainage has been achieved and that an acceptable flow rate has been attained. Inadequate venous return might indicate a poorly positioned cannula. High pressures in the aortic cannula could indicate a life-threatening aortic dissection or kink in the aortic perfusion cannula.

The surgeon should be certain that he or she is satisfied with the adequacy of venous return and that the heart is adequately emptied. In the absence of significant aortic insufficiency, the heart should be well collapsed following institution of full bypass flow. Similarly, the surgeon should feel the aorta to confirm adequacy of flow and pressure.

The anesthesiologist should confirm that the central venous pressure and pulmonary artery pressures have fallen to zero. Additionally, the anesthesiologist should examine the head for any sign of discoloration that may signify inadequate superior vena cava return or innominate artery cannulation by the aortic perfusion cannula.

The specific goals of the perfusionist in supporting the patient are discussed in Chapter 10. For our purposes, however, we are well on our way to bringing the patient to a point where the essence of the surgery will occur and which paradoxically is least under our control.

With ventilation discontinued, we will watch the electrocardiogram (ECG) and inform the surgeon of any ECG changes associated with ischemia. Such changes are not infrequent as the surgeon manipulates the heart in an effort to identify those vessels where the bypass grafts will be sewn distally. Once done, the surgeon places an aortic cross clamp, eliminating perfusion to the coronary arteries and isolating the cardiopulmonary circulation. Once the aortic cross clamp is placed, the perfusionist administers cardioplegia (see Chapter 10) via the antero-grade cardioplegia cannula (see Figure 1A-11). Next, if the surgeon so desires, additional cardioplegia solution may be administered retro-grade via a coronary sinus catheter (see Figure 1A-12). If retrograde cardioplegia is planned, the surgical technician generally passes a pressure tubing over the drape to be attached to the central venous pressure transducer, which will be connected to the coronary sinus catheter. This pressure measurement guides the perfusionist and surgeon in administering cardioplegia. A myocardial temperature probe may likewise be passed over the surgical drape so that the delivery of cardioplegia to the heart may be demonstrated by a decrease in temperature to approximately 8°C.

As cardioplegia is administered and the heart is cooled, various ECG changes (i.e., QRS widening) occur while the heart is rendered asystolic. At this point, the patient's management rests almost entirely with the perfusionist and surgeon.

During this period of bypass, anesthesia must still be maintained. Most bypass machines are equipped with a vaporizer to allow continuous administration of isoflurane or other agents during bypass. We insist that some inhalational agent be given during the bypass run. Should the patient appear to become hypertensive on bypass (i.e., mean pressure of more than 90 mm Hg), the perfusionist has but two responses. Flow may be decreased from the cardiopulmonary bypass machine, or conversely, vasodilators may be administered to the patient. Should hypertension appear to be the consequence of inadequate anesthesia, additional anesthetics (i.e., narcotics and amnestics) must be delivered. Generally, we supplement additional doses of narcotics and amnestics initially along with an increased concentration of inhalational agent should hypertension develop on bypass. If this proves ineffective, the perfusionist administers sodium nitroprusside or nitroglycerin. We prefer to maintain adequate bypass flow and perfusion during the pump run. Vasodilators are given as necessary to ensure adequate bypass flow.

Generally, the perfusionist manages the hemodynamics during the bypass run. Our formula from hemodynamics 101 may prove applicable during cardiopulmonary bypass as well as during the prebypass and postbypass periods. You will recall that blood pressure is equal to cardiac output multiplied by systemic vascular resistance. During cardiopulmonary bypass, cardiac output is determined by the flow generated by the bypass machine. Therefore, blood pressure is equal to flow multiplied by vascular resistance. As perfusionists can adjust flow at will, they can readily adjust for whatever perfusion pressure is desired. Fortunately, they, in fact, do this. If, on the other hand, blood pressure is increased, they may require additional anesthesia delivery to provide for adequate vasodilation so to maintain an appropriate blood flow. Most perfusionists, like most anesthesiologists, are very reliable and truly do not need or appreciate any unwarranted interference from the anesthesiologist. Generally, it is prudent to allow the perfusionist to practice as he or she sees fit, unless we notice some egregious error that threatens the patient's well-being.

The bypass period offers us the opportunity to reflect on the course of the patient and make plans for separation from cardiopulmonary bypass. This will be our moment, so bypass time is the time when we should be preparing to separate the patient from the pump. Generally, even separating the patient from bypass in the majority of cases requires little effort. We often have 1–3 hours simply to sit idle while the perfusionist supports the patient. Generally, it is best to sit quietly and observe as a nonintrusive presence. We let the operating room team know we are there, but do not presume to tell either surgeon or perfusionist what to do. It is hoped that by taking this approach, the surgeon, especially, will learn from this and not dictate actions to us either. Such is the basis of an effective anesthesia-perfusion-surgery team.

6

Weaning from Cardiopulmonary Bypass

If you have the pleasure of working with a skilled surgeon, only 1–2 hours or less have passed for Mr. XY for the basic three- to four-jump coronary artery bypass (CAB) to be completed. Of course, easily 3–4 hours or more may have elapsed for any number of reasons. Unfortunately, managed care providers and administrators are quick to look at anesthesia delays as the source of all intraoperative evil and yet fail to account for overly slow surgery and the problems associated with long cardiopulmonary bypass (CPB) runs.

Weaning from CPB is one of those rare pivotal moments where people actually become aware of what you are doing as an anesthesiologist. Like intubation, when all eyes turn to see if you easily place the endotracheal tube ("what a hero!") or if you fail ("what a slug!"), weaning from bypass is the same kind of defining event. Therefore, it is associated with any number of pitfalls. The patient with whom you struggle to intubate may have the most anterior larynx in the history of humankind; no matter, you are the one who will be remembered as having failed, you are the one who slowed down surgery, you are the one who is no good. Anesthesiologists know this line of reasoning is totally ridiculous, but it appears to hold sway over surgeon and nursing staff. Much the same can be said about separating the patient from bypass. The heart may have been totally underprotected by cardioplegia (see Chapter 10) or so severely damaged to begin with that successful weaning from bypass is not easy. You will still be viewed as somewhat inadequate for failing to wean the patient from bypass—that is, unless you have a clear, organized plan for addressing difficulties that occur and appear to have control of the situation. Now this advice only holds if, in fact, you have some responsibility for separating the patient from bypass. Many surgeons simply cannot allow anyone else to do the job for them. In that instance, the surgeon often directs weaning from bypass him- or herself. Indeed, the surgeon may tell you what drugs to start and what to do. Beware: These are your patients. If the surgeon's orders are foolish, one is advised not to act on them because if you carry out the act, you must be confident in the action. The "I'm just following orders" defense has no place in clinical anesthesia if we are to be considered the consultants that we are supposed to be. Fortunately, most surgeons, at least those with whom we are privileged to work, appreciate our input and leave weaning from bypass entirely to us. It is from that perspective that we discuss weaning Mr. XY from cardiopulmonary bypass.

So What Does the Heart Do Anyway?

Although many other functions may be attributed to the heart, first and foremost it is the pump providing blood flow. During CAB with CPB (and now some CABs are completed without CPB; see Chapter 19), the heart's function has been assumed by the perfusionist and the CPB machine. In fact, the heart on bypass is asystolic, electrically silent, and empty. To restore the heart to proper functioning, it first must contract, beat, and fill appropriately. Working with the perfusionist, it is our task to ensure that the conditions that are favorable to the working of the heart are present and maintained.

Restoration of Rhythm

On removal of the aorta cross clamp, in many cases sinus rhythm returns with a heart rate in the 80s or 90s. This is encouraging because an effective normal rhythm is absolutely necessary to optimize the heart's function as a pump. Of course, many other rhythms are possible as we prepare the patient for separation from bypass (Table 6-1).

In essence, we need to secure a rhythm that optimizes the heart's function as a pump. Ventricular fibrillation and tachycardias must always be corrected. Atrial fibrillation and supraventricular tachycardias likewise should receive quick correction with internal cardioversion and appropriate pharmacotherapy as previously described. A sinus rhythm or a paced rhythm of 90–100 beats per minute appears generally ideal for the patient. Some tachycardias may reflect light anesthesia and can be treated with additional doses of intravenous narcotics. If sinus tachycardia persists after weaning from bypass and the admin-

Table 6-1. A Guide to Heart Rhythm After Aortic Cross Clamp Release

Rhythm	Significance	Therapy
Sinus bradycardia, heart rate of <60 beats per minute	Sinus rhythm is OK but heart rate too slow to generate suitable cardiac output	Atrial pacing, inotropes
Sinus tachycardia, heart rate of >100 beats per minute	Is the patient adequately anesthetized? Is this a response to catecholamine administration?	Additional anesthesia, esmolol
Atrial fibrillation, supraventricular tachycardia	Was this present preoperatively?	Cardioversion, digoxin, verapamil
Atrioventricular disassociation	Very common	Atrioventricular pacing
Asystole	Common but worrisome: Is hyperkalemia present? Was myocardial protection adequate?	Atrioventricular pacing
Ventricular fibrillation/ ventricular tachycardia	Was myocardial protection adequate? Is the pulmonary artery catheter in the right ventricle?	Cardioversion; defibrillation; lidocaine, bretylium, amiodarone

istration of narcotics, small amounts of esmolol may be given, assuming that the ventricular performance as determined by cardiac output measurements and transesophageal echocardiography (TEE) is considered acceptable.

Restoration of Contractility

When you look over the drape and see a heart that's "dancing" (i.e., beating rhythmically), you can be more or less certain that right ventricular function is preserved. Remember, from our position, we cannot readily see the left ventricle, but the surgeon can often provide a visual assessment of some of the left ventricle. Similarly, assessment of ventricular function by TEE also ensures that ventricular function has been preserved. When the heart is empty, as it is during full CPB, it is difficult to assess myocardial contractility by direct inspection and TEE. To assess bypass graft length before completing the distal anastomosis to the aorta, the surgeon will often occlude venous return, permitting the heart to eject and fill. By filling the heart, the surgeon is able to assess the length necessary for the bypass graft. This is also the time when we can assess how well the heart is likely to do. If, during these trial occlusions of venous return, the heart ejects vigorously, creating pulsatile flow on the arterial trace, the ventricle will likely be vigorous on weaning from bypass. On the other hand, if the heart responds sluggishly and appears to be a distended muscular balloon in the chest, we will need to provide additional pharmacologic or mechanical support to effectively wean from bypass.

The application of the various forms of pharmacology and mechanical support in weaning from bypass is discussed in Chapter 8. At this point, however, we must assume that Mr. XY's heart is happily dancing in his chest at 90 beats per minute.

If, for whatever reason, the heart appears to function poorly, there is little reason to proceed with an attempt to wean from bypass. Such efforts only distend the heart (inflating the muscular balloon) and further deplete the heart's energy reserves. Rather, if the heart appears to function poorly before attempting to wean from bypass, we should turn to Chapter 8 and follow the guide for weaning the poorly functioning ventricle. Such methods to wean the heart require inotropic support with dobutamine, milrinone, or both, as well as vasodilators such as nitroglycerin and mechanical support (i.e., left ventricular assist device, intra-aortic balloon pump) as necessary to facilitate a successful separation from bypass.

Correction of the Myocardial Environment

While you are assessing myocardial rhythm and contractility, the perfusionist should, without instruction from you, be making certain that the appropriate environment has been established to optimize myocardial performance. In essence, the perfusionist should make the heart's world a happy, healthy place to live and to work. By this we mean that the body's core temperature should be 37°C to ensure that the patient does not become hypothermic after separation from bypass. Not only does hypothermia lead to impaired coagulation and dysrhythmias, but it can also result in increased oxygen consumption secondary to shivering as muscle relaxation is permitted to wear off in the postanesthesia care unit.

Electrolyte, acid-base, and blood glucose concentrations should be corrected prior to separation from bypass. Obvious hypokalemia and hyperkalemia can lead to dysrhythmias. Metabolic acidemia can be assumed to reflect inadequate perfusion during the bypass run or poor glucose control. Potassium chloride replacement, sodium bicarbonate administration, or both should be given as needed to correct any abnormalities (see Chapter 10).

Hyperglycemia that occurs after rewarming may require administration of intravenous regular insulin. Hyperglycemia can produce an osmotic diuresis, further contributing to potassium loss. Many patients whose diabetes has been previously managed by diet or oral hypoglycemics first need insulin at the time of rewarming from CPB. Should insulin be given, monitoring, with every 1- to 2-hour blood sugars and potassium assessments, is mandatory in the immediate postoperative period.

Last, the heart's function is to pump blood to the tissues. If the hematocrit is less than 20, this may impair oxygen delivery in the event cardiac function is depressed. The perfusionist should correct any significant anemias. Generally, the perfusionist contracts the blood volume during the bypass run if the blood volume appears large. This may well increase the hematocrit. However, should the hematocrit remain low during rewarming, packed red blood cells should be transfused by the perfusionist into the pump circuit. Additionally, the perfusionist should be aware of the platelet count before separation from bypass. If the platelet count is less than 100,000 after rewarming, you should be certain that platelets are available for transfusion because they may be necessary to control postoperative bleeding.

Thus, before separating from bypass, we have to secure an environment for the heart to pump effectively. We must be certain that the rate and rhythm are suitable to adequate function. We have attempted to assess ventricular function to see if the heart has a chance to function independently. If we suspect not, we must follow the guidelines as recommended in Chapter 8 to develop a plan by which we can assist the heart in carrying out its function. In essence, we want each heart to dance. Whether the heart has the energy for a tango or just enough for a slow waltz, the bottom line is that the heart must dance if it is to support the patient.

"Come Off"

Fortunately, Mr. XY is full of energy, and his heart dances with great energy. Full of anticipation, the heart is waiting for the surgeon to signal for separation from bypass. Once the surgeon indicates to the anesthesiologist that he or she is finished, the anesthesiologist then may instruct the perfusionist to separate from bypass. Before this, the anesthesiologist must remember to "breathe" for the patient. On more than one occasion, patients have failed to separate from bypass successfully because the anesthesiologist has failed to remember to restore ventilation.

Ventilation should be resumed initially by hand, with the surgeon watching that lung inflation does not stretch or tear an internal mammary artery bypass graft. Once the surgeon is certain that the lungs do not impinge on the grafts, several large breaths may be given. Ideally, these will expand the lungs and help to prevent atelectasis, which may develop during the bypass run, contributing to a ventilation-perfusion mismatch. Should the lungs or heart appear displaced within the chest cavity, the surgeon should look for any fluid that may have accumulated in either hemithorax during the bypass run.

Orders to Wean

With breathing restored, additional narcotics, amnestics, and muscle relaxants are administered as needed. You may tell the perfusionist to start to wean from bypass. Venous return to the bypass machine is occluded (see Chapter 10), and the heart begins to fill and to eject. Once the perfusionist has reduced bypass flow to approximately 2 liters per minute, it is wise to hold for a moment and assess how the patient is doing:

1.   Look at the heart. If it is still dancing, it should be able to complete separation from bypass.

2.   Assess ventricular filling pressures. If the pulmonary artery diastolic pressure and pulmonary capillary occlusion pressure remain relatively low (8–12 mm Hg), we can assume that the ventricle remains relatively compliant (i.e., the heart has been able to tolerate increased volume without increasing pressure). An injured myocardium tends to be poorly compliant, resulting in increased pulmonary artery pressures with only a modest increase of ventricular volume.

3.   Examine TEE images. We discuss TEE to a greater degree in Chapter 18. When CPB flow is reduced to 2 liters per minute, we have an excellent opportunity to perform a quick TEE assessment. Should the heart appear unable to successfully wean from CPB, it is wise at this point to return to full bypass flow, rest the heart, and plan to continue weaning from bypass following those guidelines described in Chapter 8. If, as in the majority of cases, ventricular performance appears adequate, the perfusionist should be instructed to discontinue bypass.

Drugs or No Drugs

Some centers advocate the use of various combinations of inotropes and vasodilators so as to maximize cardiac output and minimize ventricular distension after discontinuation of bypass. As you may recall from our previous discussion, a distended heart is hardly our goal. Obviously, a good cardiac output ensures adequate perfusion as well. Nevertheless, the application of inotropes (i.e., dobutamine, epinephrine, milrinone, and so forth) and vasodilators (i.e., sodium nitroprusside and nitroglycerin) needs to be individualized. Certainly, we must not permit the heart to become a muscular balloon—distended, ischemic, and dysfunctional. On the other hand, we do not need a racing, tachycardic pump either. In fact, experience dictates which case requires additional support and which is likely to sail off bypass dancing all the way. There is much more in Chapter 8 about how to wean the difficult patient with a simple and direct approach to pharmacologic and mechanical therapy. In fact, it really is not that difficult. It may, however, be difficult for the patient should we fail to have an organized approach to weaning from bypass in the setting of impaired ventricular function.

"We're Off"

So states the perfusionist, indicating that the patient's heart has assumed full responsibility for systemic perfusion. Table 6-2 identifies a number of questions that need to be asked immediately on weaning from bypass.

Assuming, however, that our quick assessment of myocardial performance indicates that the ventricle remains compliant, contractile, and coordinated, we may instruct the surgeon to remove the venous

Table 6-2. Questions and Answers on Weaning from Bypass

Q: Are rate and rhythm acceptable?

A: Normal rate and rhythm should be maintained after separation from bypass.

Q: Has the heart become distended like a muscular balloon?

A: It is to be hoped not. If myocardial contractility has been preserved, the heart should handle volume loading without further distention.

Q: What are the pulmonary capillary occlusion pressure and the central venous pressure?

A: Elevated pulmonary capillary occlusion pressures of >15 mm Hg may indicate impaired ventricle compliance. Elevated central venous pressure that is higher than the pulmonary capillary occlusion pressure may indicate right ventricle dysfunction.

Q: Is ventilation adequate?

A: Check end-tidal carbon dioxide, mixed venous oxygen saturation, and pulse oximetry to confirm adequacy of ventilation and oxygenation.

Q: What are the cardiac output and cardiac index?

A: Cardiac output and cardiac index should be no worse than prebypass. If cardiac index remains at <2.0 liters/min/m^2, we may well expect hemodynamic difficulty and should be prepared for reinstitution of cardiopulmonary bypass flow while we adjust the drug regimen.

cannula. The residual blood volume in the venous cannula may be returned to the reservoir after the surgical technician provides a suitable volume to chase the venous return. This permits rapid reconnection of the venous line should an unforeseen emergency dictate resumption of CPB.

With ventilation adequate and cardiac index acceptable (more than 2.5 liters per minute per m^2), we may proceed to administer protamine and reverse heparinization. Protamine administration is associated both with histamine release and hypotension as well as an idiopathic protamine reaction characterized by pulmonary hypertension and right ventricular failure. Because hemodynamic changes are frequent at the time of protamine administration, it is important that we are confident in the adequacy of our blood pressure measurement via the radial arterial cannula placed at the start of surgery. Often a significant aortic root to radial artery pressure gradient is present after separation from bypass. If the measured blood pressure appears significantly depressed, the surgeon should be instructed to feel the aortic root. Blood pressure may be measured from the aortic perfusion cannula. Measurement from the aortic cannula reflects root pressure as long as there is no flow in that perfusion cannula. If flow continues through the aorta cannula, any pressure measured is artifactually elevated. Generally, the gradient between the aortic root and radial artery pressure narrows as the time from weaning from CPB lengthens.

Assuming that cardiac function is acceptable, protamine administration may commence. Always confer with the surgeon and the perfusionist when you begin the delivery of protamine via a peripheral intravenous line. Protamine is a positively charged protein obtained from salmon sperm. Positively charged proteins interact on a one-to-one basis with the negatively charged heparin molecules. As such, dosing is generally given on a milligram per milligram basis. Heparin assays routinely employed in the operating room provide a more or less reliable measure for the amount of protamine necessary for heparin reversal.

Although protamine in excess may contribute to anticoagulation in its own right, generally slightly more protamine is administered than as determined by either heparin assay or one-to-one administration. Barring any pulmonary artery vasoconstriction, most protamine reactions are related to histamine release that occurs after too rapid administration. Should pulmonary hypertension and right ventricular failure occur, CPB may need to be resumed. Often administration of heparin in preparation for the institution of bypass may improve ventricular function secondary to interacting with protamine. Protamine-related pulmonary artery vasoconstriction is not predictable. People with a history of diabetes treated with protamine insulin may be at risk for anaphylactic reaction. The idiopathic vasoconstriction associated with right ventricular dysfunction and pulmonary hypertension may require treatment with inotropes or vasodilators as necessary. Should total hemodynamic collapse occur with equalization of pulmonary artery and systemic pressures, reinstitution of CPB may be necessary after reheparinization.

In such instances, how should the heparin be reversed? Protamine may be slowly administered by a peripheral intravenous line or alternatively, heparin reversal may be withheld awaiting heparin metabolism by the liver. Of course, administration of blood products will be necessary to compensate for the increased blood loss. Nevertheless, this is acceptable if a patient cannot tolerate protamine reversal. In our extensive practice, we have never needed to do this and have generally been able to administer protamine slowly, circumventing any recurrence of a protamine-induced pulmonary hypertension.

There Is Always Something

With successful protamine reversal and the aortic cannula removed, the surgeon obtains further hemostasis, places sternal wires, and closes the chest. Once done, we should quickly assess the patient's overall performance.

In patients with large dilated distended hearts, chest closure can increase thoracic pressures, retarding venous return and decreasing cardiac output. Additionally, a closed chest increases resistance to ventilation by positive pressure. As such, with both hemodynamic and pulmonary function potentially impaired, we must be certain that chest closure is adequately tolerated by quickly reviewing our hemodynamics, mixed venous oxygen saturation and arterial saturation. During this period, any and every potential complication can occur.

Ventricular Failure

At any time the heart may become dysfunctional, necessitating a complete reassessment of the patient. Those hearts with impaired function preoperatively are most at risk for failure postbypass. However, once we have successfully weaned from bypass and administered protamine, generally we should be able to navigate the patient through the remainder of chest closure. Ventricular failure at this time may be as a consequence of impaired venous return secondary to increased thoracic pressure. Of course, bypass grafts can become occluded or kinked, resulting in acute myocardial ischemia. Additionally, internal mammary artery vasospasm may result in inadequate blood flow and myocardial ischemia. Therapy as designed and described in Chapter 8 may be employed to attempt to correct ventricular dysfunction. Obviously, if the chest has been closed and ischemic electrocardiographic changes appear associated with ventricular dysfunction, this necessitates the surgeon re-exploring the chest and potentially replacing bypass grafts.

Vasodilation and Hypovolemia

Hypotension may present in a setting of preserved cardiac output. Often vasodilation accompanies rewarming and necessitates supplementation with modest amounts of vasoconstrictors. Hypovolemia may also present at this time secondary to inadequate volume replacement.

We administer blood scavenged from the surgical field and any residual blood left in the bypass circuit. Volume expanders such as 5% albumin and hetastarch may also be used.

Dysrhythmias

Acid-base and electrolyte imbalance may contribute to the development of both supraventricular and ventricular dysrhythmias. Mechanical causes for arrhythmia should also be considered. The pulmonary artery waveform should be confirmed as being a trace from the pulmonary artery. If the patient required temporary pacing, the pacemaker should be suspended to see if an underlying rhythm has emerged that is competing with the pacemaker. Should ventricular ectopy occur in those patients who have had recent myocardial infarction, this rhythm should be suppressed with lidocaine or procainamide before transport to the intensive care unit.

Other Conditions

Obviously, any number of other conditions may complicate this period in patient management. Metabolic acidemia may develop secondary to inadequate perfusion, diabetes mellitus, and anemia. Ensuring adequate oxygen delivery to the tissues by maintaining an acceptable cardiac index and a hematocrit of 20–25 should prevent the development of any significant metabolic acidemia. Correction of hyperglycemia with insulin prevents the development of a hyperosmolar state and diabetic ketoacidosis. Administration of sodium bicarbonate may be necessary should the pH be less than 7.1.

Impaired renal function may also be noted at this time. If urine output is minimal, we must consider the possibility of renal injury and acute renal failure. If no urine at all is produced, a mechanical source such as an occluded bladder catheter should first be considered. Once this is ruled out, if urine output remains low, we must assess the patient for both prerenal and renal sources for renal dysfunction. Chapter 15 discusses those tests that formally permit the diagnosis of renal insufficiency. However, we can be assured of a few things. If the patient is hypotensive with an inadequate cardiac output, a prerenal source for renal insufficiency may be considered. Additionally, inadequate renal blood flow subsequently leads to renal injury and the development of acute renal failure. Restoration of adequate blood flow and blood pressure is the best protection against renal injury. Still, in certain patients (particularly the elderly or those with renal insufficiency preoperatively), bypass surgery in and of itself may result in acute renal failure secondary to CPB or contrast dyes from catheterization. Thus, if blood pressure and cardiac output appear acceptable for the patient and the urine output remains low, there are few options. Furosemide, bumetanide, or both may be administered by bolus or infusion (see Chapter 15) to promote diuresis. However, such therapy does little to improve renal function per se. Nevertheless, it remains easier to treat renal failure with adequate diuresis than to deal with oliguric acute renal failure. Thus, if urine output remains low with adequate volume replacement, blood pressure, and cardiac index, administration of diuretic therapy would be in order.

Chapter 16 is devoted to the management of coagulopathy. Should the patient appear "wet"—that is, oozing (bleeding from the surgical field) after adequate heparin reversal, appropriate laboratory tests should be ordered immediately (e.g., platelet counts, fibrinogen, prothrombin time, partial thromboplastin time, and so forth). If a patient appears to be so coagulopathic that he or she is bleeding profusely, the patient's chest should not be closed but managed in the operating room with appropriate blood product therapy as described in Chapter 16. Should the patient appear only slightly wet, the patient's chest may be closed and the results of tests of coagulation awaited to specifically design replacement therapy. Obviously, an activated coagulation time and heparin assay should be rechecked to see if so-called heparin rebound has occurred. As with all patients, coagulopathy can lead to pericardial tamponade, necessitating re-exploration. Because re-exploration is undesirable, it is of paramount importance that we attempt to correct bleeding as quickly as possible.

It's Over, Isn't It?

Generally, the word "finally" crosses our minds as a case draws to a close. After a variable amount of time in the room, the prospect of ending the case and retiring to the coffee room has a certain, almost cosmic appeal for many anesthesiologists. But we must not be too complacent. We still have to move the patient to the intensive care unit, wherever that might be. For all the managerial wizards who dash about our hospitals, few have ever had the good sense to place the surgical intensive care unit, in fact, next to the operating room. As such, we must be prepared to get Mr. XY from the operating room to the intensive care unit and not have a disaster along the way.

Monitoring for the Road

We specifically monitor radial artery pressure during transport. The monitor should be placed so that we are actually able to see it. Additionally, the tone of a frequent bleep of the dancing heart is reassuring as well. An Ambu bag should be available with a full tank of oxygen. It is helpful to listen for the flow of oxygen to be certain the tank has oxygen in it and has been turned on before attaching the patient to the Ambu bag for transport. All infusion pumps must be carefully moved. Infusions should be continued on the way to the intensive care unit. Finally, in physically moving the patient, it is essential that lines be checked for ease of movement. Most anesthesiologists have had pulmonary artery lines pulled out or other cannulas disconnected at the time of transport, only to have to replace them in the intensive care unit.

Arriving in the Intensive Care Unit

We should concentrate on monitoring the patient while the nursing staff and other assistants attend to the housekeeping chores of straightening the lines and moving infusion pumps. Although nursing staff obviously would prefer us to attend to such housekeeping duties, this is an error. The anesthesiologist should focus on the monitor until the nursing staff assumes responsibility for monitoring the patient, as indicated by their attaching the intensive care unit monitors to the patient. As the respiratory therapist places the patient on the ventilator in the intensive care unit, it is imperative that the anesthesiologist confirm that adequate ventilation is occurring. Far too often, leaks in the ventilatory circuits are present and go unnoticed during the hustle and bustle of bringing the patient to the intensive care unit. We discuss in greater detail anesthesiology and intensive care unit relations in Chapter 15. For now, however, it is our job to keep an eye on the patient until the nurse monitors the patient.

Once the nurse assumes monitoring of the patient, a report is given indicating our experience with the patient. Depending on institutional protocols, anesthesiologists' involvement in postoperative management may vary from nonexistent to being in charge of total management. Before involving yourself in this arena, it is essential to know what the operating paradigm is. This too is discussed in Chapter 15. With blood pressure, ventilatory exchange, heart rate, urine output, and body temperature all acceptable, we can finally leave Mr. XY revascularized.

In the introduction, we went through the basic steps to bring an otherwise healthy patient through bypass surgery. And, you see, just as promised, we did so quite easily. In Section II, we examine those occurrences that are not quite as straightforward and that provide the additional information referred to in the preceding pages. As a follow-up on postoperative day 1, I hope you will go and visit your own Mr. XY sitting in a chair in the intensive care unit. He will look at you and say, "Oh, I think I remember you," and then you will know you have done a good job and can move on to the next case.

II

Management of Patients
Who Are Otherwise Unhealthy
for Coronary Artery Bypass

7

Reoperative Coronary Artery Bypass

In the introduction of this handbook, I promised that I would introduce you to patients with differing backgrounds and conditions as more and more complicated scenarios were presented. So far, the only patient you have met is poor old Mr. XY, whom you are probably tired of reading about. As I hope you will see, the actual knowledge base required to manage the healthy patient for coronary artery bypass (CAB) is not terribly extensive. What you will need to do now is, with the help of an experienced colleague, reacquaint yourself with patient management and protocols particular to the working rhythm of your own operating room.

That being said, we start to examine patients whose histories are less straightforward. Obviously, if you are a resident in anesthesia, these cases will require closer communication with your attending anesthesiologist. If, on the other hand, you are an established practitioner returning to cardiac anesthesia practice, these cases should be done after you have mastered the routine CAB to the point where your performance is "slick." It serves neither yourself nor the patient to attempt cases that may strain your ability and experience. Carefully building up to such challenges gives you the best chance of a successful result. As such, should the patient not do well, the surgical staff cannot say that the patient failed because he or she was not attended by some cosmically anointed anesthesiologist. In fact, if you are returning to cardiac practice or simply starting in practice after fellowship in either a private or university setting, it is far better to allow the anointed ones to deal with those types of patients until you are so designated as God's gracious gift to anesthesia by our capricious surgical colleagues. That way, when they slice through the right ventricle and the patient exsanguinates, they will assume responsibility themselves, rather than attempting to blame your inadequate volume replacement.

Unfortunately, the mention of slicing into the right ventricle brings us to our first complicated case, the reoperative CAB. And who should be our first patient but, of course, Mr. XY, naturally. Fifteen years have passed since you finished your work with Mr. XY. For better or worse, depending on your mood at this time, you remain a clinical anesthesiologist. Only now, you are no neophyte. You are your hospital's standard of anesthesia care. Once slightly insecure, you are now the cardiac anesthesiologist anointed and indispensable—that is, at least until the latest managed-care contract no longer deems you as being so worthy. But that is another story. Mr. XY did very well after his initial surgery, and he behaved well too. He watched his diet, avoided tobacco use, and even engaged in some exercise. However, time takes its toll, and now he has developed occlusions in his native vessels distal to his previous anastomosis as well as within the bypass grafts themselves. He has developed increasing angina pain and now is scheduled for a reoperative CAB.

Reoperative patients are generally at a higher risk than first-time candidates. Many have sustained additional damage to the myocardium through infarction. Often, they have diminished ventricular function. However, the problems with reoperative patients often have more to do with the actual mechanics of surgery than with their cardiac function. Many patients are 15–20 years older than when they first underwent bypass surgery. Although it is true that the type A personality who is a heavy smoker may have had bypass at 45–50 years of age, many other patients had their initial bypass at age 65–70 and now are 75–90 years of age. Taking such elderly patients to surgery increases risk merely as a consequence of the patient's general physical condition. Additionally, postoperative mobilization proves exceedingly difficult in this population. Nevertheless, the ethical, financial, and moral decisions of when to bring a patient to bypass surgery remain clouded. From our perspective, we can merely do what is best to minimize trauma to the patient during the operative course, recognizing that elderly patients are at risk for various perioperative complications.

Specifically, the reoperative CAB patient may be approached in much the same manner as the primary CAB patient. Preoperative assessment is similar, with specific attention to ventricular function. Occasionally, angiography reveals that the patient's prior bypass graft conduits have adhered to the sternum. The surgeon may approach this problem in varying ways. Occasionally, the femoral artery and vein are cannulated to initiate femoral bypass in the event that entry into the chest results in laceration of a bypass graft or the myocardium itself. Other surgeons simply explore the femoral vessels to ensure rapid cannulation should a crisis develop. Others simply go forward, occasionally having to hurry to obtain femoral bypass if the ventricle is compromised by the sternal saw. Because the heart frequently adheres to the sternum, surgeons may approach the heart via thoracotomy or minithoracotomies. In this instance, the surgeon may plan a CAB without institution of a cardiopulmonary bypass. A double-lumen endotracheal tube may be requested to facilitate surgical exposure should bypass surgery via thoracotomy be planned.

Generally, however, most reoperations proceed similarly to the primary bypass surgery. Of course, the possibility of injury from the sternal incision is always present. Should the heart be lacerated, femoral cardiopulmonary bypass is begun and the patient resuscitated appropriately. We must be prepared to expeditiously administer heparin to the patient should this become necessary. Additionally, before surgical incision, it is prudent in all reoperative cases to have blood products available, including fresh frozen plasma, platelets, and cryoprecipitate in addition to packed red blood cells.

Perioperative Bleeding

Because reoperations are associated with a higher incident of perioperative bleeding, steps must be taken to minimize perioperative blood loss. Although no pharmacologic intervention totally prevents perioperative bleeding, we can attempt to limit blood loss through the administration of aminocaproic acid, tranexamic acid, or aprotinin.

Epsilon-aminocaproic acid and tranexamic acid inhibit fibrinolysis. The dosage schemes for administration of these agents is variable from surgical group to surgical group. We routinely administer 5–10 g of ε-aminocaproic acid before bypass, in the bypass circuit, and after bypass. Generally, there has been no increased incidence of thrombotic complications of either bypass grafts or other vascular structures after administration of antifibrinolytics. Still, with a patient with a history of pulmonary embolism and deep vein thrombosis, we are concerned about the administration of antifibrinolytics.

Aprotinin (Trasylol) is a protease inhibitor. The exact mechanism of action of aprotinin is unclear, but has been attributed to aprotinin's inhibition of plasmin and kallikrein. Aprotinin is administered by a continuous infusion via central line.

Aprotinin, 280 mg (2.0 million KIU), is given as a loading dose followed by an infusion of 70 mg per hour (500,000 KIU per hour). An additional 2.0 million KIU is given in the bypass pump prime. A test dose of 1 ml of aprotinin (10,000 KIU) is given before the loading dose. However, the dosage regimen is subject to continuous revision. Aprotinin inhibits activation of the intrinsic pathway by contact with a foreign surface; therefore, partial thromboplastin time and activated clotting time may be elevated. We must be certain that our heparin response is adequate to institute cardiopulmonary bypass in the setting of aprotinin delivery. In this instance, an activated coagulation time in excess of 800 seconds is preferred. Obviously, as inadequate heparinization can lead to coagulopathy, we prefer to err on the side of caution when using aprotinin and run an activated clotting time in excess of 800 seconds. Of course, the dosage requirement changes so frequently with both epsilon aminocaproic acid and aprotinin that we must alter our approach fairly frequently.

We administer a test dose of 1–2 ml of aprotinin before commencing a loading dose to observe for an allergic response. So far, based on our clinical experience and current thought, vessel thrombosis remains a minimal risk with aprotinin use. As always, should excessive bleeding be noted postbypass, judicious administration of blood products is indicated before transporting the patient from the operating suite.

Ventricular Function

We describe in detail the management of the patient with poor ventricular function in Chapter 8. Many patients for reoperative CAB may be included in this group as a consequence of a poor ventricular performance preoperatively. Additionally, there is always the risk of embolization of atherosclerotic material through the previous bypass grafts in patients undergoing redo surgery. This can result in areas of the heart that are unprotected on bypass, resulting in poor ventricular function and occasionally an inability to wean from bypass and patient death.

Femoral Bypass

If femoral bypass is contemplated either electively or emergently, it is important that close communication be maintained, with the perfusionist regarding the degree of venous return to the pump and the flow generated by the bypass machine. It is possible that a significant amount of blood flow will continue to be delivered to the heart. Therefore, we must be certain that ventilation and oxygenation continue as pulmonary blood flow continues so that the patient continues to be adequately oxygenated.

Postoperative Complications

In addition to bleeding, other complications, such as renal dysfunction and pulmonary insufficiency, can present in the reoperative patient (see Chapter 15). Therefore, the patient for reoperative CAB presents a number of additional challenges. Fortunately, as mentioned at the start of this text, our patients, at least, will always do well: Mr. XY has survived you once again. Whether he reappears for a third reoperative CAB remains as much dependent on political and economic forces affecting medical practice as perhaps any cardiology advances that may occur within the next several years. We are often presented with relatively elderly patients for third and fourth reoperations. Whether this continues in the future will be a source of continued medical, legal, and ethical debate.

8

Patients with Poor Ventricular Function

Having successfully taken patients with relatively good ventricular function through surgery, cardiac anesthesia looks relatively easy. Alas, not every patient has the kind of ventricular function that makes this task so easy. Every so often we encounter a patient who, for whatever reason, has a heart that is impaired as a pump.

Generally, this impairment in the coronary bypass population is secondary to previous myocardial infarctions in either the recent or distant past. Additionally, patients with long-standing valvular heart disease may have dysfunctional ventricular performance even after the valvular lesion has been corrected. Finally, some patients present to surgery with relatively preserved ventricular function, only to sustain myocardial damage during the surgery. Inadequate cardioplegia during cardiopulmonary bypass can result in a severely dysfunctional heart after release of the aortic cross clamp. Patients undergoing reoperative bypass surgery are at risk for embolization of atheromatous material down their previous bypass grafts, leading to inadequate delivery of anterograde cardioplegia. Also, in those instances where the heart is open to facilitate valvular repair or ventricular aneurysmectomy, the possibility of air embolization via the native coronary vessels can also lead to postoperative pump failure. Last, bypass graft vasospasm, improperly sewn bypass grafts, and graft kinking can impair blood flow to the myocardium while attempting to wean from cardiopulmonary bypass.

Thus, poor ventricular function can be encountered in two distinct patient populations at the time of coronary revascularization. Patients with significant preoperative ischemic cardiomyopathy, obstructive cardiomyopathy, or dilated cardiomyopathy can obviously present challenges from the moment they present for surgical revascularization or valvular repair. Often these patients require support of the circulation either before induction of anesthesia or during the prebypass period.

The second type of patient requiring inotropic support is the patient who everyone expects to do well but who, for whatever reason, does not. This patient creates incredible tension in the operating room, as individuals worry how a patient undergoing routine surgery can appear to be in life-threatening jeopardy.

In reviewing management of the patient with poor ventricular function, two cases are presented. Imagine both of these patients undergoing coronary revascularization at the same time, maybe in adjacent operating rooms. These cases illustrate management of patients with both predictable and unpredictable ventricular dysfunction. Patient 1, Ms. YY, is a 70-year-old diabetic woman with a history of inferior myocardial infarction some years ago. She had been taking an occasional sublingual nitroglycerin for unspecified chest discomfort for the past several months. A few weeks before surgery she awakened from sleep acutely dyspneic with fulminant pulmonary edema. She was taken to the emergency room, intubated, and ventilated. Diuresis with furosemide was commenced. A pulmonary arterial flotation catheter was placed after admission to the intensive care unit. Her cardiac index was 1.9 liters per minute per m^2, with a pulmonary arterial pressure of 45/25 mm Hg and a pulmonary capillary occlusion pressure (PCOP) of 23 mm Hg. After treatment with dobutamine, nitroglycerin, and furosemide, her cardiac index increased to 2.5 liters per minute per m^2 and her PCOP decreased to 12 mm Hg. She was successfully extubated 1 day after her admission. A creatine kinase–MB measurement indicated that she had suffered a myocardial infarction. Echocardiography demonstrated inferior akinesis and anterolateral hypokinesis. Her ejection fraction was estimated at 25%. Cardiac catheterization revealed three-vessel occlusive disease and poor ventricular function. No valvular heart disease was noted. She was scheduled for elective surgery. Patient II, Mr. ZZ, is a 35-year-old man with a history of increasing angina. He has a strong family history of coronary disease and familial hyperlipidemia. He has never had a myocardial infarction. Ejection fraction was estimated at 65% by echocardiography. Catheterization reveals three-vessel occlusive disease. He is scheduled for surgery.

Here, then, we have two patients with essentially the same surgery next door to one another. Both are at risk for significant ventricular failure during the course of the surgery. But before we place them at risk for perioperative mortality, we briefly review what ventricular function is about.

The Heart as a Pump

Heart failure at its most basic is the inability of the heart to meet the oxygen supply needs of the tissues. Simply put, the pump does not pump that well. Although any number of etiologies can lead to ventricular dysfunction (e.g., viral myocarditis, alcoholic cardiomyopathy, and so forth) these are examples of chronic heart failure. The patient with chronic ventricular dysfunction attempts to compensate for inadequate ventricular performance. The compensatory mechanisms result in increased catecholamine release. This increases heart rate, myocardial contractility, and vascular tone (to preserve blood pressure).

The renin-angiotensin-aldosterone system augments plasma volume, often resulting in peripheral edema in the setting of right ventricular failure or pulmonary edema in the setting of left ventricular failure. Each of these compensatory responses to ventricular dysfunction attempts to improve stroke volume by increasing volume load to the heart or by improving myocardial contractility. Increasing heart rate, as previously mentioned, increases cardiac output (cardiac output = stroke volume × heart rate), thereby improving blood delivery to the tissues. Both impaired systolic function (i.e., contractility) in the setting of a myocardial infarction and reduced diastolic ventricular relaxation (as occurs in patients with ventricular hypertrophy) can result in reduced ventricular performance. In the case of Ms. YY and Mr. ZZ, acute events may quickly impair ventricular function.

Although physiologists may question the simplicity of this analysis, from a clinical perspective it remains useful to focus on stroke volume as our measure of ventricular performance. Recall that stroke volume = left ventricular end-diastolic volume – left ventricular end-systolic volume. Stroke volume = cardiac output ÷ heart rate. The determinants of stroke volume are (1) the volume load presented to the heart (preload), (2) the resistance opposing ventricular contraction (afterload), and (3) myocardial contractility (Table 8-1).

Alterations in any of these three determinants can both exacerbate and ameliorate ventricular dysfunction in the acute and chronic setting.

Table 8-1. Stroke Volume

Stroke volume = left ventricular end-diastolic volume – left ventricular end-systolic volume

Stroke volume = cardiac output/heart rate

Determinants of stroke volume

1. Volume load presented to the heart (preload)
2. Resistance opposing ventricular contraction (afterload)
3. Myocardial contractility

How anesthesiologists manipulate these parameters will determine our success in managing both the patient with chronic ventricular dysfunction and the patient with acute decompensation after cardiopulmonary bypass.

Volume loading of the heart may be estimated by the PCOP. As mentioned earlier, the PCOP is an approximation of left ventricular end-diastolic pressure. A pressure is not a volume, however, and it is the volume load to the heart that determines the stroke volume. Nonetheless, the PCOP is a convenient measurement that, barring significant mitral valvular disease, provides an estimate of left ventricular end-diastolic pressure, and by extension, left ventricular end-diastolic volume.

The relationship between pressure and volume in the ventricle is determined by ventricular compliance. Compliance relates changes in ventricular volume with ventricular pressure. In a normally compliant heart, increased ventricular volume is accommodated with only minimal changes in ventricular pressure (Figure 8-1).

For patients such as Ms. YY who have sustained ventricular damage, the ventricle may be significantly less compliant than the healthy heart. In such instances, small changes in volume can lead to significant increases in ventricular end-diastolic pressure that subsequently can lead to pulmonary edema. The effects of volume loading on the stroke volume are expressed by the Frank-Starling relationship (Figure 8-2).

As the familiar Starling curve indicates, increasing ventricular volume augments stroke volume to a point. Excessive volume overload fails to increase the stroke volume. Indeed, volume overload can subsequently lead to stroke volume reduction as a consequence of ventricular distention, increased ventricular wall tension, and increased myocardial oxygen demand resulting in myocardial ischemia and ventricular failure.

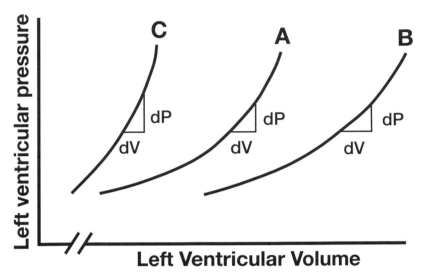

Figure 8-1. *Ventricular compliance curves. Left ventricular diastolic pressure-volume relationships: normal (A), increased volumes and compliance (e.g., effect of chronic volume overload) (B), and decreased volumes and compliance (e.g., effect of chronic pressure overload or pericardial tamponade with pressure measured relative to atmosphere) (C). For a given change in volume (dV), the change in pressure (dP) varies inversely with compliance. (Modified from WJ Hoffman, JD Wasnick [eds]. Postoperative Critical Care of the Massachusetts General Hospital. Boston: Little, Brown, 1992;157.)*

Although in general we are concerned with volume overload in the failing heart, it is possible to have inadequate ventricular function as a consequence of inadequate loading of the heart. Mitral stenosis can retard flow to the left ventricle, resulting in a diminished stroke volume. Impaired diastolic relaxation as a consequence of ventricular hypertrophy or myocardial ischemia can similarly reduce volume loading to the left ventricle with an associated reduction in stroke volume. Pericardial disease can also reduce ventricular volume loading by impairing venous return to the heart. The interventricular septum can shift left in patients with elevated right ventricular pressures as a consequence of pulmonary hypertension into the left ventricular cavity, thereby reducing left ventricular filling and stroke volume.

The second determinant of stroke volume that we must consider before we attempt to take Ms. YY or Mr. ZZ to surgery is the effect of afterload on the heart. Afterload may be considered to represent

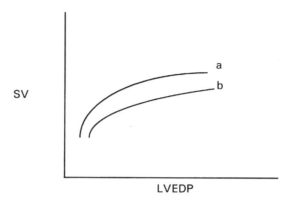

Figure 8-2. *Frank-Starling curve. Curves a and b reflect differing contractile states of the heart. The contractile state of the heart represented by curve a is greater than that represented by curve b. LVEDP approximates left ventricular end-diastolic volume. Increasing ventricular volume and pressure (LVEDV and LVEDP) improves stroke volume. (SV = stroke volume; LVEDP = left ventricular end-diastolic pressure.)*

those forces that oppose ventricular contraction. Generally, we approximate these forces through the calculated value known as the systemic vascular resistance. Systemic vascular resistance = [(mean arterial pressure – central venous pressure) ÷ cardiac output] × 80. The afterload contributes to the development of myocardial wall tension (recall LaPlace's law: Wall tension = [ventricular radius × ventricular pressure] ÷ ventricular wall thickness). As you may recall, increasing myocardial wall tension contributes to increased myocardial oxygen demand. Therefore, increases in afterload can increase myocardial oxygen supply and demand imbalances and promote ventricular failure.

The final determinant of stroke volume to consider is myocardial contractility. Contractility reflects the shortening of the individual myocardial fibers. Although it is possible to measure myocardial contractility in vitro, a clinical assessment has not readily found its way into routine practice. Assessments of stroke volume and cardiac output are always dependent on the loading conditions presented to the heart—that is, preload and afterload. Echocardiography, although still influenced by loading conditions, provides a quick assessment of ventricular function that may be an acceptable approximation for measures of myocardial contractility.

Myocardial contractility is augmented by catecholamines, calcium, and other inotropes. It is retarded by beta blockers and calcium antagonists, as well as other drugs, including many inhalational and intravenous anesthetic agents.

What then can cause reduction in stroke volumes? The answer is obvious: decreased contractility, inadequate preload, or excessive afterload. These determinants of stroke volume must be sought in the ventricular failure patient in the surgical suite. How the determinants of stroke volume can affect ventricular performance is clear. The patient experiencing volume loss secondary to inadequate replacement or continued bleeding is likely to have reduced stroke volume as a consequence of inadequate preload. Volume replacement generally restores stroke volume and the cardiac output.

Although volume loss may be the most obvious source of decreased stroke volume as a consequence of reduced preload, it is by no means the only etiology of decreased stroke volume resulting from inadequate loading of the heart. Restrictive pericarditis can impede blood return to the right ventricle, reducing the volume presented to the left side of the heart for ejection into the systemic circulation. Likewise, pericardial tamponade of many etiologies can retard blood return, resulting in an underloaded heart.

In patients in whom pericardial processes retard the return of blood to the right side of the heart, care must be taken at the time of induction of anesthesia that the surgical team is available to open the chest and relieve pericardial pressure. Institution of positive pressure breathing can further reduce blood return to the heart, potentially leading to a dramatic reduction of stroke volume and hemodynamic collapse.

The second determinant that can lead to perioperative ventricular failure is increased afterload. Generally, patients at risk from failure as a consequence of increased afterload will be known prior to surgery. Such patients include those with aortic stenosis and a hypertrophic left ventricle. The patient with idiopathic hypertrophic subaortic stenosis also can present an increased resistance to ventricular contraction resulting in heart failure. Those instances in which a patient's decreased preload or increased afterload can result in ventricular failure will be most likely known before taking the patient to surgery. If the patient has tamponade or valvular heart disease, we will most certainly be aware of it and can expect reductions in stroke volume secondary to changes in preload or afterload at the time of induction of the anesthesia.

The vast majority of patients in whom ventricular failure is a concern simply have poorly contracting hearts secondary to ischemia, cardiomyopathy, or recent myocardial infarction. In this population, the cause of the heart's failure is less likely to be as immediately corrected as volume administration in inadequate preload. Although it may be true that some patients perform better once taken to surgery and revascularized, patients who have had much myocardial damage and an ejection fraction of less than 35% can prove exceedingly difficult to manage perioperatively. The expected improvement in ventricular function after surgical revascularization may not be immediate in patients who have required prolonged cardiopulmonary bypass runs and numerous administrations of cardioplegia. We discuss the precise management of patients with ventricular failure secondary to valvular heart disease and pericardial processes in Chapter 14. Next, we want to bring our patients Ms. YY and Mr. ZZ out of the operating room by attempting to maximize their myocardial performance. The question is simple: How can the anesthesiologist improve cardiovascular function so that patients with poor ventricular contractility can be optimized at the time of surgery and successfully weaned from cardiopulmonary bypass?

Assessment of Ventricular Function

In attempting to optimize ventricular performance in those at risk for perioperative heart failure, we must carefully gather the appropriate information to supplement our understanding of hemodynamics 101. The pulmonary artery flotation catheter measures cardiac output, PCOP, and right atrial pressure. These measurements are essential in guiding our perioperative management. In spite of recent warnings about pulmonary artery catheter use, the pulmonary arterial catheter is helpful in assessing ventricular function perioperatively. New studies of pulmonary artery catheter use in the coronary artery bypass (CAB) population will, it is hoped, be readily forthcoming.

Pulmonary Capillary Occlusion Pressure

PCOP provides an approximation of left atrial pressure that further approximates left ventricular end-diastolic pressure. The left ventricular end-diastolic pressure provides a rough approximation for left ventricular end-diastolic volume. It is the left ventricular end-diastolic volume that determines the volume load of the left ventricle before contraction. In patients with a normally compliant left ventricle, changes in volume load result in only minimal changes in left ventricular end-diastolic pressure. However, in patients with poor left ventricular function, ventricular compliance is likely reduced. In this setting, small changes in volume may result in significantly increased left ventricular end-diastolic pressure (estimated by a PCOP of more than 20 mm Hg).

Right Atrial Pressure

Right atrial pressure provides an approximation of right ventricular pressure and volume. Elevation of the right atrial pressure of more than 20 mm Hg, especially if the right atrial pressure is significantly greater than the PCOP, may suggest right ventricular failure leading to inadequate volume loading of the left side of the heart and the potential for cardiovascular collapse.

Cardiac Output

The pulmonary capillary flotation catheter provides a measure of cardiac output using the thermodilution technique. Cardiac output reflects the product of stroke volume and heart rate. Cardiac output or cardiac index can be misleading taken by themselves. Because tachycardia may increase overall cardiac output, we can have a false sense of security if ventricular function is impaired. Tachycardia is a compensatory mechanism for the failing heart. As such, an elevated heart rate can provide an acceptable cardiac output. When the stroke volume is calculated, however, we can appreciate that myocardial function is significantly impaired. (Normal stroke volume is approximately 60–80 ml per beat.)

Right Ventricular Ejection Fraction

A pulmonary artery flotation catheter equipped with a rapid-response thermistor can assess right ventricular ejection fraction. A decrease in right ventricular ejection fraction can indicate right ventricular failure. Right ventricular failure can lead to underloading of the left ventricle and a reduced cardiac index.

Transesophageal Echocardiography

Transesophageal echocardiography (TEE) provides a visual assessment of both left and right ventricular function. With little experience, the anesthesiologist is able to determine from TEE a rough assessment of ventricular performance and contractility.

Clinical Observation

Although measures of cardiac output, pulmonary artery flotation catheter pressures, and TEE provide a definitive assessment of ventricular performance, clinical observation is often very useful to determine if a given cardiac index or stroke volume is acceptable in a given patient. We should not expect a stroke volume of 80 ml per beat in a patient who is at most 50 kg by weight. Assessments of capillary refill, color, urine output, acid–base balance, and mental status in the awake patient provide clues as to the adequacy of cardiac index and stroke volume. In the patient undergoing surgery, direct observation of the beating heart often provides an effective assessment of right ventricular function. Thus, as we think about the heart failure patient, we must gather information from clinical observation, TEE, hemodynamic profiles, and physical signs.

Thinking About Heart Failure in the Surgical Candidate

The patient presenting to the emergency room in pulmonary edema may have many causes for heart failure. The patient may be volume overloaded secondary to renal failure. Perhaps he or she has retained too much fluid from eating too many salt-laden foods. The patient may be having an acute myocardial infarction or may simply have forgotten to take medication. Although these may be causes encountered by the internist, they are hardly our concern when we face the patient with a failing heart in the operating room, where two scenarios predominate: the expected and the unexpected. In Ms. YY we expected to have difficulty with ventricular function perioperatively. She had sustained previous damage to her heart and has a reduced ejection fraction. Despite revascularization and, it is hoped, good cardioplegia, it is likely that her ventricular performance will be impaired at the time of weaning from cardiopulmonary bypass. In patients such as Ms. YY it is also likely that she may have a stormy course up to the point of placing the bypass cannulas. On one hand, induction of anesthesia may unload the heart as a consequence of vasodilation, leading to improved myocardial performance. On the other hand, vasodilation can lead to hypotension and hypoperfusion, resulting in ischemia and progressive ventricular dysfunction up until the time bypass is initiated. Whatever course occurs, it is clear that in patients with a history of significant ventricular damage we should expect the expected, namely, a potentially rocky intraoperative course.

On the other hand, Mr. ZZ, by all accounts, should be the perfectly healthy CAB patient with which any anesthesiologist should ideally be comfortable. Unfortunately, he is also one of those patients with whom things have not gone well. Due to an underprotected ventricle during the aortic cross clamp as a consequence of inadequate cardioplegia delivery, his heart is injured at the time of surgery, leading to a poorly contractile state at the time of weaning from bypass support. In a case such as his, the anesthesiologist who encounters ventricular dysfunction can make a difference. How we manage ventricular dysfunction in this setting can well determine the outcome for this otherwise healthy individual. As always, whenever we encounter unexpected ventricular dysfunction, we must be aware of the emotional stress that this places on the entire operating room team. The prospect of an otherwise healthy patient not doing well is particularly threatening to the surgeon currently when morbidity and mortality reports frequently find their way into the mass media. An ideal performance as an anesthesiologist is absolutely essential for two reasons. On one hand, the patient deserves it so that he or she has a chance to wean from bypass. Second, anesthesiologists need to protect themselves so that the surgeons cannot blame them for failing to wean the patient from bypass. Generally, surgeons rarely acknowledge that they have inadequately protected the heart.

So what can we do? Obviously, when we encounter ventricular dysfunction, we must be cognizant of the three determinants of stroke volume that we have already discussed—namely, preload, afterload, and contractility because these are the variables that we can manipulate. Whether we do so pharmacologically or mechanically constitutes our therapy so that patients may survive the surgical suite.

Before attempting to apply our drugs and mechanical assist devices in the heart failure patient, we must be certain that the myocardial environment is such that effective myocardial contractility is possible.

If we are at the point of weaning from bypass, we must be certain that a regular rhythm has been restored. This can either be a regular paced rhythm or preferably a normal sinus rhythm. Acid–base and electrolyte balances and temperature should be corrected to normal. Never forget to check that ventilation is adequate. From time to time, a rare patient has failed to come off the bypass machine because the anesthesiologist has forgotten to reinflate the lungs and ventilate the patient. High inspiratory pressures during positive pressure ventilation can retard right ventricular filling and thereby decrease cardiac output. As such, bronchodilator therapy may be necessary at the time of restoring ventilation in patients with significant pulmonary disease. Also, it is important to be aware that if positive end-expiratory pressure is being used to improve oxygenation, it may result in the intraventricular septum being dislocated into the left ventricle, thereby distorting left ventricular volume and reducing cardiac index. Finally, we must be certain that valvular function has not been altered (i.e., acute mitral regurgitation in the setting of an ischemic heart). If we are certain that there are no other precipitants of ventricular dysfunction, we can proceed to manipulate the determinants of stroke volume to optimize cardiac performance.

An ordered and composed approach is necessary to address these determinants in the patient with either expected or unexpected poor ventricular function. With the heart cannulated, if we fail to wean from bypass we can quickly escape by restarting bypass flow and then adjusting our therapy. It is prudent to retreat to bypass rather than to force a heart incapable of meeting the perfusion needs of the patient to struggle for any protracted length of time. Depleted of energy reserves, the failing, distended heart will progressively worsen, further impairing perfusion. Thus, should the heart appear to struggle, it is far wiser to retreat to cardiopulmonary bypass for a period of rest than to continually force the failing heart to attempt to meet the patient's perfusion needs.

In general, the failing heart after cardiopulmonary bypass is poorly contractile, poorly compliant, and readily distended. The ideal goal in weaning a patient from circulatory support is to have a heart that is contractile, compliant, and nondistended. How we manipulate the determinants of stroke volume can go a long way toward achieving desired ventricular performance.

Although dated, the Frank-Starling model still provides a quick conceptualization of how our therapy can be directed toward this end. Although not as elegant as left ventricular pressure volume loops, the Starling curve is readily reproduced in the surgical suite should it be needed. Of course, clinical anesthesiologists do not employ models when treating patients. They know how to make the heart contract and

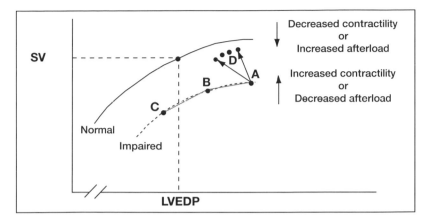

Figure 8-3. *A Frank-Starling approach to ventricular failure. Each curve describes the relationship between ventricular end-diastolic pressure (LVEDP; a correlate of end-diastolic volume [LVEDV] or preload) and stroke volume (SV) for a given contractile state and afterload. Point A corresponds to a failing ventricle with high LVEDP and low SV. Reduction in LVEDP from A and B along the flat portion of the curve results in little change in SV; further reduction in LVEDP as from B and C along a steeper portion of the curve causes a much greater decrease in SV. Points labeled D indicate possible responses to enhanced contractility, afterload reduction, or both; the resultant increase in SV is often associated with a concomitant decrease in LVEDP (LVEDV). (Modified from WJ Hoffman, JD Wasnick [eds]. Postoperative Critical Care of the Massachusetts General Hospital. Boston: Little, Brown, 1992;166.)*

keep it from becoming distended. The Frank-Starling curve merely provides us a graphic representation of therapy in action (Figure 8-3).

Mechanisms of Ventricular Dysfunction and Therapy After Cardiopulmonary Bypass

Preload

Obviously, if too little volume is presented to the heart, stroke volume will be reduced, lowering cardiac output and blood pressure. So what is the right volume with which to load the left ventricle? This is by no means an easy question to answer. Too little ventricular volume and the stroke volume is unacceptably low. Too great a volume load can lead to myocardial distension, ischemia, and pulmonary edema. There is no ideal PCOP as a guide for ventricular volume loading. Although some may establish arbitrary ideal numbers such as a PCOP of 15–20 mm Hg, these are not universally applicable. Impaired ventricular compliance secondary to ischemia or myocardial infarction can result in a significantly higher left ventricular end-diastolic pressure needed to adequately load the left ventricle. Ideally, the lowest filling pressure to achieve an acceptable stroke volume, cardiac output, and blood pressure should be the goal in adjusting volume preload.

Infusions of nitroglycerin or nitroprusside vasodilate the capacitance vessels to reduce volume return to the heart. Beta agonists and phosphodiesterase (PDE) inhibitors (i.e., amrinone and milrinone) have a vasodilatory capability as well. Additionally, ongoing blood loss from the surgical field as well as increased urine output from mannitol included in the cardioplegia have the tendency to decrease the volume load to the heart immediately postbypass. Obviously, should volume to the heart be inadequate, blood pressure and stroke volume will decrease. The aortic perfusion cannula provides a reliable conduit by which large amounts of volume can be administered relatively quickly following separation from bypass. Administration of small volumes (50–100 ml) of blood via the aortic perfusion cannula compensates for blood volume loss, vasodilation, or both after weaning from cardiopulmonary bypass.

Observation of the heart provides an excellent assessment of both ventricular volume and myocardial contractility before and after separation from the bypass machine. Although from the anesthesiologist's perspective, only the right side of the heart is visible, this nonetheless can assist in guiding ventricular volume adjustments. A small, snapping, dancing heart is generally healthy, contractile, and adequately loaded. A large, poorly contractile muscular balloon is generally overloaded, distended, and in need of both volume reduction and inotropic support. TEE is helpful in assessing both myocardial contractility and volume loading perioperatively. However, TEE may not be indicated in routine bypass surgery, although some advocate its frequent use as a screen for an atheromatous aorta.

Impaired Ventricular Contractility

The second determinant of stroke volume that we must consider in dealing with the failing heart is inadequate contractility. In the patient with poor ventricular function, institution of therapy with inotropes augments myocardial contractility. However, inotropic agents often produce tachycardia that can shorten diastolic filling, thereby reducing loading to the heart and decreasing stroke volume. Additionally, in patients at risk for ischemia, increasing heart rate and contractility may increase myocardial oxygen demand. Of course, this is a particular concern when inotropes are needed before myocardial revascularization. In that setting, inotropes may or may not produce a favorable oxygen supply and demand balance. Impaired ventricular contractility increases myocardial wall tension, which can augment oxygen demand. By reducing ventricular volume, oxygen demand may, in fact, be reduced. It is a balancing act as to whether one improves ischemia or promotes it by using inotropes in the ischemic patient. Once revascularized, the application of potential tachycardia-producing inotropes should be less of a concern. Thus, in this regard, we have the advantage over the emergency room physician who must be concerned whether inotropes will exacerbate myocardial ischemia or improve it. We will assume that in the postbypass patient, myocardial oxygen supply has been improved. We must also be aware that bypass grafts can become kinked and that air and other particulate emboli can produce profound ischemia even after the heart has been revascularized. If we suspect at any time that impaired myocardial contractility is a consequence of an embolic phenomenon or graft dysfunction, it is most prudent to maintain cardiopulmonary bypass until the surgeon has been able to review the anatomy and is certain of bypass graft patency. Should air embolization be considered, the perfusion pressure should be augmented by the perfusionist with phenylephrine in an effort to clear air emboli from the myocardium. Once corrected, resting the heart on the bypass circuit for some time should give the injured myocardium the chance to replenish energy so that a successful separation from bypass can be attempted. Nonetheless, the heart may often appear poorly contractile even after the surgeon is confident that all obvious causes of myocardial ischemia or dysfunction have been corrected. At this point, we must begin to consider inotropic, mechanical, or both kinds of support for the patient.

Afterload Reduction and the Failing Heart

The last determinant to consider is afterload reduction. By decreasing ventricular wall stress (recall LaPlace's law), we can improve the oxygen supply-to-demand ratio. By reducing the calculated systemic vascular resistance and the forces that constitute the impedance against which the heart must contract, we can increase the stroke volume and improve the cardiac output. In so doing, we must also be aware that arterial impedance does contribute to the generation of blood pressure along with cardiac output. Reducing vascular tone can lower blood pressure sufficiently that our perfusion is inadequate in spite of an adequate cardiac output. Renal azotemia, acidemia, and ischemia may result as a consequence of inadequate perfusion pressure.

Various drugs are available to reduce vascular tone, including nitroglycerin, nitroprusside, angiotensin-converting enzyme inhibitors, beta agonists, and PDE inhibitors. All can reduce arterial impedance, lessen wall tension, and improve stroke volume. Many of the agents for treating the failing ventricle affect two or all of the determinants that constitute a stroke volume. Inotropes that vasodilate can reduce both preload as well as arterial impedance while simultaneously improving ventricular contractility. One key to weaning the patient from cardiopulmonary bypass with an impaired ventricle is balancing the effects of these various medications.

Pharmacologic Approach to the Failing Heart

Any number of inotropic drugs are available to reduce preload and afterload and to improve contractility. The exact choice of drugs employed depends less on the particular properties of that agent and more so on the experience and prejudices of the institutions where that drug is to be employed. Although epinephrine may be considered a first-line agent in low doses for inotropic support at cost-conscious institutions, in others, epinephrine may be considered the drug of the dying. Namely, only moribund patents are associated with its use. Although such an outlook is obviously faulty, it is important that the anesthesiologist be aware of the local myths and prejudices that are encountered. After all, the last thing one needs is a panicked surgeon worrying about a poor mortality report in *The New York Times* simply because the patient has been placed on epinephrine, which that surgeon considers a drug of desperation. That being said, any number of drugs are available both to improve myocardial contractility and adjust the loading conditions of the heart (Table 8-2).

As can be seen from Table 8-2, the various inotropes have different effects on stroke volume, peripheral resistance, arrhythmogenicity, and so forth. Although science may delineate these many properties, it is the

Table 8-2. Frequently Used Inotropes

Drug	Dose	Effect
Epinephrine	0.5 µg/min titrated upward to effect	Beta agonist, alpha agonist Increases heart rate, contractility, and SVR Increases or decreases CO Arrhythmogenic
Norepinephrine	0.5–20.0 µg/min titrated upward to effect	Alpha agonist more than beta agonist Causes vasoconstriction Increases or decreases heart rate and CO
Dopamine	2–10 µg/kg/min	Beta agonist, alpha agonist Causes vasoconstriction at higher doses ? Renal vasodilator Arrhythmogenic Increases or decreases SVR
Dobutamine	5–10 µg/kg/min	Beta agonist Causes vasodilation Increases myocardial contractility Decreases SVR Increases or decreases blood pressure Arrhythmogenic
Amrinone	0.75 mg/kg load, then 5–10 µg/kg/min	PDE inhibitor Increases CO, vasodilation, cellular cAMP; and Ca^{2+} uptake into cells Decreases SVR Increases or decreases heart rate Increases or decreases blood pressure May impair platelet function
Milrinone	50 µg/kg load, then 0.50–0.75 µg/kg/min	Similar to amrinone Greatly increases vasodilation Fewer platelet effects than amrinone

SVR = systemic vascular resistance; CO = cardiac output; PDE = phosphodiesterase.

art of practice by which they are successfully employed in combination with vasodilators to effectively manage the patient with impaired stroke volume and ventricular function. In our sample patients, we examine how these drugs are employed both actively and reactively to respond to the failing heart at weaning from cardiopulmonary bypass.

Mechanical Assist Devices

The failing heart most frequently responds to any number of combinations of inotropes, vasopressors, and vasodilators. Unfortunately, in some patients ventricular function is so impaired that even combined aggressive pharmacologic support is unable to generate an adequate stroke volume to ensure suitable organ perfusion. In such settings, rather than continuing the administration of ever-increasing quantities of vasoconstrictors and arrhythmogenic inotropes, mechanical assistance can be helpful to maintain the cardiac output and relieve myocardial ischemia. Mechanical assistance of the failing ventricle includes both intra-aortic counterpulsation to reduce arterial impedance and improve diastolic coronary blood flow, as well as ventricular assist devices (VADs) that can more or less assume the function of either the left or right ventricle. Certainly, there is a significant difference in the kind of support a VAD provides (e.g., HeartMate [ThermoCardiosystems, Woburn, MA], Abiomed [Abiomed, Inc., Danvers, MA]) versus simple aortic counterpulsation. Institution of support with a VAD depends on both the surgeon's assessment of the ventricle's recovery of function and the possibility of myocardial transplantation. Without either possibility, the placement of VADs is merely an exercise to avoid intraoperative mortality for legal or statistical reasons.

Intra-Aortic Balloon Pump

The intra-aortic balloon pump is no substitute for a contracting left ventricle (Figure 8-4). Its name defines its purpose. It is an assist device designed to aid the circulation. For it to be effective, intra-aortic balloon counterpulsation requires a beating heart. Either normal sinus rhythm or a paced rhythm is acceptable to coordinate balloon inflation and deflation. The aortic balloon itself is little more than a balloon-tipped catheter placed into the descending thoracic aorta via the femoral artery. It works through the principles of counterpulsation in that it is inflated by an electrocardiogram or a pressure trigger during diastole and then deflated before systole. The intra-aortic balloon pump

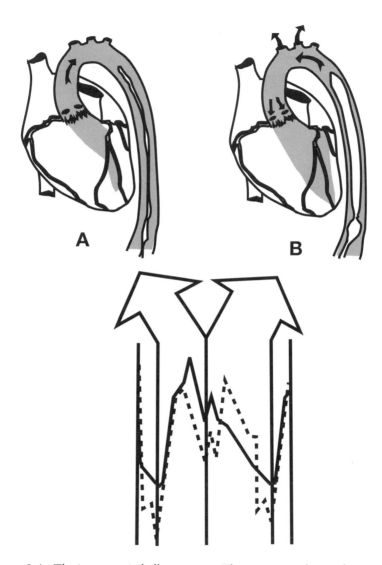

Figure 8-4. *The intra-aortic balloon pump. The continuous line is the arterial pressure waveform without circulatory assistance. The dotted line is the arterial pressure with the intra-aortic balloon pump on. (A) Balloon deflation just before ventricular systole enhances left ventricular ejection by reducing end-diastolic pressure. Peak systolic pressure is reduced. (B) Balloon inflation occurs early in diastole, causing an increase in diastolic pressure and coronary blood flow. (Modified from TE Oh. Intensive Care Manual [4th ed]. Oxford: Butterworth–Heinemann, 1997.)*

therefore augments diastolic pressure, improving left coronary perfusion while also decreasing systolic wall tension, thereby reducing myocardial oxygen demand. As a consequence, the balloon augments stroke volume. This is done in two ways. First, by improving the oxygen supply demand ratio to the left heart it may improve contractility. Second, by lowering arterial impedance through systolic deflation, the intra-aortic balloon improves the ejection of the left ventricle. Therefore, the intra-aortic balloon pump provides an effective assistance to the heart with failing ventricular function.

The cardiac anesthesiologist is likely to encounter the intra-aortic balloon pump in three ways. Patients with ischemia refracting to medical therapy are occasionally placed on intra-aortic balloon counterpulsation to improve the myocardial oxygen supply to demand ratio while they are awaiting surgery. Other patients present to surgery in cardiogenic shock, often after failed angioplasty, with an intra-aortic balloon pump in place. But generally, the cardiac anesthesiologist encounters the intra-aortic balloon pump after the failure of pharmacotherapy to wean the patient from cardiopulmonary bypass. Balloon pump complications include arterial dissection, ischemia in the lower extremities, obstruction of vessels of the aortic arch, and hemorrhage on catheter withdrawal.

The intra-aortic balloon pump is relatively contraindicated in patients with aortic regurgitation and peripheral vascular disease. Direct placement of the balloon into the thoracic aorta is possible when peripheral disease or previous aortic femoral grafts makes femoral placement impossible. Once placed, timing of the intra-aortic balloon pump inflation and deflation requires some patience. For the anesthesiologist renewing his or her familiarity with the intra-aortic balloon pump, it is often helpful to turn to the intensive care unit nurse for assistance. Intensive care unit staff literally, by spending hours and hours with patients equipped with intra-aortic balloon pumps, become quite facile at adjusting balloon timing to optimize counterpulsation. In reality, timing of the balloon pump inflation and deflation is quite simple once an acceptable trigger is established and a relatively regular rhythm is secured. Intra-aortic balloon pump inflation should occur at the time of the dicrotic notch on the arterial pressure tracing as measured from the balloon tip. Deflation should occur before the onset of systole.

Although the intra-aortic balloon pump is a useful device, it is only an assist device. If the ventricle does not contract and eject blood, the intra-aortic balloon pump is useless. The balloon console is equipped with an internal setting in which the balloon inflation and deflation occur independent of any trigger. Although this may be used to provide pulsatile flow during cardiopulmonary bypass, it has no function in a heart that is unable to eject blood from the left ventricle. In this instance, the patient must be considered either dead, or a VAD must be placed to substitute for the function of a noncontractile ventricle or ventricles.

Ventricular Assist Devices

Having exhausted our pharmacologic armamentarium and still having failed to wean the patient from cardiopulmonary bypass with the assistance of an intra-aortic balloon pump, the decision comes as to whether a VAD should be placed. These devices, such as the Abiomed or Heart-Mate, replace the function (of the ventricle) by providing a complete substitute for ventricular function. Of course, in deciding to place a VAD, questions must be asked of the surgeon who proposes such an action. Namely, if the patient is not a candidate for heart transplant, can the myocardium recover? What other systemic illnesses are present?

If the patient is not a candidate for transplant, implanting a VAD can lead to significant consumption of materials and human resources in a futile gesture to avoid an intraoperative death. Indeed, as anesthesiologists, we can often tell if the surgeons with whom we work possess sound judgment or not in their ability to discern whether a VAD is warranted in a patient who fails to wean from cardiopulmonary bypass. Anesthesiologists are likely to encounter the VAD placement in two settings. First, the most common setting was alluded to previously—that is, the VAD is an escape from an intraoperative death for patients who cannot be weaned from cardiopulmonary bypass. The second setting in which VADs may be encountered is in patients with severe cardiomyopathy who are in danger of hemodynamic collapse while awaiting transplant. Implantable VADs—for example, the HeartMate—can provide prolonged support to patients as they await a donor heart.

It is the left ventricle that routinely first fails. However, right ventricular dysfunction can often accompany left ventricular dysfunction as well. Naturally, isolated right ventricular failure can occur, resulting in the need for a right VAD. Generally, however, it is the left ventricle that is assisted first, with a right ventricular assist added should right ventricular failure ensue.

The types of VADs are numerous and each institution may acquire a different device to treat ventricular failure. Various types of centrifugal and roller head pumps have been attached to vascular cannulas to assist a given ventricle. These require heparinization and a perfusion team to manage the flow of blood. Other pumps, such as the Hemo-

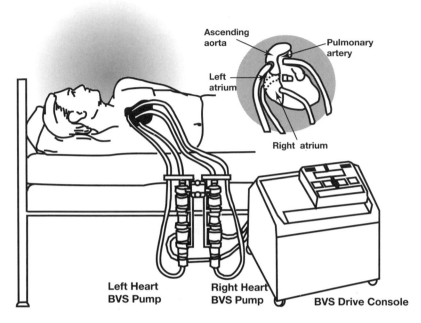

Figure 8-5. *The Abiomed BVS 5000 ventricular assist device. The inset shows the placement of the cannulas. (Reprinted with permission from Abiomed, Inc. Danvers, MA.)*

pump (Nimbus Medical, Rancho Cordova, CA), assist the ventricle by literally propelling blood from the left ventricle into the systemic circulation via a catheter placed across the aortic valve into the left ventricle. Whether one device or another becomes available depends on the preferences of the cardiologists and the surgeons with whom the anesthesiologist is likely to work. As this technology changes, anesthesiologists will have to become accustomed to those devices that are available in their institution. Currently, VADs that have proved popular in practice are those that require less intense supervision and no systemic heparinization. Pneumatically driven pulsatile VADs have been employed both as bridges to transplantation and to provide temporary support in patients with ventricular dysfunction in hopes that stunned myocardium can recover following ischemic insult. Both the extracorporeal Abiomed device and the implantable HeartMate can be used to replace left ventricular function (Figures 8-5 and 8-6).

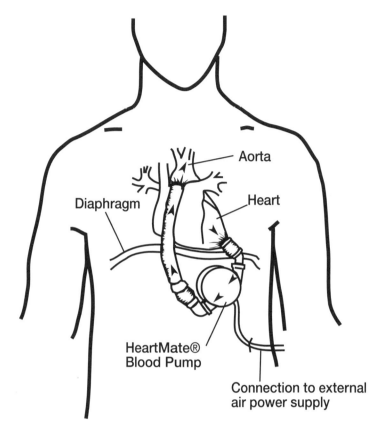

Figure 8-6. *The HeartMate ventricular assist device. (Modified from ThermoCardiosystems, Woburn, MA. Reprinted with permission.)*

    To employ a left ventricular assist using an extracorporeal pneumatic device, cannulas are placed in the left atrium as well as in the aorta to bypass left ventricular function. As blood is drained from the left side of the heart, left ventricular end-diastolic pressure and left atrial pressure decrease to values potentially lower than right atrial pressure and right ventricular end-diastolic pressure. TEE is employed to rule out any patent foramen ovale or atrial septal defect that might lead to right-to-left shunting of blood. Once cannulas are placed, the surgeon confirms that no air is in the device or the cannula tubing. The patient is weaned from cardiopulmonary bypass, and the assist device ejects blood in a pulsatile fashion, replacing the function of the bypassed ventricle. This pumping activity is generally not coordinated with the heart's intrinsic contraction, but this should not create a false sense of security. Simply because the left VAD assumes the function of the left ventricle in no way diminishes the need for the anesthesiologist to continue careful pharmacologic support. The right ventricle must deliver blood through the pulmonary circulation to the left atrium so that it may enter the assist device. Thus, right ventricular contraction provides the driving force that delivers oxygenated blood to the VAD. Inadequate volume replacement or right ventricular failure can impair blood return to the assist device, lowering left ventricular output and leading to systemic hypoperfusion and cardiogenic shock.

Should right ventricular failure that is unresponsive to inotropes or pulmonary vasodilators occur, a right-sided VAD must be placed as well. Right-sided VAD involves placement of cannulas in the right side of the heart and in the pulmonary artery. Adequate volume replacement is essential to load the right-sided VAD. With both ventricles bypassed, perfusion then becomes more or less independent of rhythm and myocardial function.

If the heart appears capable of resuming function, the patient can be taken to the operating room, the ventricular function assessed, and the cannulas removed.

The implantable HeartMate device can be used as both a left-sided VAD and a right-sided VAD, but has generally been used for left ventricular support. Draining blood from the left ventricular apex, the HeartMate can provide prolonged ventricular assist while patients await donor heart availability. Patients supported with either an extracorporeal or implantable VAD are at risk for hemorrhage, embolic stroke, and systemic hypoperfusion. Any or all of these may complicate VAD placement and postoperative management. Ultimately, VAD placement and management remain a surgical decision. Nevertheless, the anesthesiologist has a key role to optimize the pharmacologic therapy of the unbypassed ventricle, as well as to ensure that adequate volume replacement has been given. Correction of coagulopathy also remains the task of the anesthesiologist at the time of VAD placement. In those instances in which patients awaiting heart transplant deteriorate to the point where VAD placement becomes necessary, the anesthesiologist must manage the patient for elective VAD placement as he or she would any patient with exceptionally poor ventricular function. Manipulating inotropes, vasodilators, and vasoconstrictors may be time consuming as the anesthesiologist attempts to stabilize the patient until initiation of cardiopulmonary bypass for VAD placement. Generally, a combination of inotropes, vasodilators, narcotics, and muscle relaxants can effectively manage the patient for elective VAD placement. Nevertheless, as patient deterioration can occur quickly, the surgical team should be ready at the time of induction of anesthesia to expedite vascular cannulation for cardiopulmonary bypass should ventricular function deteriorate once anesthesia has been induced.

Pulling It All Together: A Comprehensive Approach to Weaning the Patient with Poor Ventricular Function from Bypass

Having now reviewed the pharmacologic and mechanical means available to us, we can attempt to wean our two sample patients from cardiopulmonary bypass. Remember Ms. YY is the elderly diabetic woman with poor ventricular function. In contrast, Mr. ZZ is a relatively healthy 35-year-old man who has had a particularly difficult time in surgery and now has a poorly contractile left ventricle as a consequence of inadequate delivery of cardioplegia. Thus, both patients ZZ and YY, although dramatically different at the start of surgery, have similar problems as we attempt to wean them from cardiopulmonary bypass.

Weaning the sick patient from cardiopulmonary bypass is another one of those pivotal moments as an anesthesiologist when people actually pay attention to what you do. How we choose drugs and mechanical assist devices at this time can well determine whether our patients start off on a smooth recovery or whether they have a prolonged time in the intensive care unit suffering from multisystem failure as a consequence of hypoperfusion.

When Is the Heart Failing?

Obviously, if the heart cannot generate a cardiac index to perfuse the tissue, the heart is failing in its mission. The causes of ventricular failure are many. In the postbypass patient, however, generally right or left ventricular dysfunction is a consequence of ischemia, inadequate myocardial protection, or both. For the sake of this discussion we assume that acid–base balance, ventilation, and oxygenation have been corrected before any attempt to wean from bypass. Likewise, we assume that either sinus rhythm or atrioventricular sequential pacing has been instituted to ensure regular rate and rhythm. Obviously, in patients with a history of chronic atrial fibrillation, patients may not be restored to sinus rhythm after coronary revascularization. Nevertheless, it is important that even if the patient has chronic atrial fibrillation that the ventricular response be controlled—that is, heart rate approximately 100 beats per minute at the time of weaning from bypass. Should patients who have not been previously in atrial fibrillation present in atrial fibrillation at the time of weaning from bypass, synchronized cardioversion should be initiated before an attempt at weaning bypass flow. Thus, before we even attempt to wean the impaired heart from cardiopulmonary bypass, we must be certain that we give the heart every advantage possible. Acid–base abnormalities, electrolyte problems, and rhythm disturbances must all be corrected. Ventilation must be restored and the lungs expanded. Only once routine housekeeping chores are attended to should we concentrate on how we are going to address poor ventricular function.

The first question is to consider if the patient is likely to perform poorly or at all. We know that patients such as Ms. YY are likely to have difficulty in weaning from bypass based on experience. Having sustained previous damage to the left ventricle, she clearly is likely to have difficulty following prolonged cardioplegia and bypass surgery. Still, patients sometimes surprise us. In patients who have been well protected by cardioplegia during the time of the aortic cross clamp, revascularized patients can often improve considerably when compared with their prebypass function. Thus, sometimes patients we think will be quite difficult, in fact, turn out to be rather easy to wean from bypass once they have been effectively revascularized.

Patient ZZ, however, demonstrates the opposite phenomenon. Patients we occasionally expect to do well can often perform quite poorly at the time of separation from bypass. We must ask, "How do we know which patients will do well and which ones will not? What tools are available to assist in guiding our therapy?"

Direct Observation

Although we can generally see only the right ventricle from our vantage point, if the patient has a poorly contractile right ventricle we might expect some difficulty in weaning from cardiopulmonary bypass. We discuss right ventricular failure later in this chapter. Right ventricular dysfunction is a frequent accompaniment of left ventricular failure as well. Thus, if we determine that the right side of the heart is poorly contractile we may assume that weaning from bypass will be difficult.

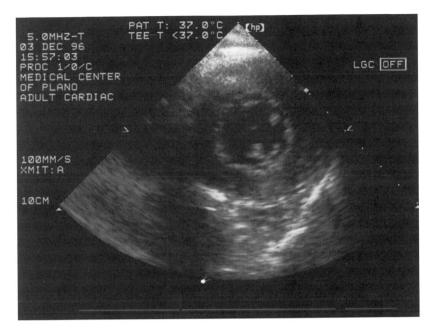

Figure 8-7. *Transesophageal echocardiography view of the left ventricle in cross section.*

Transesophageal Echocardiography

As volume is returned to the heart from the cardiopulmonary bypass machine, TEE provides an assessment of both left and right ventricular contractility. A quick look at the left ventricle as seen on a cross-sectional view (Figure 8-7) provides a rapid assessment of ventricular function.

Electrocardiography and Pressure Monitors

Last, low pulmonary arterial pressure as a patient is weaned from bypass also indicates a relatively strong ventricular performance. If pulmonary arterial pressure increases significantly as bypass flow is reduced to 2–3 liters per minute, left ventricular compliance is impaired, significant mitral regurgitation is present, or both. In such a setting, it is likely that left ventricular function is impaired. Observation of the electrocardiogram is also helpful, although not specific. ST-segment elevation and broad electrocardiographic complexes often are signs of ventricular ischemia. Clearly, should ischemia be present the surgeon must be confident that the bypass grafts are functioning adequately.

If we suspect poor ventricular function from observation, TEE examination, or hemodynamic signs of poor ventricular compliance, we believe it better to initiate therapy before attempting a trial at weaning from bypass. Simply turning off the pump and forcing the heart to struggle only results in ventricular distension, increased myocardial work, and depletion of myocardial adenosine triphosphate. It is far more prudent to initiate therapy with vasodilators and inotropes before attempting to wean from bypass to give the ventricle a fighting chance of meeting the body's perfusion needs.

Some surgeons simply do not wish to initiate therapy before they see that the heart fails. Indeed, you may encounter such a "show-me" surgeon. If this is the case, it is wise for the perfusionist to reduce bypass flow to 2 liters per minute, at which point the surgeon and you can assess myocardial performance. If the heart distends and the pulmonary artery pressure is increased or there is no ejection of blood from the ventricle as measured by a pulsatile flow on the arterial pressure tracing, it is safe to say that the heart has failed and full bypass flow should be instituted while inotropic therapy is initiated. While drugs are infused, the heart is rested on bypass in a collapsed manner to give the ventricle time to replete energy stores before asking it to resume its pumping function. In this instance, we must remember that some surgeons and anesthesiologists simply are incapable of taking the proactive steps necessary to give the heart a fighting chance. Many just insist that the patient come off the bypass pump irrespective of how the heart does. Indeed, some surgeons are so confident of their abilities that the use of drug therapy represents some form of failure. Should we encounter such an individual, although we may advise inotrope therapy before attempting to wean from bypass, sometimes we simply have to turn the pump off and see how the patient does. We do not recommend this course. Obviously, if this is done and a cardiac index of less than 2 liters per minute per m² is measured, it is clear that ventricular function is inadequate and bypass should be restarted and inotropic drugs begun.

Once we separate from cardiopulmonary bypass, if the heart distends and the cardiac index decreases, we must remember that the pump remains as the quick escape for the patient. Rather than attempting to initiate therapy for ventricular failure for a struggling heart, it is prudent to resume bypass flow and rest the heart while drugs are administered.

Generally, we assess ventricular function before attempting to wean from cardiopulmonary bypass through direct observation, TEE, or both. We are able to assess how the patient performs by gradually weaning bypass flow. Through a slow wean we have enormous opportunity to see exactly how the patient will perform. On the contrary, for those surgical teams who reduce flow quickly, there is little time to assess ventricular function. Thus, whether we expect patients to have ventricular dysfunction or not, we should always attempt to wean from bypass support carefully and slowly so we can observe ventricular function and to initiate therapy as indicated.

Once we have determined that the heart is dysfunctional, we must attempt to provide the correct mixture of vasodilators, inotropes, vasoconstrictors, and mechanical assistance to free the patient from the bypass machine.

Figure 8-3 provides a schematic approach using Frank-Starling curves to represent the therapeutic goals in treating the ventricular failure patient. Decreasing impedance against ventricular contraction (afterload) and improving contractility augment stroke volume. In this sense, the goals of therapy for the patient with a dysfunctional ventricle postbypass are no different than the goals of therapy in any other patient who presents with ventricular dysfunction. Improving myocardial contractility and reducing arterial impedance lowers left ventricular end-diastolic pressure and left ventricular end-diastolic volume, which subsequently lead to reductions in left atrial pressure and PCOP. Thus, we try to improve cardiac output while reducing ventricular volume. This is never as easy as the simple schematic indicates. Remember that vasodilators and inotropes may improve cardiac index and stroke volume but at the same time may lower blood pressure too greatly and impair organ perfusion. Hypotension can lead to hypoperfusion, resulting in renal injury or myocardial ischemia. Thus, we must always balance the need for an acceptable perfusion pressure with the necessity for a suitable cardiac index. This is not an even balance by any means, however. If we assume a relatively normal baseline blood pressure, the absence of carotid occlusive disease, adequate urine output, and no evidence of ischemia on the electrocardiogram or as determined by TEE, the cardiac index may be maximized in the setting of a relatively low blood pressure (mean, approximately 60 mm Hg). By allowing a lower systemic pressure, impedance is reduced and stroke volume is maximized. In patients with normally high systemic pressures, those with concomitant carotid disease, and those failing to produce urine, higher systemic pressures may be needed at the expense of cardiac index to secure an adequate pressure for organ perfusion.

Approach to Drug Therapy for Failure to Wean from Cardiopulmonary Bypass

First-Wave Therapy

Once we have determined that the left ventricle requires support, we can initiate a first-wave approach. Generally, both a vasodilator and an inotrope are employed to maximize reductions in arterial impedance and to improve myocardial contractility. The exact choice of drugs is much less important than the way in which the drugs are used. Although in our practice we employ dobutamine because of its beta-agonist effects, this is by no means the only suitable choice. Epinephrine and dopamine can be employed as first-line inotropes if necessary. Care must be taken when using either dopamine or epinephrine because of the possibility of vasoconstriction at higher doses. Cost containment, however, may dictate the choice type of inotrope used from institution to institution. Obviously, epinephrine is a most cost-effective inotropic agent. However, if this choice is made, we must be prepared to treat any arrhythmias that present as well as to avoid vasoconstriction that could reduce stroke volume and cardiac index at higher doses.

Nitroglycerin provides a suitable vasodilator to use with first-line inotropic therapy. Generally, poor ventricular function is accompanied by elevated pulmonary arterial pressures. Increases in pulmonary arterial pressure can lead to right ventricular dysfunction, further compromising ventricular performance. Nitroglycerin (starting at 50 µg per minute) may be titrated to lower pulmonary arterial pressures and reduce ventricular wall tension to a degree. Naturally, nitroglycerin may lower systemic blood pressure as well. In attempting to reduce pulmonary arterial pressures, we must be careful not to overshoot with vasodilators so that systemic hypotension develops. Beta effects from dobutamine and epinephrine may similarly cause reductions in systemic and pulmonary arterial pressures in those patients being treated for a low cardiac index. For many patients, the combination of an inotrope plus nitroglycerin significantly reduces the loading conditions of the heart while increasing myocardial contractility, thereby facilitating weaning from cardiopulmonary bypass.

Second-Wave Therapy

Should this combination fail, a PDE inhibitor (milrinone, amrinone) may be administered as well. Generally, if failure to wean occurs after initiation of therapy with a vasodilator and one inotrope, full bypass flow should be resumed and a PDE inhibitor loaded and an infusion begun. PDE inhibitors in combination with other drugs may lead to significant vasodilation. Although cardiac index and stroke volume may improve dramatically, systemic pressure may be seriously reduced. When blood pressure decreases, small doses of phenylephrine may be administered to partially restore vascular tone. If systemic pressure remains low and cardiac index is appropriately corrected, supplemental volume administration may be given to more adequately volume load the heart. Of course, volume administration in a patient with a PCOP much greater than 20 mm Hg is only likely to lead to volume overload, pulmonary edema, and right ventricular failure. In this instance, volume administration is not appropriate. If, however, after administering nitroglycerin, an inotrope, and a PDE inhibitor the PCOP is reduced to less than 10 mm Hg, volume replacement would be acceptable in restoring blood pressure. Vasodilation-producing infusions may need to be decreased as well. If volume administration fails to secure an appropriate systemic pressure, an infusion of norepinephrine may be titrated to provide vascular tone. Like phenylephrine, norepinephrine produces vasoconstriction. Nonetheless, in small doses vasoconstriction provides an acceptable blood pressure without sacrificing many of the beneficial effects of vasodilator and inotropic therapy. The overwhelming direction of therapy for the poor ventricle is to reduce pulmonary hypertension, improve stroke volume, and increase cardiac index. Vasoconstrictors should be used sparingly to offset hypotension, which on a case-by-case basis is thought to threaten organ perfusion.

The Art of Weaning the Failing Heart from Cardiopulmonary Bypass

We now examine how we will wean patients YY and ZZ from bypass flow employing the modalities that we have discussed. These patterns provide a pattern of action that can be employed for most patients irrespective of operative course and surgical repair when a poor ventricle is encountered, be it after bypass surgery, valvular replacement, arrhythmia surgery, or another surgery. These are appropriate pathways to successfully wean the failing heart from bypass flow. Patient YY gives us a perfect example to illustrate our approaches.

1. We note the following before separation from bypass: TEE demonstrates poor contractility, pulmonary arterial pressure is 45/25 mm Hg at 2 liters of bypass flow, and blood pressure is 40 mm Hg at 2 liters of bypass flow.

2. We resume full flow, administer dobutamine, 4 µg per kg per minute, and nitroglycerin, 50 µg per minute.

3. TEE demonstrates improved contractility. Pulmonary arterial pressure is 20/15 mm Hg at 2 liters bypass flow. Blood pressure is approximately 70 mm Hg systolic at 2 liters of bypass flow.

4. We come off the pump. TEE shows left ventricular distension. The pulmonary arterial pressure is 50/25 mm Hg, and the cardiac index by thermodilution is 1.5 liter per minute per m^2. Blood pressure is 85 mm Hg systolic. The right ventricle is distended on direct observation.

5. We resume full bypass flow and infuse amrinone, 0.75 mg per kg load and at 5 µg per kg per minute. TEE demonstrates vigorous contractility. Pulmonary arterial pressure is 20/10 at 2 liters of bypass flow. Blood pressure is 90/60 at 2 liters of bypass flow. We come off the pump. TEE shows a contractile left ventricle. The pulmonary arterial pressure is 20/12, and the cardiac index is 2.8 liters per minute per m^2. Blood pressure is 60 mm Hg systolic. The right ventricle vigorously contracts.

6. We correct hypotension. Norepinephrine is begun, and volume from cardiopulmonary bypass circuit administered. TEE shows left ventricle contractile, the pulmonary artery is 22/15 mm Hg, and the cardiac index is 2.8 liters per minute per m^2. Blood pressure is 80 mm Hg systolic. The right ventricle is contractile. The venous cannula is discontinued. Protamine is administered via peripheral intravenous line. The chest is closed, and the patient is returned successfully to the intensive care unit.

Patient YY demonstrates the use of combination drug therapy to wean from cardiopulmonary bypass. What we should note is that at no time during administration of inotropes, vasodilators, or vasoconstrictors is drug therapy static. For example, as vascular tone is restored, perhaps by decreasing inhalation anesthetics, the need for vasoconstrictors to offset the vasodilatory effect of PDE inhibitors is lessened. Similarly, if a patient becomes tachycardic (a heart rate of more than 120 beats per minute), dobutamine may need to be reduced. The development of ventricular ectopy may call for a reduction in beta agonists and the institution of antiarrhythmic therapy with lidocaine, procainamide, or bretylium.

What is the key to weaning a patient from the pump? Minute-to-minute, second-to-second adjustments are made to match the patient's pharmacologic need with drug therapy. How do we make these adjustments? Eventually, experience guides the anesthesiologist in the use of the drugs selected at his or her institution. In the beginning, however, careful attention should be paid to maximizing stroke volume and maintaining adequate perfusion pressure. Ultimately, direct observation of the beating heart can provide one of the best guides to success or failure in patient management. A distended right ventricle is an obvious sign of impending hemodynamic distress. The heart should always be small and contractile and never the boggy muscular balloon so characteristic of ventricular failure.

Patient YY was successfully weaned from bypass with multiple drug therapy because even though her heart was poorly functioning preoperatively, it managed do better postbypass. The restoration of blood flow improved myocardial performance even though she had previously damaged the heart.

Our second patient, ZZ, is not nearly as fortunate. Every now and then a patient actually does worse after surgery than we expect. Although rare, inadequate cardioplegia can lead to ischemic injury during aortic cross clamp. In reoperative patients, embolization of material down previous bypass grafts can also lead to myocardial damage during cardiopulmonary bypass. Finally, inadequate revascularization in patients with poor distal runoff can also lead to poor ventricular performance at the time of surgery. Such is the case for Mr. ZZ. A young, basically healthy patient taken to surgery for simple angina is now presenting with ventricular failure. For whatever reason, his heart has become poorly contractile at the time of weaning from bypass. Even after drug therapy is applied as in the case of Ms. YY, the left ventricle remains completely dysfunctional as assessed by TEE, and the right ventricle is grossly distended. Separating this patient from bypass requires us to employ not only the pharmacologic therapy we used for patient YY, but to consider mechanical assistance to wean the patient from bypass flow.

1.   Dobutamine, amrinone, nitroglycerin, and norepinephrine are infused as in the previous case.

2.   TEE shows poor left ventricular contraction, inferior akinesis, no mitral regurgitation, and anterior hypokinesis. The pulmonary artery pressure at 2 liters of flow is 50/25 mm Hg. The blood pressure at 2 liters of bypass flow is 50/30 mm Hg.

3.   Intra-aortic balloon pump is placed and one-to-one ballooning is initiated. TEE shows intra-aortic balloon pump confirmed in the

aorta. The pulmonary artery pressure at 2 liters of flow is 30/20 mm Hg. The blood pressure at 2 liters of flow is 70/40 mm Hg. An attempt is made to wean from bypass. The cardiac index is 1.8 liters per minute per m². The pulmonary artery pressure is 50/37 mm Hg. Systemic pressure is 70/40 mm Hg.

4.   Dobutamine, amrinone, nitroglycerin, and norepinephrine are adjusted, and epinephrine is added. The cardiac index is now 1.5 liters per minute per m². The pulmonary artery pressure is 50/35 mm Hg. The blood pressure is 55/45 mm Hg. Cardiopulmonary bypass is resumed. The heart is rested. Repeat attempts to wean from cardiopulmonary bypass failed. Cannulas are placed for left VAD (Abiomed).

5.   The Abiomed is placed. Bypass flow is reduced. Dobutamine and amrinone are continued, and norepinephrine and epinephrine are discontinued. Left ventricle assist is engaged as cardiopulmonary bypass is reduced. The left VAD is in place.

6.   The cardiac index is 2.2 liters per minute per m². TEE demonstrates a contractile right ventricle. The pulmonary artery pressure is 30/20 mm Hg. The blood pressure is 70/50 mm Hg. Volume is administered. The cardiac index is 3.0 liters per minute per m². The central venous pressure is 15 mm Hg. The pulmonary arterial pressure is 30/22 mm Hg. The blood pressure is 90/60 mm Hg. Right ventricle is contractile by TEE. The patient is moved to the intensive care unit with the left VAD in place. Dobutamine and amrinone are administered to support right ventricular contractility. Vascular tone is maintained with norepinephrine with 1 µg per minute. The left ventricle recovers in the intensive care unit as assessed by TEE over 48 hours. The patient is returned to the operating room 48 hours later and the Abiomed is discontinued. The patient recovers.

As promised at the outset, no patient ever dies in this text. Of course, in those cases in which VADs are necessary because of poor perioperative performance, death is not an infrequent occurrence. Nevertheless, it is possible for a so-called stunned myocardium to recover so that an otherwise healthy patient like Mr. ZZ might survive surgery because of left VAD placement.

A left VAD may provide the only viable approach to wean the patient from bypass flow. If the surgeon does not consider the patient a candidate for a VAD, there is no choice but to drain the blood volume into the pump and discontinue perfusion, resulting in patient death. Although this is naturally highly undesirable, in those patients who are not likely to recover, an intraoperative death may be preferable to a protracted demise of a patient supported by an extracorporeal left VAD. Naturally, the ability of the myocardium to recover is often unknown by the surgeon, and it is thus likely that as VADs become more and more available, they will be placed in patients who would not otherwise be successfully weaned from cardiopulmonary bypass. How changes in health care economics and managed care will affect the use of these costly devices remains unclear. At the very least, we can expect health insurers to limit the use of such devices to those patients with the greatest possibility of survival or those most likely to be candidates for transplantation. As technology improves, permanent biVADs may replace heart function altogether. It is certainly likely that the technology to maintain a patient with a total artificial heart will continue to be refined over the course of the next century. Whether this technology becomes available for use in the general population remains as much a social and ethical question as it does one of mere medical management. Figure 8-8 provides a schematic for weaning the patient with left ventricular dysfunction from cardiopulmonary bypass.

Right Ventricular Failure

We have focused primarily on weaning the patient with left ventricular failure from cardiopulmonary bypass. Left ventricular dysfunction often leads to right ventricular dysfunction as well, so we have generally been attempting to treat biventricular failure. Nonetheless, isolated right ventricular failure occurs independent of left ventricular dysfunction. Right ventricular dysfunction frequently accompanies pulmonary arterial hypertension. As pulmonary arterial pressures increase—that is, secondary to idiopathic pulmonary hypertension, pulmonary disease, or mitral stenosis—the impedance to right ventricular ejection increases. As a result, right ventricular failure ensues. A right ventricular infarction can likewise reduce right ventricular ejection, potentially leading to the underloading of the left ventricle. Rather than being the passive conduit for blood as the right ventricle was once believed to be, it is now clear that the right side of the heart actively contributes to the loading of the left ventricle. If right ventricular output decreases, so will left ventricular output. Thus, as left ventricular failure often leads to right ventricular dysfunction, so too does right ventricular failure lead to systemic hypotension and reduced

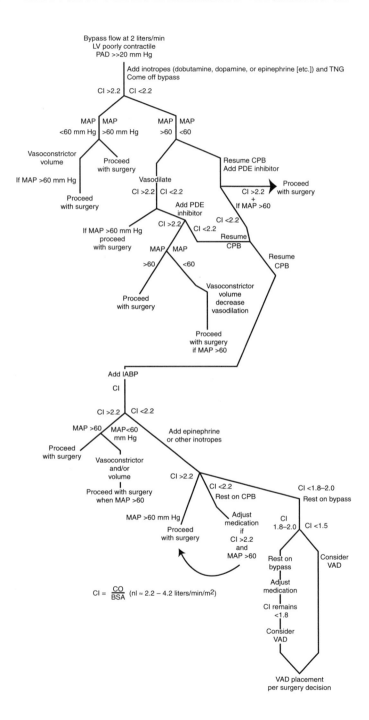

left ventricular output. Additionally, right ventricular enlargement often produces a septal shift that distorts left ventricular anatomy, reducing left ventricular filling. Patients who have chronic right ventricular dysfunction demonstrate the classic signs of right-sided volume overload. Elevated right atrial pressures, peripheral edema, and hepatic engorgement are all characteristic of chronic right ventricular failure. Atrial fibrillation and paroxysmal atrial tachycardia can accompany right ventricular dysfunction.

In the cardiac surgery suite, right ventricular failure may be encountered in three primary ways. First, right ventricular failure may be chronic secondary to high pulmonary arterial pressures from either respiratory disease or mitral valvular disease. Second, right ventricular failure may occur as a consequence of a perioperative right ventricular infarction. Third, right ventricular failure may appear secondary to acute pulmonary arterial hypertension in a classic protamine reaction.

A decreased right ventricular ejection fraction may be measured by an appropriately equipped Swan-Ganz catheter in the patient with right ventricular dysfunction. TEE may demonstrate a dilated, noncontractile right ventricle. Hemodynamic monitoring reveals an elevation of the right atrial pressure. A right atrial pressure that is greater than PCOP is suspicious of right ventricular failure. In the patient with an open chest, observation of a distended right side of the heart can give a clear picture for right ventricular dysfunction.

Generally, therapy for right ventricular failure in the postbypass patient is directed toward improving delivery of blood to the left ventricle. Volume loading can provide increased flow through the right ventricle. However, it is clear that the right ventricle is not simply a passive conduit. Inotropes such as dobutamine, amrinone, milrinone, or isoproterenol may be used to increase right ventricular contractility. Of course, these drugs are not specific to the right ventricle. Systemic hypotension and tachycardia may occur with these agents, potentially limiting the application of inotropic therapy. Vasodilators such as nitroglycerin and nitroprusside may likewise be employed. But again, the

◀ Figure 8-8. *Weaning the patient with poor ventricular function from cardiopulmonary bypass. (LV = left ventricle; PAD = pulmonary artery diastolic pressure [mm Hg]; TNG = nitroglycerin; CI = cardiac index [liter/minute/m²]; MAP = mean arterial pressure [mm Hg]; CPB = cardiopulmonary bypass; PDE = phosphodiesterase; IABP = intra-aortic balloon pump; VAD = ventricular assist device; CO = cardiac output; BSA = body surface area.)*

effects are not specifically directed to the pulmonary vasculature. In the past, prostaglandin E_1 has been infused to decrease pulmonary arterial resistance to improve right ventricular ejection. Norepinephrine frequently was administered via a left atrial line into the systemic circulation to maintain vascular tone during prostaglandin E_1 infusion.

Nitric oxide has been shown to be a potent dilator of the pulmonary vasculature. Administered by inhalation, nitric oxide does not result in systemic vasodilation to any degree. Although nitric oxide delivery equipment has not yet appeared routinely in the cardiac operating room, it is available in many institutions should right ventricular failure be encountered with pulmonary hypertension. However, its use is still under investigation.

Should all else fail to improve right ventricular function, a right VAD may be placed. Right VAD flow must be carefully monitored so as not to overload the left ventricle in case it has not been bypassed. Extracorporeal right VAD placement such as the Abiomed may provide support to the right ventricle until right ventricular function improves.

The obvious lesson in considering right ventricular failure is not to dismiss the right ventricle as being somehow unimportant to the patient's survival.

Let us return to our favorite patient, the otherwise healthy Mr. XY. As you recall, for his first bypass procedure, he had a relatively uneventful course. Suppose, however, at the time of administration of half of his protamine dose, as estimated by heparin analysis, we note a rapid increase in pulmonary arterial pressure equal to systemic pressure at approximately 60/40 mm Hg. Direct observation of the heart shows a massively distended right ventricle. TEE likewise demonstrates right ventricular dilation.

Protamine reactions include both classical anaphylaxis as well as milder histamine-induced vasodilations. In these instances, the blood pressure and pulmonary arterial pressures may decrease. Occasionally, however, protamine administration leads to a profound pulmonary vasoconstriction and right ventricular failure. Believed to be mediated by thromboxane, this type of protamine reaction leads to rapid circulatory collapse. What is clear is that, as pulmonary pressures increase and the right ventricle becomes dysfunctional, it no longer adequately loads the left ventricle, leading to systemic hypotension. There are relatively few options available to us at this point. Occasionally, administration of a small amount (2,000–5,000 U) of heparin interacts with the protamine, inhibiting pulmonary vasoconstriction. At the same time, small amounts of nitroglycerin may be administered via the pulmonary arterial catheter to promote pulmonary arterial relaxation. PDE inhibitors, dobutamine, and other inotropes may be administered to support the circulation. If these maneuvers do not restore ventricular function and hemodynamic stability, full heparinization is essential and resumption of cardiopulmonary bypass is necessary. Once right ventricular function is restored, the patient may then be weaned from bypass flow. Reversal with protamine could again lead to circulatory collapse. Although not yet readily available, the enzyme heparinase I may soon provide an alternative to protamine for heparin reversal. At present, however, if necessary, protamine reversal may not be possible and blood product replacement may be needed until heparin is metabolized.

Conclusion

We have now encountered two patients with poor left and right ventricular function in addition to the healthy patient undergoing cardiopulmonary bypass. We have attempted to provide a praxis approach to managing both the patient with impaired ventricle function and those with normal myocardial contractility. As we encounter other disease states and other surgical procedures—for example, valve replacement, ventricular septal defect repair, and so forth—as anesthesiologists we will return to these basic approaches to manage the patient. Whatever the surgeon does, we must return to these same therapies, pharmacologic or mechanical, to respond to the patient at the time of weaning from bypass flow. What the surgeon does is important, especially if he or she contributes to myocardial failure. However, no matter what the surgeon does, if the patient is on bypass, we still must find some way to wean that patient from bypass flow. Whether the patient has undergone repair of a ventricular septal defect, a ventricular aneurysm, a mitral valve, or an excised arrhythmogenic focus, when it comes to weaning, either the patient has good ventricular function or not. If he or she does, we can proceed as we did with Mr. XY. If not, we need to follow the pharmacologic or mechanical approaches employed for patients YY or ZZ. Thus, although an operation may appear novel from a surgical standpoint, the anesthesia approaches should become quite routine even in the sickest of patients.

We must remember that the final common pathway for adult patients depends on the success with which the repaired ventricle is able to meet the pumping needs of the patient. How we manipulate ventricular function will determine how successful we are as cardiac anesthesiologists.

9

Patients with Heart Structure Defects

Generally, we encounter patients with distortions in the heart's structure in two populations. First, we know that congenital heart disease can lead to a variety of defects in the heart. Atrial septal defects (ASDs), ventricular septal defects (VSDs), tetralogy of Fallot (right ventricular outlet obstruction, right ventricular hypertrophy, VSD, and an overriding aorta), transposition of the great vessels (aorta from the right ventricle, pulmonary artery from the left ventricle), and truncus arteriosus (common path for right ventricular and left ventricular outflow) all distort the basic structure of the heart.

Although many aggressive surgical repairs are possible for neonates afflicted with these anatomic distortions, we do not focus on them. Entire texts have been written on both pediatric and neonatal cardiac anesthesia, and the readers are referred to these sources for specific guidelines for pediatric anesthesia care for the pediatric heart patient. Because these surgeries generally are not performed in community cardiac anesthesia practice, they are not included in this text.

Nevertheless, it does not mean that patients with distortions in the heart's anatomy are not seen in the adult population. Patients with long-standing VSDs and ASDs may present for repair at any time. Chronic volume overload of the right ventricle in patients with a VSD and an associated left-to-right shunt can lead to right ventricular failure, pulmonary hypertension, and even right-to-left shunt with hypoxemia should left ventricular pressures decrease. Acute VSDs and ventricular aneurysms can also appear in patients after myocardial infarction, requiring emergency surgical repair. This chapter reviews these anatomic abnormalities in the adult patients.

Shunts

Defects of the heart can lead to an inappropriate flow of blood following pressure gradients from one ventricle to another. What is certain about the shunting of blood is that physics rules. Pressure gradients dictate blood flow in the heart. If a VSD is present with low right ventricular pressures, blood will flow from the left side of the heart to the right. The right ventricle is volume overloaded, possibly leading to pulmonary edema. On the other hand, should right ventricular pressures be elevated in excess of the left-sided pressure as a consequence of pulmonary hypertension (Eisenmenger's syndrome), this blood can flow across the defect into the systemic circulation, leading to hypoxemia. Right-to-left shunting is a frequent characteristic of congenital heart disease (tetralogy of Fallot) but is encountered less frequently in the adult patient afflicted with acute defects in the structural integrity of the heart. Nonetheless, the occasional patient with a VSD and increased pulmonary resistance can present with right-to-left shunting in the setting of decreased systemic vascular tone and increased pulmonary vascular resistance.

Rarely, a patient presents for isolated ASD closure in later life. Generally, right ventricular function is preserved and pulmonary vascular resistance unaffected. Of course, over time, pulmonary arterial pressures may increase, leading to pulmonary hypertension. Anesthetic choice depends on individual preference. Should a right-to-left shunt be present, increases in pulmonary resistance can lead to hypoxemia. All ASDs must be corrected in patients requiring left ventricular assist devices (VADs). Right-to-left shunting occurs in left VAD placement if a patent ASD is present. Drainage of blood from the left ventricle into the assist device subsequently reduces left atrial pressure, giving the opportunity for right-to-left shunting should a conduit be present. Additionally, whenever an ASD is present, the possibility of air embolism, however unlikely, exists. Care must be taken to clear all intravenous tubing of air prior to connecting to the patient.

An occasional unrepaired VSD from childhood may be encountered in the adult patient. If significant flow has occurred across the defect, it is possible that pulmonary vascular resistance has increased to the extent that a right-to-left shunt could occur should pulmonary resistance be further augmented (i.e., as a consequence of hypoxia or hypercarbia) or if systemic vascular tone and left ventricular end-diastolic pressure decrease. Ensuring adequate gas exchange and systemic vascular tone should prevent the development of a right-to-left shunt and systemic hypoxemia. Of course, acute VSD with perioperative myocardial infarction is far more likely to be encountered in a community anesthesia practice. Infarction of the intraventricular septum can result in septal rupture, leading to a left-to-right shunt, right ventricular and subsequent left ventricular failure, pulmonary edema, and cardiogenic shock. Angiography and echocardiography will have confirmed the extent of the VSD before taking the patient to surgery.

Acute Ventricular Septal Defect

The patient taken to the operating room for repair of an acute VSD is likely to be in cardiogenic shock. Patients most often already have an intra-aortic balloon pump in place to support the systemic circulation. Many patients already have been intubated as a consequence of pulmonary edema. Various combinations of inotropes and vasoconstrictors are likely to have been administered to preserve blood flow and systemic pressure. Although increases in left ventricular end-diastolic pressure tend to increase left-to-right shunting, the use of vasopressors (i.e., norepinephrine) may be essential to maintain a suitable systemic perfusion pressure. Transesophageal echocardiography is useful to identify the defect and assess the adequacy of the surgical repair.

As always, the choice of anesthesia is less important than being able to respond to changes in patient behavior. Although anesthetics that lower peripheral vascular resistance may reduce left-to-right shunting, thereby reducing right ventricular failure and pulmonary blood flow, the patient may become too hypotensive to ensure adequate coronary perfusion. If a patient presents with significant hypotension (systolic pressure of less than 60 mm Hg), anesthetic management consists of the administration of muscle relaxants and scopolamine with small amounts of narcotics and benzodiazepines added as the patient's condition stabilizes. Once the patient is placed on cardiopulmonary bypass, additional anesthetics may be given.

After the VSD is repaired and any bypass grafts completed, the patient with acute VSD must be weaned from cardiopulmonary bypass like any other patient. Right ventricular dysfunction is common in this setting, and poor left ventricular function should likewise be expected. A multiple drug regimen with intra-aortic balloon counterpulsation may well be necessary to successfully separate the patient from cardiopulmonary bypass. Right VAD, left VAD, or bi-VAD placement may prove necessary if the heart fails to wean from bypass support. As always, before preceding with VAD placement, the surgeon must be confident that the patient has some potential to recover ventricular function or that the patient is a candidate for heart transplantation. If significant multisystem failure is present before surgery, the chances for survival after acute VSD are at best extremely limited.

Left Ventricular Aneurysm and Ventricular Rupture

After myocardial infarction, it is possible for necrotic myocardium to break down, leading to a myocardial rupture and aneurysm formation. Generally, these patients do not appear in the surgical suite, having expired long before the operating team can be mobilized. Nonetheless, occasionally patients with adherent pericardium may form a ventricular pseudoaneurysm as the pericardium walls off the area of ventricular perforation. These patients may well be taken to surgery. Patients with acute deterioration are most likely to be in cardiogenic shock, receiving both pressor support and intra-aortic counterpulsation. Anesthetic administration is dependent on the overall hemodynamic management of the patient. Once the aneurysm is repaired, the patient will need to be weaned from cardiopulmonary bypass and no doubt will require mechanical and pharmacologic assistance.

True ventricular aneurysms are areas of infarcted, akinetic myocardium that have not ruptured but that can harbor ventricular thrombus and fail to contribute to ventricular contractility. Ventricular aneurysmectomy involves removing the aneurysm and associated clot and then sewing the ventricle together after the excision. Theoretically, the smaller ventricle free of aneurysmal dilation should perform more efficiently, leading to improved ventricular ejection fraction. Recently, surgeons have begun to excise myocardium in patients with profound ventricular failure to produce smaller and theoretically more efficient pumps. Whether or not the heart, after ventricular aneurysmectomy, becomes more efficient or not depends not only on the success of the surgery but also on the time it takes the surgeon to complete the task. Protracted bypass runs can be expected in such settings, and ventricular performance may be quite impaired when an attempt is made to wean from bypass. Once again, a combination of mechanical assistance and pharmacologic support will likely be necessary to wean the patient from cardiopulmonary bypass.

Cardiac Masses

Atrial myxomas, organized clots, or other tumor masses may occlude either the left or right ventricular inflow. Right atrial myxomas can lead to an underloaded right ventricle. Similar masses of the left atrium can lead to an underloaded left ventricle, pulmonary hypertension, and right ventricular dysfunction. Should such lesions be encountered, the heart will need to be opened and the patient placed on cardiopulmonary bypass to facilitate excision of the mass. As in other conditions in which right ventricular inflow is occluded (i.e., restrictive pericarditis), positive pressure ventilation can result in a reduction of venous return, leading to a catastrophic hemodynamic collapse at the induction of anesthesia. The surgical team should be readily available to open the chest and institute cardiopulmonary bypass should this prove necessary. If the right atria is occluded by a mass, pulmonary artery catheter placement may not be possible or prudent. Anesthetic management is directed at preserving blood return to the heart. The exact choice of agents is an individual selection.

Should the surgeon have to remove a cardiac tumor, varying amounts of healthy myocardium may be sacrificed as well. The structural integrity of the heart may be compromised, leading to new valvular disease at the time of surgery (i.e., mitral regurgitation). Loss of myocardium can make the heart pump inadequately, making separation from cardiopulmonary bypass quite difficult. Transesophageal echocardiography is helpful in managing these patients.

10

Cardiopulmonary Bypass

With Tom Rawles, CCP*

As important as cardiac anesthesia is, it remains true that the essence of the surgical repair is completed at the time when the anesthesiologist is least involved in the care of the patient, namely, during cardiopulmonary bypass. For the most part, the bypass period is under the direction of the surgeon (who places the bypass cannulas) and the perfusionist (who assumes the functions of respiration and circulation). With respiration and circulation under the perfusionist's control, there is little that the anesthesiologist necessarily needs to do during the bypass period, except to be observant to the needs of the patient and the surgical team. Certainly, even if the perfusionist has assumed the responsibility for cardiac and respiratory function, the anesthesiologist must be certain that at the very least the perfusionist and surgeon have not forgotten one essential point in management—that is, to keep the patient asleep. Inhalational anesthetic vaporizers are a part of most bypass circuits, allowing for administration of inhalational anesthesia while the patient is on cardiopulmonary bypass. The anesthesiologist, in addition to being certain that the patient is adequately anesthetized, must also be confident that sufficient nondepolarizing muscle relaxants have been administered to prevent thermogenesis (shivering) during hypothermic cardiopulmonary bypass. That said,

---

*Perfusionist, Cardiothoracic Surgery Associates of North Texas, Dallas

however, the anesthesiologist may involve himself or herself in the actual management of cardiopulmonary bypass to varying degrees. With an experienced perfusion and surgery team, the need for the anesthesiologist's involvement in the actual management of cardiopulmonary bypass is probably unnecessary. Still, it is important that the anesthesiologist be aware of how anesthesia and related drug therapy can affect the bypass run.

Hemodynamics 101 remains in effect for the patient on bypass as well as for the patient supported by the native heart: Blood pressure = systemic vascular resistance × cardiac output. During the bypass run, the perfusionist adjusts flow of the bypass machine, thereby generating the cardiac output. Generally, a cardiac index that would be considered acceptable for a patient off bypass is equally acceptable for a patient on bypass (i.e., cardiac index of 2.2–3.0 liters per minute per m^2). Increases in vascular tone can lead to hypertension on bypass (mean arterial pressure of more than 100 mm Hg), requiring a reduction in bypass flow (i.e., cardiac output). Often, vasodilator therapy with sodium nitroprusside is needed to offset increases in vascular tone, assuming that the anesthesia and perfusion team is confident that the patient is adequately anesthetized. On the other hand, vasoconstrictors (i.e., phenylephrine) may be needed if systemic pressure decreases too low and the venous volume is inadequate to increase bypass flow (i.e., inadequate venous return to the bypass machine results in reduced pump flow lest the perfusionist run the reservoir dry). Certainly, anesthesiologists can alter the hemodynamic picture of the patient on bypass. Administration of anesthetics, vasopressors, and vasodilators by the anesthesiologist can alter the perfusionist's plan for management. Additional doses of benzodiazepines or narcotics can easily lead to vasodilation during cardiopulmonary bypass. The administration of inotropes and vasodilators before weaning a patient from bypass can likewise result in the patient's becoming either vasodilated or vasoconstricted, altering the perfusionist's ability to adjust bypass flow. Close coordination and communication between the perfusionist and anesthesiologist are essential during the bypass period so that they do not work at cross purposes with one another. The perfusionist needs to be aware of any additional drugs the anesthesiologist might administer during the bypass run.

As to the actual bypass machine itself, the handling of the machine is generally best left to the perfusionist without any anesthesia interference. Of course, it is helpful to know what the perfusionist is doing and be able to assist the perfusionist as necessary should trouble develop. This chapter examines the bypass circuit as well as the goals of the perfusionist in managing the patient during the period of cardiopulmonary bypass.

Cardiopulmonary Bypass from the Perfusionist's Perspective

First, it must be remembered that cardiopulmonary bypass is not a homeostatic process ("during cardiopulmonary bypass pulseless diluted blood circulates over vast areas of plastic and metal at abnormal temperatures and pressures . . . homeostasis is in chaos").* What more can be said of cardiopulmonary bypass than it is not a "natural" process? Thus, the perfusionist's goal is not to maintain a normal physiology. Rather, the perfusionist tries to do what is necessary to minimize any trauma from this nonhomeostatic method of circulation. Like anesthesia, nobody comes to the hospital for perfusion services. It is merely a necessary evil to facilitate a greater good—the surgical repair. Perfusion, again like anesthesia, makes surgery possible. So the perfusionist's goal is to facilitate the surgical repair with as little impact on the patient as is possible. Obviously, in one sense, the best bypass run would be no run. In this regard, one of the advantages of minimally invasive coronary artery bypass (CAB) (see Chapter 19) is the ability to avoid the use of cardiopulmonary bypass. Of course, cardiopulmonary bypass cannot nor should not be avoided for the vast majority of patients who require CAB. Thus, the goals of the perfusionist as well as the surgeon and anesthesiologist should be to make the cardiopulmonary bypass run as safe as possible, as efficient as possible, and as timely as possible.

The essence of cardiopulmonary bypass is really quite simple: Venous blood is drained by gravity (that is why the pump is so low to the floor) from cannulas placed in the inferior and superior vena cava or in the right atrium. The deoxygenated venous blood is drained into a reservoir and then returned through a gas exchanger (oxygenator) and various filters and then pumped back to the patient via either a cannula placed in the aorta or the femoral artery (Figure 10-1).

---

*From LH Edmunds. Systemic Inflammatory Responses Secondary to Cardiopulmonary Bypass. In AS Wechster (ed), Systemic Effects of Cardiopulmonary Bypass. New York: Cahners, 1993.

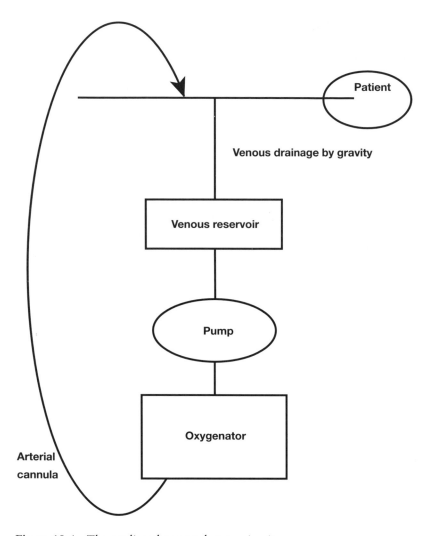

Figure 10-1. *The cardiopulmonary bypass circuit.*

This sounds simple, doesn't it? In many ways, cardiopulmonary bypass is relatively routine. Still, significant morbidity and mortality are associated with its use. In the past, the inattentive perfusionist could let the venous reservoir "run dry," pumping a massive air embolism into the arterial circulation. Today, as a consequence of the numerous filters, detectors, bells, and whistles, the possibility of this occurrence

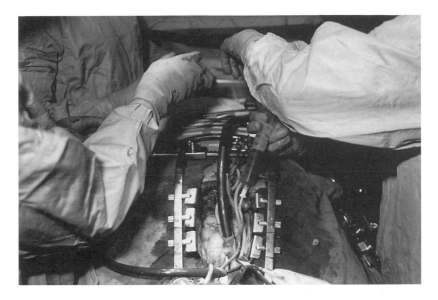

Figure 10-2. *Venous cannula drains deoxygenated blood from patient.*

is small. Still, morbidity from bypass can be great and includes coagulopathy, neurologic defects, renal failure, and vascular injuries.

Bypass Circuit

Figures 10-2 to 10-7 present a typical bypass circuit, identifying key features in the layout of the cardiopulmonary bypass machine. Although the anesthesiologist should never have to do anything with this equipment, some familiarity is helpful nonetheless.

Gas Exchange on Cardiopulmonary Bypass Circuit

The principal component of the cardiopulmonary bypass circuit is the oxygenator. The oxygenator provides the surface area over which gas exchange occurs during cardiopulmonary bypass. In other words, the oxygenator is the lung of the bypass circuit. In the past, both bubble- and membrane-type oxygenators (gas exchangers) were available. Today, membrane oxygenators are preferred as the pump's gas exchange system.

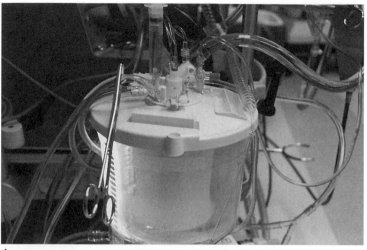

A

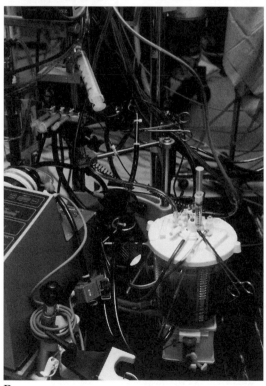

B

Figure 10-3. *Venous reservoir (A) before bypass flow and (B) holding venous blood during cardiopulmonary bypass.*

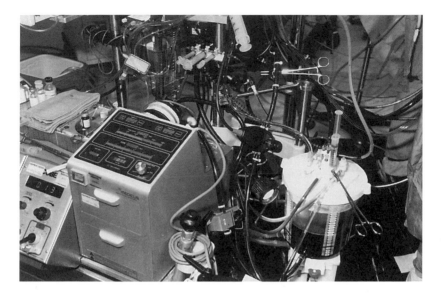

Figure 10-4. *Oxygenator and venous reservoir and pump. The pump, venous reservoir, and gas exchangers are visible.*

The bubble oxygenator exposed desaturated venous blood to the pump's oxygen supply. By bubbling oxygen directly into the blood, the venous blood became oxygenated. However, this also resulted in hemolysis with associated hemoglobinuria during the bypass run. An increased incidence of coagulopathy was also noted with the bubble device.

Oxygenation During Cardiopulmonary Bypass

The membrane oxygenator employs a microporous membrane that separates the ventilating gas in the bypass circuit from the deoxygenated blood. The membrane reduces both the development of gas embolization and the blood trauma associated with bubble oxygenators. Gas exchange occurs by diffusion. An air and oxygen gas mixture is employed that adjusts for the desired arterial oxygen tension (PaO_2). Increasing inspired oxygen concentration (FiO_2) increases the systemic PaO_2. Arterial carbon dioxide tension ($PaCO_2$) is adjusted by controlling the total gas flow in the oxygenator (sweep gas). Increasing gas flow decreases the partial pressure of carbon dioxide in the patient. This is not significantly different from the lungs, where increasing ven-

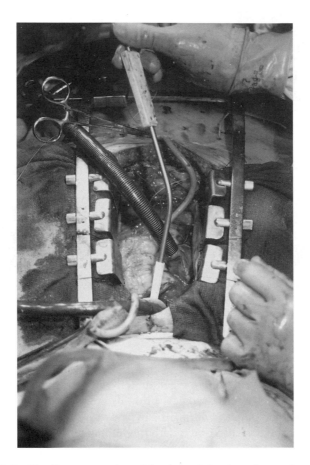

Figure 10-5. *Cardiotomy suction. After heparinization, the suction scavenges blood from the surgical field.*

tilation results in a reduction of arterial carbon dioxide. So, if a patient such as Mr. XY becomes hypercarbic on bypass, only two possible causes should be considered. Either ventilation is inadequate (i.e., there is inadequate gas flow in the bypass circuit) or the patient has increased carbon dioxide production (i.e., malignant hyperthermia, shivering, or thyrotoxicosis). Oxygenation of the patient is dependent on the FiO_2 as adjusted by the oxygen and air blender. Generally, a PaO_2 of 150–250 mm Hg is desired during the bypass run.

The measured PaO_2 gives an indication of the performance of the oxygenator. However, it reveals little about the adequacy of perfu-

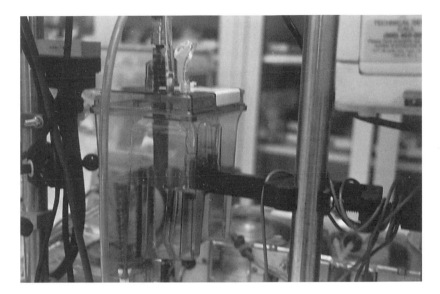

Figure 10-6. *Cardioplegia reservoir.*

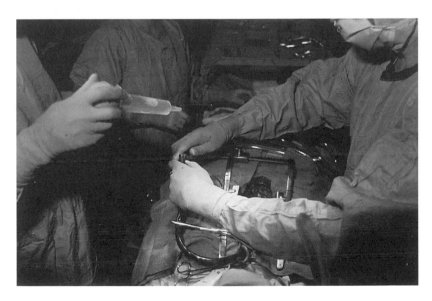

Figure 10-7. *Arterial cannulas. The arterial cannula returns oxygenated blood to the patient. The surgeon carefully checks that air bubbles are absent from the arterial perfusion cannula.*

sion. The mixed venous oxygen tension (PvO_2) and a mixed venous oxygen saturation (SvO_2) serve as far better indicators of the adequacy of tissue perfusion. It is key to ascertain that oxygen is being delivered to the tissues to an acceptable degree to ensure cellular survival. The perfusionist's goal is to obtain a mixed venous oxygenation saturation of approximately 65–80% (PvO_2 of approximately 40 mm Hg, assuming normal hemoglobin). Profound anemia, reduced bypass flow, and increased oxygen consumption (as in shivering) can all lead to reductions in PvO_2 and SvO_2. Thus, reductions in SvO_2 indicate a greater extraction than normal of oxygen from the blood being delivered to the tissues. If the oxygen demands of tissues are not adequately met, anaerobic glycolysis ensues, leading to tissue acidemia and tissue ischemia. Decreasing temperature, increasing bypass flow, increasing hemoglobin, and administering muscle relaxants are among the maneuvers to reduce oxygen consumption or improve oxygen delivery.

Thus, it is important to remember that oxygenating the blood is relatively easy. The pump oxygenator will reliably do this. What is not as guaranteed is the certainty of oxygen delivery to the tissues. Observing SvO_2 and PvO_2 measurements helps to confirm that tissue oxygenation is acceptable during the bypass run.

Ventilation During Cardiopulmonary Bypass

The ideal $PaCO_2$ during bypass has been a hotly debated issue. Certainly, there are those of you who, while studying for the anesthesia boards, recall the agony of trying to remember the difference between a pH-stat gas management and an alpha-stat management for determining the ideal $PaCO_2$ during cardiopulmonary bypass. Well, here we go again. But do not worry; in actual practice you do not have to think much about this. Clearly, the surgeon and the perfusionist will have their own practice for bypass management, and these days it is almost surely an alpha-stat management scheme.

The question of pH-stat versus alpha-stat $PaCO_2$ management arises because of the use of hypothermia during cardiopulmonary bypass. During hypothermia, the solubility of oxygen and carbon dioxide is increased, thereby reducing the measured gas tension. Increases in carbon dioxide solubility result in a decreased $PaCO_2$ and an increased pH—an alkalosis. pH-stat management corrects for this alkalosis by adding carbon dioxide to the bypass gas mixture in an attempt to compensate for the hypothermia-induced reduction in $PaCO_2$. If we were to manage Mr. XY using a pH-stat approach, we would place him on bypass and begin cooling to reduce oxygen consumption. The perfusionist would next obtain a blood gas sample to assess the adequacy of gas exchange. The blood gas would naturally be measured at 37°C (normal body temperature). Once these values for pH and $PaCO_2$ are obtained, the perfusionist would then determine what the actual pH and $PaCO_2$ are depending on the patient's core temperature. The calculated values would reveal a pH greater than that noticed at 37°C and would determine a $PaCO_2$ less than that obtained when measured at normal body temperature. At this point, the perfusionist would add carbon dioxide to the bypass gas mixture to increase $PaCO_2$ in the hopes that there would be increased cerebral blood flow. Recall that as $PaCO_2$ increases, so does cerebral blood flow. By increasing cerebral blood flow, the perfusionist using pH-stat management hopes that there is a reduction in neurologic injury associated with cardiopulmonary bypass.

As you may recall, at one time hypercarbia was advocated for the same reasons during carotid endarterectomy. Although it is true that carbon dioxide may be a cerebral vasodilator, it can impair cerebral blood flow autoregulation, leaving the brain without a protective mechanism to ensure adequate distribution of cerebral blood flow.

Ultimately, pH-stat management was not found to be useful for the management of hypothermic cardiopulmonary bypass. Alpha-stat management, on the other hand, simply accepts the $PaCO_2$ and pH measurements as determined at 37°C. It appears that in living tissue $PaCO_2$ and pH decrease and increase according to temperature. The dissociation of water into protons and hydroxyl ions also changes during hypothermia—that is, there is less dissociation of water, with a resultant decrease in protons. Therefore, there is an increase in pH as temperature decreases. The imidazole group of histidine, an amino acid, provides a buffering mechanism by which pH gradients are maintained between the intracellular and extracellular environment. In other words, the buffering system of the body provides for changes in pH associated with hypothermia. In essence, the body is prepared to function at lower temperatures. Alpha-stat management acknowledges these buffering systems so that additional carbon dioxide is unnecessary. Thus, today temperature correction has no part in the routine management of cardiopulmonary bypass.

$PaCO_2$ is maintained between 35 and 45 mm Hg by adjusting the sweep gas flow rate. Increasing gas flow decreases $PaCO_2$. Frequent arterial blood gases and in-line measures of arterial gas tension ensure the adequacy of oxygenation and ventilation during cardiopulmonary bypass.

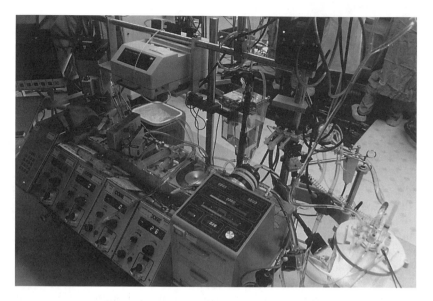

Figure 10-8. *The bypass machine with roller pumps is shown on the left.*

Perfusion During Cardiopulmonary Bypass

The Pump

Going on bypass, putting the patient on the pump, is really just that. A mechanical pump replaces the body's natural pump, namely, the heart. The pumps found on the bypass machine are of two types (Figure 10-8): the arterial pump (i.e., the one that pumps blood through the oxygenator and back to the patient) and the nonarterial pumps. The nonarterial pumps provide for surgical field suction, delivery of cardioplegia, and other uses in the management of cardiopulmonary bypass.

Pumps are either of a roller or centrifugal design. Roller pumps are positive-displacement pumps that push blood through the tubing ahead of the roller. They ideally occlude the tubing just enough to effect pumping without producing trauma to the blood. If they compress the tubing too greatly, they can contribute to hemolysis and hemoglobinuria during bypass.

Centrifugal pumps are composed of concentric cones or impeller-like fins that spin in a plastic housing through a magnetic link with the pump's motor. Spinning fins generate a pressure differential that results in the movement of blood. Because centrifugal pumps are nonocclusive pumps, if the pump should stop, blood can drain from the aorta back into the circuit. Thus, the arterial line must be occluded when the pump is not in motion. Since the centrifugal pump is not occlusive, it is sensitive to increased pressure in the arterial tubing. Decreased flow of the centrifugal pump can alert the perfusionist to a kink in the line or a poorly positioned aortic cannula. A decrease in pump flow may provide a warning that arterial flow from the pump is impaired. The occlusive roller-type pump does not provide this type of feedback, possibly resulting in either a ruptured arterial line or an aortic dissection in the event of kinked tubing or a malpositioned aortic cannula, respectively. The centrifugal pump is also unlikely to pump more than 35 ml of air at any one time should air enter the circuit. This is not the case with the occlusive roller type pump.

What Constitutes Adequate Flow and Pressure During Bypass?

Like so many other things in medicine, there is debate regarding what constitutes adequate flow and pressure. At its most obvious, adequate bypass flow is that which meets the oxygen needs of the tissue. Because hypothermia, anesthesia, and muscle relaxants all lower metabolic needs, acceptable bypass flow is dependent on the degree to which hypothermia and other measures reduce oxygen consumption. Hemodilution that is associated with cardiopulmonary bypass can reduce the oxygen-carrying capacity of the blood, further potentially complicating an assessment of the adequacy of blood flow. It is clear, however, that if bypass flow is inadequate patients are at risk for tissue ischemia and the development of metabolic acidemia.

Monitoring mixed venous oxygen saturation provides a convenient method by which to assess the adequacy of perfusion in a given patient. A decreasing mixed venous oxygen saturation below 65–70% is a good indication that oxygen delivery to the tissue is inadequate for a given flow, temperature, and hemoglobin concentration. An increase in cardiopulmonary bypass flow, a decrease in temperature, or an increase in hemoglobin concentration can restore oxygen delivery to the tissue or decrease oxygen demand.

Inadequately anesthetized or paralyzed patients may have increased oxygen demand. Generally, a pump flow of 2.2–3.0 liters per minute per m^2 is acceptable to provide organ perfusion. Flows may be reduced to less than 2 liters per minute per m^2 in those patients in whom tissue oxygen delivery is confirmed to be adequate. Monitoring of mixed venous oxygen saturation and a venous blood gas measurement will determine if reduced blood flows are acceptable for any given patient.

Much as the bypass flow is adjusted based on individual performance, so too is the mean arterial pressure required during bypass flow. Although autoregulation is maintained over a wide range of pressures during hypothermic bypass (as low as 20 mm Hg mean pressure) during alpha-stat acid–base management, few surgical teams actually permit such low perfusion pressures. Surgeons remain concerned that patients with coexisting arterial disease or long-standing hypertension may not tolerate such pressure reductions and continue to provide for organ perfusion. Mean arterial pressure at 60–70 mm Hg or greater may be requested by the surgical team in those patients with long-standing hypertension.

Just as with the patient whose heart is beating, blood pressure during the period of cardiopulmonary bypass may be conceptualized by understanding hemodynamics 101. Blood pressure = cardiac output × systemic vascular resistance, where cardiac output is equivalent to the bypass flow. Blood pressure may be increased during cardiopulmonary bypass by increasing peripheral vascular tone or by increasing cardiac output, namely, bypass flow. Perfusionists generally employ small bolus doses of phenylephrine (20 mg in 250 ml of 5% dextrose in water) to augment peripheral vascular resistance as necessary. If additional vasopressor support is necessary to maintain vascular tone during cardiopulmonary bypass, norepinephrine or phenylephrine may be administered by continuous infusion into the bypass circuit. Both bypass flow and the mean arterial pressure during cardiopulmonary bypass must be individualized by the perfusionist during the pump run. This does not mean that the anesthesiologist cannot have a say in this as well. Generally, a consensus must be reached between perfusionist, surgeon, and anesthesiologist as to what constitutes adequate mean arterial pressure and bypass flow for a particular patient. Low mean arterial pressures in patients with atheromatous aortas may be at increased risk of stroke.

Other Pumps, Filters, and Suckers

A discussion of cardiopulmonary bypass circuits would not be complete without at least a cursory mention of the myriad hoses and roller pumps that adorn the bypass machine. Although the anesthesiologist is likely to have little responsibility for this device, it is important to have

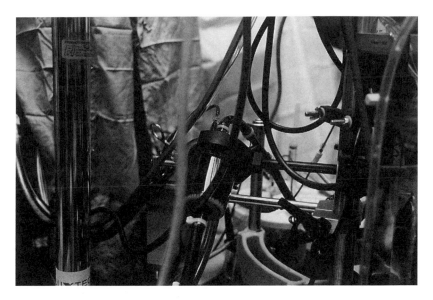

Figure 10-9. *The arterial filter guards against air or particulate arterial emboli during cardiopulmonary bypass.*

some sense of what the perfusionist is up to and why things are where they are.

Filters

Heparinized blood is scavenged from the surgical field by the pump sucker. Particulate material collected with the blood is then filtered to prevent it from entering the venous reservoir. Filters are also placed in the arterial line to provide a last line of defense against particulate and gaseous emboli. A purge line is found in the housing of the arterial filter proximal to the filter media. The port is left open and connected by tubing to the venous or cardiotomy (suction) reservoir. This provides a continuous purge against air emboli in the arterial circuit. A bypass loop around the filter that is clamped during routine cardiopulmonary bypass allows the filter to be excluded or changed if it becomes necessary during the pump run (Figure 10-9).

Reservoir

Reservoirs hold the blood volume of the patient during cardiopulmonary bypass. Venous reservoirs accept the blood drained by gravity from the cannula placed in the inferior and superior vena cava or the right atrium during cardiopulmonary bypass. The cardiotomy reservoir contains blood suctioned from the surgical field after heparinization. (An autotransfusion sucker should always be used to scavenge blood prior to systemic heparinization.) Many systems in use incorporate both reservoirs into one large blood storage tank. The reservoir may be either open or closed. Open reservoirs permit an air and blood interface, whereas closed systems do not. Reservoirs may be a hard shell construction or a plastic bag. The hard shell device is an open system in which both the venous reservoir and the cardiotomy reservoirs may be combined. Thus, there is one blood reservoir that drains blood from the venous cannulas and from the field sucker. The closed-bag system requires two reservoirs: one for drainage from the field sucker and the other to contain the venous return. Whichever system is used is simply a matter for the perfusionist to decide and is of little concern to the anesthesiologist.

Some argument can be made for providing a separate cardiotomy reservoir. If the cardiotomy reservoir becomes obstructed, it can be easily changed without interfering with pump flow. The cardiotomy filter generally does not get loaded with clot or other debris under routine circumstances. Nonetheless, if inadequate heparin anticoagulation occurs for whatever reason, a separate reservoir permits the rapid change of the cardiotomy reservoir should it become clotted.

After discontinuation of bypass, some surgeons have protamine administered while the cardiotomy sucker is used to scavenge blood from the field until approximately one half of the protamine dose is administered as estimated by a heparin analysis machine. Because it is possible to overshoot, protamine reversal might lead to clotting of the cardiotomy reservoir. A two-reservoir system permits any blood exposed to protamine to be isolated from the venous reservoir should emergency reinstitution of cardiopulmonary bypass prove necessary.

Myocardial Preservation and Cardioplegia Systems

In order to isolate the heart from the circulation to make the necessary surgical repairs, it is necessary for the surgeon to place a clamp across the ascending aorta to interrupt coronary blood flow. Although not all repairs require the administration of cardioplegia (some surgeons prefer to operate on a fibrillating heart in spite of ventricular fibrillation's high oxygen demand), it is essential to protect the myocardium from ischemic injury if coronary blood flow is to be interrupted. Inadequate myocardial protection leads to ventricular dysfunction and an untimely intraoperative death. The successful delivery of cardioplegia is essential to patient survival. The perfusionist and the surgeon must communicate with one another to be certain that the delivery of cardioplegia is adequate, timely, and correct.

Fortunately or not, depending on your perspective, the anesthesiologist has virtually nothing to do with cardioplegia administration in the clinical setting. Delivery of cardioplegia is a problem for the perfusionist and the surgeon. It does not routinely involve the anesthesiologist. The results, however, of poor cardioplegia are a great concern to the anesthesiologist. Failure to provide adequate cardioplegia can lead to a struggle to wean the patient from bypass and the potential for intraoperative death, which can certainly reflect on the anesthesiologist as well as the surgeon and perfusion team.

Cardioplegia solution in its simplest form consists of a crystalloid solution or blood with various additives. The principal ingredient in cardioplegia is a relatively high potassium concentration to produce electrical silence in the heart. This fluid most likely is cooled and may be oxygenated by the perfusionist and then delivered either in an anterograde or retrograde fashion. Anterograde cardioplegia is given via an aortic cannula. After application of the cross clamp, cardioplegia is administered via the aortic cardioplegia cannula. If an aortic valve is competent, pressure develops in the aortic root proximal to the site of the cross clamp, delivering cardioplegia down the coronary vascular tree. In those patients with aortic valvular incompetence, inadequate pressure may be generated in the aortic root to produce electrical silence and to provide suitable cardioplegia. Additionally, in aortic regurgitation the delivery of cardioplegia may lead to significant left ventricular distention.

Retrograde cardioplegia is given via a cannula placed in the coronary sinus. A balloon cuff seals the outflow of the coronary sinus, allowing the development of pressure in the venous drainage vessels of the heart. Coronary sinus pressure is measured and cardioplegia infused retrograde through the venous system into the coronary vasculature. Generally, pressure in the coronary sinus should not exceed 45 mm Hg as measured at the tip of the coronary sinus catheter. The surgeon and perfusionist determine both the amount and timing of cardioplegia delivery. Generally, myocardial temperature is followed to determine the adequacy of cardioplegia delivery. (Myocardial temperatures of 8–10°C indicate adequate delivery of cool cardioplegia to the myocardium.) The exact composition and temperature of the cardioplegia solution and the delivery system, as well as the timing of cardioplegia, remain a choice of the surgical team. Aortic root pressures of 60 mm Hg are generally adequate for anterograde delivery, assuming there is aortic valve competency. Retrograde pressures, as previously mentioned, should not exceed 40–45 mm Hg with retrograde flows of approximately 250 ml per minute. If vein bypass grafts are to be employed, once the distal anastomosis is completed, the surgical team may administer additional doses of cardioplegia directly into the coronary vasculature via the bypass graft. In our practice, cardioplegia is routinely administered every 20 minutes. The electrocardiograph is continuously monitored to ensure electrical silence. Myocardial temperature is followed to ascertain appropriate cooling of the myocardium. Reappearance of any electrical activity warrants the immediate administration of additional doses of cardioplegia.

In those cases in which the aorta is opened (e.g., for aortic valve replacement), direct infusion of cardioplegia may be given in the right and left coronary ostia. Retrograde cardioplegia should be given as well to ensure adequate myocardial protection. Additionally, retrograde cardioplegia can remove any air that may have embolized down the coronary vasculature in the event that air embolism into the coronary vasculature is of concern.

Vents and Suckers

In addition to the field sucker, the bypass machine also may provide for venting of the ventricle. In spite of venous drainage into the cardiopulmonary bypass machine, the heart can nevertheless become quite distended during cardiopulmonary bypass. Because a flaccid, empty heart is desirable during bypass, a vent may be placed so that blood may be drained from the left ventricle under suction. Left ventricular venting can be accomplished through the aortic cardioplegic cannula or a catheter can be placed into the left ventricle via the right superior pulmonary vein through the mitral valve into the left ventricle. A roller-type pump provides suction to evacuate blood from the left ventricle.

Safety Devices and Other Concerns

The bypass circuit is equipped with numerous alarms to alert the perfusionist to the presence of air bubbles and a low blood volume in the

Table 10-1. Specific Concerns for the Anesthesiologist During
Cardiopulmonary Bypass

---

1. The anesthesiologist should supervise the administration of anesthetics during the bypass run.

2. The anesthesiologist ensures maintenance of muscle relaxation to decrease oxygen consumption.

3. The anesthesiologist monitors anticoagulation and protamine reversal.

4. The anesthesiologist communicates with the surgery and perfusion team should drugs be administered before attempting to wean the patient from cardiopulmonary bypass.

5. The anesthesiologist is available for consultation with the perfusionist and surgeon regarding intraoperative management. The anesthesiologist confirms the adequacy of perfusion, blood replacement, glucose, and electrolyte management during the bypass run in cooperation with the perfusionist.

---

venous reservoir. An alert perfusionist generally is the key to successful bypass management. Similar to anesthesia, perfusion requires a high degree of vigilance to be certain of the adequacy of delivery of oxygen to the patient during cardiopulmonary bypass. Generally, the anesthesiologist should be available to the perfusionist as necessary to assist in whatever way he or she may desire during the bypass run. It is unwise for the anesthesiologist to interfere with the management of cardiopulmonary bypass because this is generally most adequately handled by the surgery and perfusion team. Specific concerns of the anesthesiologist during cardiopulmonary bypass are presented in Table 10-1.

11

Patients for Arrhythmia Surgery

Anesthesiologists are frequently required to assist both cardiologists and cardiac surgeons in the treatment of chronic arrhythmias. Generally, we are asked to assist in the therapy of these patients in three distinct ways: (1) sedating patients for electrical studies of the heart in the catheterization or electrophysiology (EP) laboratories, (2) providing anesthesia for implantable cardioversion-defibrillation devices, and (3) managing patients during surgery for the correction of arrhythmic foci. This chapter briefly examines specific anesthesia-related concerns for arrhythmia surgery that might be encountered in a community practice. Treatment of postoperative arrhythmias is discussed in Chapter 15.

Sedating Patients for Electrical Studies of the Heart

There are few things that can cause as much distress among anesthesia personnel as having to leave the operating room to provide anesthesia "off floor." Although none of the places where we go out of the operating room are ever particularly inviting (e.g., the magnetic resonance imaging suite, the emergency room, or the catheterization laboratory), none is as distressing as the EP laboratory. There we stand in heavy lead gowns. The anesthesiologist sits with the patient, generally at some distance, awaiting the cardiologist's successful completion of an electrical study of the heart. Cardiologists do EP studies by placing catheters into the heart to locate those foci responsible for arrhythmia generation. This task is quite time consuming and may require several hours. As such, the anesthesiologist must be prepared for a prolonged course in the laboratory, where the patient may need several hours of sedation.

A fully ready anesthesia machine should be available to the anesthesiologist wherever he or she goes off floor, be it the catheterization laboratory or EP laboratory. A full armamentarium of anesthesia drugs must also be available. Patients need to be monitored in the same manner as they would be for a surgical procedure. In patients undergoing an EP study of the heart, transcutaneous defibrillation pads should be applied by the catheterization laboratory staff and confirmed by the anesthesiologist. The patient needs to be connected to a defibrillator. Once full monitoring is established and supplemental oxygen provided, the patient may be sedated in a manner consistent with the skill and particular practice of the anesthesiologist. Propofol, midazolam, and fentanyl are frequently used to sedate patients during these procedures. Adequate analgesia of the catheter introducer site is essential before placing the catheter sheaths. Patients scheduled for EP studies should be given nothing by mouth before coming to the catheterization laboratory, and the ease of airway management should be assessed. In addition to intubation equipment, an appropriate sized laryngeal mask airway should be available in case general anesthesia becomes necessary or in the event the patient requires resuscitation. The anesthesiologist must always be certain that he or she has clear access to the patient before the cardiologist begins work. Remember, many cardiologists have little idea of what an anesthesiologist needs or what an anesthesiologist's concerns are. Few realize that sedation requires careful monitoring and management skills. Careful sedation should permit both a successful mapping of ectopic foci and ablation of any aberrant conduction pathways in the EP laboratory should they be discovered. If fibrillation needs to be induced electively, deeper levels of sedation with propofol can be administered and a mask airway maintained during cardioversion. Obviously, if there is any question as to the ease of airway management, it is preferable to have a secure airway prior to providing heavy sedation. In this regard, induction of a general anesthesia should be considered only after a reasoned approach to airway management has been considered.

Providing Anesthesia for Implantable Cardioverter Defibrillators

Until recently, implantable cardioverter defibrillators (ICDs) required exposure of the heart for placement of epicardial defibrillation patches.

Currently, ICDs are often placed with great ease by cardiologists in the EP laboratory. Using a transvenous catheter system, the ICD has been reduced to requiring little more effort than a pacemaker insertion. Although the device was once quite large, requiring the creation of an abdominal pocket, the ICD has been successfully reduced to only slightly larger than a typical pacemaker. Placed transvenously in the EP laboratory, the current ICD often requires only careful sedation. Previously, general endotracheal anesthesia with arterial line monitoring was used in the operating room for surgical placement of the ICD. As always, exact anesthesia selection varied according to a patient's particular medical condition. Because many patients for ICD placement have had previous myocardial infarctions, coronary artery bypass grafts, ventricular aneurysms, as well as ventricular failure, careful selection of anesthesia was necessary to avoid congestive heart failure at the time of ICD placement. The precise selection of drugs chosen to avoid hemodynamic collapse was less important than the fact that the anesthesiologist took actions to ensure hemodynamic stability. Arterial line monitoring was frequently employed to carefully monitor hemodynamic performance during the procedure. If general anesthesia was required, careful titration of propofol, fentanyl, inhalation agents, and muscle relaxants supplemented by close monitoring and inotropes provided suitable hemodynamic stability and a rapid emergence for patients undergoing surgical placement of an ICD. As always, the anesthesiologist needed to be able to respond to sudden hemodynamic collapse or the development of lethal arrhythmias.

As cardiologists have taken this procedure away from cardiac surgery, the placement of ICDs occurs more frequently in the EP laboratory. Here the anesthesiologist must be as cautious as in the operating room. General anesthesia can be employed for patients as needed; however, implantation of these small ICD devices can often be managed with sedation such as that used for an EP study. The one problem in using sedation for ICD placement is that the patient undergoes three to four periods of ventricular fibrillation followed by defibrillation shocks as the device is tested. As this is the case, airway management in the event of refractory ventricular fibrillation presents some concern. Obviously, if the patient develops ventricular fibrillation refractory to defibrillation, many anesthesiologists might prefer to have an endotracheal tube in place to be guaranteed airway management. Still, because the majority of patients quickly convert from ventricular fibrillation to a rhythm consistent with life in the EP catheterization laboratory, it is possible to manage these patients with mask ventilation and propofol sedation during testing of the device. Of course, if patients present particular problems in airway anatomy, prudence dictates securing the airway before proceeding with general anesthesia and testing of the ICD.

Managing Patients for Arrhythmia Surgery

The expansion of EP studies and the growth of services offered by most EP laboratories has reduced the frequency with which patients are taken to the operating room for excision of foci responsible for arrhythmia generation. Additionally, the ease with which ICDs are placed also lessens the urgency with which patients are taken to surgery to correct potentially life-threatening arrhythmias. Still, a number of patients are brought into the operating room for intraoperative mapping of ectopic foci and for cryoablation (freezing) or surgical excision of ectopic foci.

From a practical standpoint, when a patient is brought to surgery for open chest electrical mapping of the heart, the operating room is even more crowded with material and people than in a routine cardiac case. Other than this, little else differs in surgery for EP mapping of the heart than in routine coronary artery bypass surgery. Patients are taken to the operating room and placed on cardiopulmonary bypass in the usual fashion. The heart is mapped using a variety of techniques, and foci are either cryoablated or excised. Because many of these patients have had previous cardiac surgery, myocardial infarctions, and ventricular aneurysms, excision of an ectopic foci is often but one part of a surgery that includes valvular repair, excision of a ventricular aneurysm, or bypass surgery. Anesthetic management is as routine as for any patient requiring cardiopulmonary bypass. The patient is heparinized and placed on cardiopulmonary bypass. The electrophysiologist and surgeon map the heart with a variety of nets and catheters in a search for arrhythmogenic foci. The heart is opened, and the endocardium or a ventricular aneurysm is resected or cryoablated. The inability to induce further arrhythmias is considered a sign of success. Once completed, the heart is sewn together and air is removed. The patient is weaned from cardiopulmonary bypass.

Although this sounds relatively straightforward, we must be cautious. Often these patients present with relatively poor ventricular function to begin with and spend several hours on cardiopulmonary bypass, often in ventricular fibrillation. Because EP studies are performed in a nonarrested, non–cross-clamped heart, prolonged bypass runs can result in further difficulties for the patient. Excision, cryoablation, or both of myocardium may impair both right and left ventricular function, potentially leading to difficulty in weaning from cardiopulmonary bypass. Of course, ventricular aneurysmectomy, by reducing the size of the heart, may make the heart a more efficient pump. Because the heart is opened to facilitate arrhythmia surgery, the possibility of air embolization via either bypass grafts or down the native coronary vasculature raises the possibility of acute ventricular dysfunction. Should air embolism into the coronary vasculature occur, elevated perfusion pressures as well as administration of retrograde cardioplegia may dislodge air or particulate emboli from the myocardial capillary bed. After resection of arrhythmia foci, patients often require extensive pharmacologic or mechanical support as described in Chapter 8.

The Maze procedure is available to correct chronic atrial fibrillation. Numerous incisions are made in the atria to impair any possible pathway for aberrant rhythm conduction. Cardiopulmonary bypass is employed in this procedure, therefore necessitating the same concerns as in any bypass patient.

Pacemakers

We could not review arrhythmia surgery and implantable devices without mentioning pacemakers. In general, the anesthesiologist should not be required to assist with routine pacemaker placement. If called on, sedation and local infiltration is all that is required to render a patient comfortable for placement of a permanent pacemaker. Settings for pacemaker placement are the responsibility of both the pacemaker representative and the surgeon. A far greater concern to the cardiac anesthesiologist is the use of temporary pacing with either esophageal, transvenous, epicardial, or transcutaneous modes in patients in acute deterioration in either the preoperative, intraoperative, or postoperative settings. Of the modes discussed, it is generally epicardial pacing with which most cardiac anesthesiologists are most familiar. Atrial and ventricular sequential pacing can be established with a temporary pacer with a dual-chamber pacing ability and epicardial pacing wires (Figure 11-1).

In atrioventricular pacing (DOO) both the ventricle and atria are paced. The DOO code implies dual-chamber pacing without the ability to sense or inhibit the pacer by the innate cardiac rhythm. Such a pacing mode may lead to ventricular fibrillation if a pacer beat occurs at a vulnerable period should the heart have its own rhythm. The DDD mode is frequently employed in many temporary pacemakers. In this setting, both chambers of the heart are paced and sensed while the pacer is inhibited should a native rhythm compete with the pacer settings. In DVI

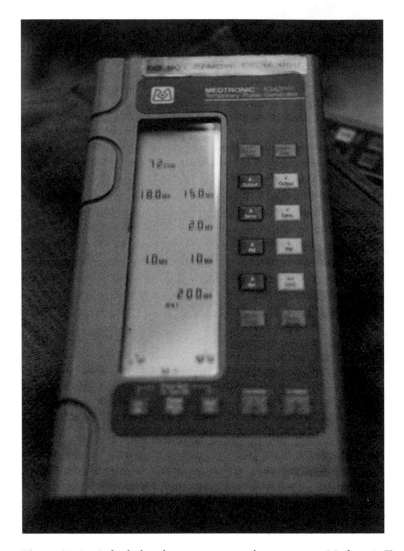

Figure 11-1. *A dual-chamber temporary pulse generator (Medtronic Temporary Pulse Generator from Medtronic, Minneapolis). A temporary pacer set in DVI mode.*

pacing both chambers are paced while the device senses the ventricles and inhibits the pacemaker should a native ventricular signal occur.

In VVI pacing the ventricle is paced, sensed, and inhibited by a native beat. This setting is occasionally used postoperatively, especially in patients who are incapable of atrial contraction, namely those in chronic atrial fibrillation with a slow ventricular response. Atrial pacing alone, either AOO in which the atrium alone is paced or AAI pacing in which the atrium is paced, sensed, and inhibited, can provide for rapid increases in sinus rhythm should the patient develop sinus bradycardia. This setting is often useful in patients who have a slow sinus bradycardia when weaned from bypass.

In the period immediately after bypass, dual-chamber pacing is employed as necessary with a sensing capability (DVI pacing). Atrial pacing may also be employed should a slow sinus rhythm be present. Often dual-chamber pacing is necessary immediately after the discontinuation of cardiopulmonary bypass but is no longer needed at the end of the procedure. Many patients require no pacing at all after cardiopulmonary bypass, particularly if they have received adequate cardioplegia and return to sinus rhythm following release of the aortic cross clamp. Often in this situation surgeons will leave only epicardial ventricular pacing wires in place.

Transvenous temporary pacing may be encountered in patients taken from the catheterization laboratory either electively or emergently. Generally, such pacing tends to be of the VVI mode in which the ventricle is paced, sensed, and inhibited. Postoperatively epicardial pacing is preferred to eliminate the possibility of pacing wire migration inhibiting pacing.

Pacing pulmonary arterial catheters and pacing port pulmonary arterial catheters can provide pacing capability as well as the routine information expected from a pulmonary arterial catheter. Often patients at risk for the development of a heart block in the period before cardiopulmonary bypass may benefit from placement of a pacing Swan-Ganz catheter so that transvenous pacing is available until the surgeon can provide for epicardial pacing. A transvenous pacing ability may be of use in patients undergoing reoperation in which access to the heart may be limited for some time due to the presence of adherent adhesions. A pacing Swan-Ganz catheter can provide transvenous pacing should sinus bradycardia develop after induction of anesthesia. Previous myocardial infarctions and scarring may impair effective pacing in the transvenous pacer.

Transcutaneous pacing may be employed in emergency situations after cardiac arrest. Although not routine in the operating room, it is possible that patients could be delivered to surgery while being paced transcutaneously. Obviously, the establishment of transvenous pacing or epicardial pacing by the anesthesia and surgical team is necessary if the patient is pacemaker dependent. After cardiopulmonary bypass, the surgical team places epicardial pacing wires. Care must be taken to connect them appropriately to the atrial and ventricular ports on the pacemaker device. Generally, atrial wires are handed over the surgical drape to the right of the anesthesiologist, whereas the ventricular wires tend to be handed to the left. Many times the pacer wires are labeled as atrial or ventricular. However, in many operating rooms these have become mixed to the degree that a pacing cable may say ventricle when in fact it has been connected to the atrium. Care must be taken in establishing pacing to ensure that the circuit is correctly attached (Table 11-1 and Figure 11-2).

Table 11-1. Pacemaker Modes

Code		Common Designation	Comment
VOO	Paces the ventricle No sensing	Fixed rate Asynchronous	Obsolete except for pacemaker testing
VVI	Paces the ventricle Senses ventricular activity Ventricular activity inhibits the pacemaker	Ventricular demand	Most commonly used in life-threatening bradycardia
AAI	Paces the atrium Senses atrial activity Atrial activity inhibits the pacemaker		Indicated in sinus bradycardia with intact AV condition
VAT	Paces the ventricle Senses atrial activity Atrial activity triggers ventricular pacing	Atrial synchronized P-wave triggered	Obsolete Replaced by VDD and DDD
DVI	Paces both atrium and ventricle Senses only ventricular activity Ventricular activity inhibits atrial and ventricle pacing	AV sequential	Dual-chamber pacing mode commonly used in intensive care unit
VDD	Paces the ventricle only Senses atrial and ventricular activity	Atrial synchronous Ventricular inhibited	May be useful when normal sinus rhythm is present with a high degree of AV block

Code	Common Designation	Comment
DDD	Paces and senses both atrium and ventricle Atrial activity triggers ventricular pacing	—	—
DDI	Paces and senses both atrium and ventricle Atrial activity not tracked; thus, atrial tachyarrhythmias do not trigger rapid atrial pacing	—	Useful for sinus bradycardia with AV block and paroxysmal supraventricular tachyarrhythmias

AV = atrioventricular.
Source: Modified from TE Oh. Intensive Care Manual (4th ed). Oxford: Butterworth–Heinemann, 1997.

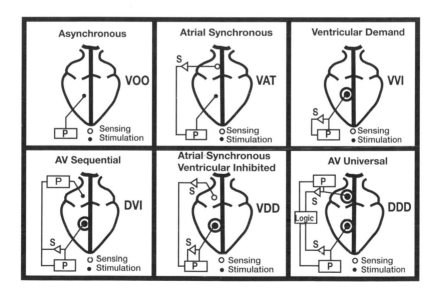

Figure 11-2. *Pacemaker modes II and their three-position (letter) codes. (AV – atrioventricular; P – pacemaker; S = sensing.) (Modified from TE Oh. Intensive Care Manual [4th ed]. Boston: Butterworth–Heinemann, 1997.)*

12

The Surprise Patient

Occasionally, patients are brought to the cardiac surgery operating room for emergency bypass after either failed interventions by cardiologists or other acute deteriorations. The increasing numbers of multiple angioplasties and other interventional procedures being undertaken in the catheterization laboratory (e.g., angioplasty, atherectomy, and so forth) indicate that more and more patients with an increasingly severe cardiac disease are receiving their primary intervention in the catheterization laboratory. As the acute nature of these patients' disease increases, so too does the risk that they will present in significant distress should cardiology-mediated interventions be unsuccessful. As cardiologists become more aggressive in managing these patients in the catheterization laboratory, incidences of failed intervention may increase as well. In general, the surprise patient from the catheterization laboratory presenting to surgery occurs in the following ways:

1. The patient scheduled for elective catheterization has been discovered to have a significant critical left main disease. The patient is placed on the list for immediate, urgent surgery. Although the patient may be in no distress, the lesion so panics the medical staff that surgery is booked immediately.

2. The patient arrives for elective catheterization but develops ischemia in the catheterization laboratory.

3. The patient for angioplasty and atherectomy has developed myocardial ischemia after failure to open the diseased artery.

4. Patients scheduled for angioplasty and atherectomy are sent to surgery in cardiogenic shock from the catheterization laboratory.

5. Patients in full arrest are delivered from the catheterization laboratory for an attempt at salvage.

Obviously, the various histories with which patients arrive in the operating room contribute to the great differences in their outcomes. Although the patient with critical left main disease may be at risk for sudden death if that left main becomes occluded, he or she is not actively ischemic. In this instance, the patient may be transferred to the operating room in an urgent but not emergent fashion. Nevertheless, if patients become ischemic, an intra-aortic balloon pump and other anti-ischemic therapies may be necessary to stabilize the patient's condition while taking them to the operating room emergently. As patients develop cardiogenic shock or enter full arrest, they are frequently rushed to the operating rooms at times with cardiopulmonary resuscitation in progress. Occasionally, the chest is open and open chest massage is necessary until the patient can "crash" onto bypass. Of course, in this setting patient outcome after revascularization usually is quite poor. Even if a patient is successfully revascularized and weaned from cardiopulmonary bypass, after prolonged periods of cardiopulmonary resuscitation in the catheterization laboratory, renal and neurologic injury may ensue, leading to a protracted death in the intensive care unit.

Rarely will a cardiologist permit a patient to die in the catheterization laboratory. As such, patients, no matter how moribund they are or how futile may be the gesture, are sent to cardiac surgery so that they will not die in the catheterization laboratory. Because cardiac surgeons cannot say "no" to a cardiologist (if they wish to continue to receive referrals), the cardiologist always manages to send the dead and dying to heart surgery for an attempt, however futile, at patient salvage. In this setting, the anesthesiologist becomes responsible for continuing the resuscitative effort until the patient is placed onto cardiopulmonary bypass. Often, the operating room, catheterization laboratory, and medical staff can become very distressed should a failed angioplasty patient require emergency surgery. This can complicate our management. It is incumbent on the anesthesiologist to attempt to provide some degree of calm and to provide the necessary monitors and lines that he or she would normally require to successfully manage a patient in the operating room. Of course, the anesthesiologist must be flexible. Considering that the situation is probably less than ideal if a salvage is to be attempted, the anesthesiologist may need to make do with what is available until additional vascular access and other monitors can be applied.

Anesthesia for Angioplasty

Cardiologists frequently provide their own sedation for angioplasty. Angioplasty standby has routinely come to mean just that—the anesthesiologist stands by in case of an operating room emergency, rather than being intimately involved in patient management in the catheterization laboratory. Although some may argue that the anesthesiologist should manage all sedation for invasive procedures, the cardiologist can routinely manage sedation for angioplasty patients without the additional expense of an anesthesiologist.

Various levels of standby have been developed to categorize the potential need for a surgery and anesthesia team should angioplasty fail. How human resources are employed in standby angioplasties must be continually reviewed as new procedures are introduced. By assigning a risk level to each angioplasty, operating room personnel need not be needlessly standing by for low-risk procedures. Nonetheless, an operating room team must be available on short notice should the patient require emergency surgery, even for a low-risk procedure. In large institutions where many "heart rooms" are available, a heart team can be assembled quickly if needed. In smaller hospitals, however, where the operating room team may be the only team to perform both elective and emergency cases, the catheterization laboratory must be clear before elective surgery can be undertaken, even if the risk of a given angioplasty procedure is quite low.

One of the great concerns of any anesthesiologist in the care of the angioplasty patient is the cry, "we need more sedation." This happens when the anesthesiologist is called by the cardiologist because the angioplasty patient has become disoriented or combative as a consequence of either oversedation, hypoxemia, or a neurologic event. If an anesthesiologist is called to assist with sedation in a procedure already in progress, it is most important that the anesthesiologist be able to quickly assess the patient's status. Attention to the ABCs (airway, breathing, and circulation) needs to be addressed first because patients may be combative because they have been oversedated and are somewhat hypoxemic. Also, as cardiologists frequently administer benzodiazepines to elderly patients, many patients become dysphoric in the catheterization laboratory. Because embolization from catheters is not unheard of, the anesthesiologist must be certain that no focal lesion has occurred, involving him or her in a situation in which stroke must be managed as well. Once the anesthesiologist becomes involved in the case he or she may proceed with sedation with whatever drugs are necessary. A propofol infusion provides a relatively short-acting sedative that can be readily titrated to effect.

Should a patient in the cardiac catheterization laboratory require emergent or urgent surgery as described previously, the anesthesiologist needs to respond promptly. The patient with critical left main disease may be managed in the usual fashion with particular care in maintaining the tenuous balance between myocardial oxygen supply and demand. Patients who present from the catheterization laboratory with active ischemia but who are not yet in cardiogenic shock require careful titration of anti-ischemic therapy with nitroglycerin and anesthetic agents. At times, induction of anesthesia can help to relieve myocardial ischemia. At other times, the development of hypotension associated with anesthesia induction may exacerbate the imbalance in myocardial oxygen supply and demand, leading to cardiogenic shock. The combination of nitroglycerin and phenylephrine can often be employed to provide for vasodilation of the capacitance vessels while maintaining systemic pressure. Often placement of an intra-aortic balloon pump by the cardiologist before transporting the patient to surgery provides significant relief from ischemia and makes the induction of anesthesia considerably more stable. The surgeon then has the time to carefully place the patient on cardiopulmonary bypass. As always, when using an intra-aortic balloon pump, it is important that an effective trigger be available to time the counterpulsation effectively.

In the event that the patient is in full arrest or profound cardiogenic shock, cardiopulmonary resuscitation or aggressive resuscitative measures may be in progress. If the patient has fibrillated, efforts no doubt will already have been made to defibrillate the patient several times prior to moving the patient to the operating room. Cardiopulmonary resuscitation and advanced cardiac life support will be in progress on the way to the surgical suite from the catheterization laboratory. After repeated attempts at cardioversion and administration of epinephrine, there may be little choice but to continue cardiopulmonary resuscitation until the patient can be placed on cardiopulmonary bypass. In some instances, cardiologists may be concerned that the patient has experienced a myocardial rupture secondary to catheter erosion of the heart. In this instance, the patient's chest may well be open and the pericardium incised to relieve any potential pericardial tamponade. If this is the case, the surgeon will most likely be providing open chest cardiac massage on the way to the operating suite. As the patient is taken to the operating room, the anesthesiologist must be certain that the airway is secured and that breath sounds are bilateral. In the patient who is in full arrest, little anesthesia is required other than to successfully administer a paralyzing dose of muscle relaxants, heparin, and oxygen. Additional doses of narcotics, muscle relaxants, and amnestics may be employed as necessary once the patient is successfully on cardiopulmonary bypass. For patients in cardiogenic shock, induction of anesthesia can be somewhat difficult. Judicious administration of narcotics, amnestics, and muscle relaxants can provide anesthetic induction. Often, however, even small doses of anesthetic drugs can reduce peripheral vascular resistance, leading to hypotension at the time of surgery. Administration of small boluses of phenylephrine may be necessary at surgery to maintain systemic pressure. Generally, once the patient is on cardiopulmonary bypass, larger doses of narcotics may be administered so an effective level of anesthesia is achieved. Invasive monitors are placed as tolerated. Often, a femoral line is necessary to provide effective blood pressure monitoring. If an intra-aortic balloon pump has already been placed, this is available. Arterial pressure monitoring can be achieved using the femoral line without having to locate the radial artery. Central line placement is also necessary at this point. Patients often have a femoral venous catheter in place that at least permits the administration of drugs while other access is sought. As always, when patients are transported from one location to another we must be certain that the endotracheal tube has not been dislodged or that a right main stem intubation has occurred.

When a patient from the catheterization laboratory arrives in the surgical suite in full arrest, he or she will no doubt be equipped with multiple drug infusion and innumerable tangled intravenous lines. Once the patient is safely delivered to the operating room and placed on cardiopulmonary bypass, the anesthesiologist is well advised to transform the collected mass into something with which he or she is familiar, namely, take the cardiologist's mess and make it your own. At least this way we can be certain that appropriate access and monitors are in place where we expect them to be and that infusions are available for an attempt to wean from cardiopulmonary bypass if the patient is capable of survival. If the patient has poor ventricular function following an attempt at revascularization or surgical repair, the question next arises whether the patient can be successfully weaned from cardiopulmonary bypass. After attempting to wean the patient according to the protocols described earlier in this text, it is quite possible that a left ventricular assist device or a biventricular assist device may be necessary so that the patient can be weaned from cardiopulmonary bypass. Surgical teams should carefully consider the length of cardiopulmonary resuscitation at this point to be certain that the patient has a possibility of survival before commencing support with a left or right ventricular assist device.

Patient from the Emergency Room

Patients encountered directly from the emergency room by the cardiac anesthesiologist generally present after having been diagnosed with a dissecting thoracic aneurysm (Chapter 15). Injuries to the heart constitute another group seen by the cardiac anesthesiologist. Often patients with stab injuries or gunshot wounds to the heart will have died long before being delivered to the emergency room department, much less the operating room. Nevertheless, every now and then a patient with a stab wound to the heart presents with pericardial tamponade. In patients in whom impaired ventricular filling is a concern, the operating room team should be available to quickly open the chest and relieve pericardial tamponade on the institution of positive pressure ventilation. Ketamine and muscle relaxants provide the basis for induction of anesthesia should the patient remain conscious. Narcotics or other inhalational agents may be titrated to effect as the patient's condition improves. As with all trauma patients, close observation for other injuries (e.g., head, lungs, abdomen) is essential because they may have been overlooked in an effort to take the patient to surgery for the release of pericardial tamponade and the repair of an injury to the heart. Generally, however, most patients with injuries to the heart die in the field and therefore are not routinely encountered in community cardiac anesthesia practice. However, at trauma centers the possibility of dealing with patients with tamponade after a knife injury to the great vessels or the heart is a more likely possibility.

Re-Exploration in the Patient from the Intensive Care Unit

The postoperative patient may develop various amounts of mediastinal bleeding after surgery. A blood loss of more than 300 ml per hour is suspicious for surgical bleeding, necessitating re-exploration. Should excessive blood loss be noted from both mediastinal and chest tubes, it is important first and foremost that any degree of coagulopathy be corrected. Tests of coagulation (prothrombin time, partial thromboplastin time, and fibrinogen) as well as heparin concentration analyses and platelet count should all be reviewed and appropriate therapy given (e.g., additional protamine, platelet transfusion, and so forth) should patients have excessive postoperative blood loss. Blood product replacement may be necessary as guided by laboratory tests. Nonetheless, if hemorrhage continues with normal laboratory test results, it must be concluded that a surgical site of bleeding is present. If patients are returned to the operating room before extubation, induction of anesthesia may be undertaken with judicious administrations of narcotics, amnestics, and muscle relaxants. If already extubated, care must be taken to avoid vasodilation on induction, especially if pericardial tamponade appears to be present. Pericardial tamponade should be suspected in any patient in whom the central venous pressure and pulmonary arterial pressure become equivalent and the cardiac index steadily decreases. The increasing need for vasopressors and inotropes is also a warning that the patient's myocardial function may be impaired due to elevated pericardial pressure. As always, the exact choice of anesthetic for inducing a patient who is awake and extubated is at the discretion of the individual anesthesiologist. Ketamine and other short-acting agents may be employed for anesthetic induction. In those patients who are intubated and partially paralyzed from the intensive care unit, having not yet awakened from surgery, doses of anesthetics, narcotics, amnestics, and induction agents may be titrated to effect with careful monitoring. Once the patient is taken to the operating room, the chest is exposed and prepared. The surgical team should stand by to intervene and release any pericardial tamponade.

During the surgical re-exploration, the surgeon often "mugs" the heart—that is, lifts the heart out of the chest cavity to inspect grafts sewn on the part of the heart not routinely visible. This often results in arrhythmias and decreased cardiac output. Inotropes and vasopressors may be necessary to support the circulation if this maneuver is frequently repeated by the surgeon. If the patient is unable to sustain a blood pressure consistent with adequate tissue perfusion for the time it takes for additional sutures to be applied to grafts visualized by lifting the heart, it may be necessary to reinstitute cardiopulmonary bypass. If the patient must again be placed on cardiopulmonary bypass, coagulopathy should be expected after repair of the bleeding site. Blood products should be ordered and readily available to correct coagulopathy after weaning from cardiopulmonary bypass.

Patients Presenting Emergently to the Operating Room from the Intensive Care Unit After Routine Surgery

If a patient arrests in the intensive care unit, it is quite possible the chest has been opened to inspect the heart and to release any pericardial fluid in an effort to resuscitate the patient. Often, these patients are transferred to the operating room with the chest open and cardiac massage in progress. Much like the crash in the catheterization laboratory, bringing the patient directly from the intensive care unit requires that the anesthesiologist assume control of the situation to provide appropriate access, monitoring, and airway management so any attempt at salvage is possible. In the patient who is in full arrest, there is little need for anesthetic agents; muscle relaxants may be given and various amounts of narcotics and other sedatives titrated to effect should the resuscitation be successful. Cardiopulmonary resuscitation and epinephrine administration constitute the resuscitative effort. Occasionally, the patient who deteriorates acutely will have suffered from an occluded graft due to graft vasospasm or kinking. In this instance, the patient is placed on cardiopulmonary bypass for repair of the bypass graft. Any patient transported to surgery undergoing cardiopulmonary resuscitation has a high risk for renal and neurologic injury perioperatively. Additionally, ventricular function may be impaired if ischemia has resulted from an occluded graft. Placement of a ventricular assist device may be considered by the surgical team if the surgeon considers the patient's chance for survival good. Generally, in patients who have survived the initial operation only to present to surgery in an arrest situation, aggressive therapy will be undertaken by the surgical team, including the use of an extracorporeal ventricular assist device.

Conclusion

Patients are taken to emergency surgery for a variety of reasons. The anesthesiologist's role is principally to continue the resuscitation attempted by the cardiologist or intensive care physician until the patient is placed on cardiopulmonary bypass. In patients who are in full arrest, the main goal is to quickly and effectively place the patient on cardiopulmonary bypass. Those patients with active ischemia but not yet in arrest likewise generally benefit from cardiopulmonary bypass, particularly if they remain ischemic after intra-aortic balloon pump placement. Last, patients who are taken to surgery emergently because of dangerous anatomy (e.g., left main disease) must be approached with great care, but careful preparation should help to manage the patient with critical anatomy as well as the patient with less acute coronary disease.

13

Patients for Repair of the Ascending Thoracic Aorta

Repair of the ascending thoracic aorta for either aneurysm resection or acute aortic dissection can be particularly challenging for even the most experienced cardiac anesthesiologist, let alone the trainee or the experienced anesthesiologist returning to cardiac practice. Such cases should be undertaken only after management of the routine coronary artery bypass graft (e.g., patients such as Mr. XY) has been accomplished. This is not because there is anything so remarkably different about anesthesia management per se, rather the emergency nature of the surgical repair subjects the patient to any number of potential complications including stroke, heart failure, coagulopathy, renal dysfunction, and spinal cord injury. This chapter presents the anesthetic management of patients with ascending aortic disease as well as briefly reviewing management schemes for deep hypothermic circulatory arrest.

Patient AA is a 72-year-old man who presents in the emergency room with severe pain of a tearing quality in the chest. This is accompanied by signs of congestive heart failure. Physical examination reveals the murmur of aortic regurgitation and a pulseless right radial artery. Neurologic examination is otherwise within normal limits. Chest radiography reveals an enlargement of the mediastinum. Echocardiography demonstrates ascending aortic dissection. Patient AA has obviously developed an acute aortic dissection with aortic regurgitation. This presentation represents one of the few times when a cardiac anesthesiologist may be required to transport a patient from the emergency room to the operating room directly. Transesophageal echocardiography, magnetic resonance imaging, and computed tomographic scans may all be used to make the evaluation of acute aortic dissection. Although arteriography and angiography may be helpful in new-onset aortic insufficiency and congestive heart failure, patients may need to be transported to emergency surgery directly without the information provided by cardiac catheterization. In addition to the development of ventricular dysfunction as a consequence of aortic regurgitation, if the coronary ostia becomes occluded by a dissection flap, electrocardiography may reveal signs of myocardial ischemia. The patient will likely develop fulminant ventricular dysfunction. Congestive heart failure and hemodynamic collapse ensues both from acute aortic insufficiency and myocardial ischemia.

Much has been written about varying types of aortic dissections that can be encountered emergently (Figure 13-1). Generally, in the cardiac operating room we most frequently manage the anesthesia for patients undergoing repair of type A (ascending dissection), such as Mr. AA is experiencing.

The diagnosis having been made by emergency and cardiology staff, the anesthesiologist will find the patient already receiving medical management. Supportive care will be in place as necessary (e.g., mechanical ventilation, reduction of blood pressure with sodium nitroprusside, and possibly beta blockade). Should the patient become profoundly hypotensive, cardiac tamponade may be suspected as a consequence of aortic dissection. This may have already been relieved in the emergency room prior to taking the patient for surgical exploration. Surgical therapy remains the definitive treatment for ascending aortic dissections. Medical therapy with blood pressure reduction is more likely to be employed in dealing with those dissections distal to the subclavian artery.

Anesthetic Management of Emergency Proximal Aortic Dissections

Careful assessment of Patient AA and those like him should be completed quickly before taking the patient to surgery. In particular, it is important to know that the patient is neurologically intact or if there are any absent pulses. Dissections involving the innominate artery and the aortic arch may subject the patient to varying degrees of neurologic injury or leave them without a pulse in the extremities. After estab-

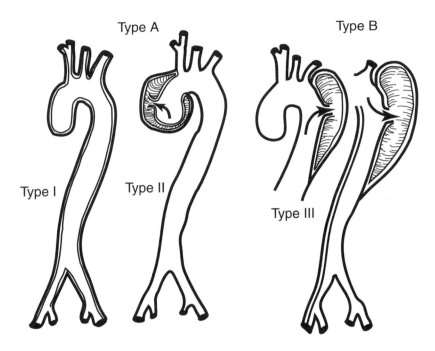

Figure 13-1. *Location of aortic dissections. The Stanford system classifies aortic dissections based on involvement of the ascending aorta (type A) or noninvolvement (type B). The DeBakey system classifies dissections into type I, II, or III. (Modified from ME DeBakey, et al. Surgical management of dissecting aneurysms of the aorta. J Thorac Cardiovasc Surg 1965;49:130.)*

lishing a brief baseline neurologic examination (it may not be possible if the patient is intubated and sedated), the patient can be taken to surgery. The choice of induction agents must be determined based on the patient's particular situation. The awake hypertensive patient with an acute dissection may be induced with the usual combination of narcotics, amnestics, and muscle relaxants. On the other hand, the patient with acute aortic insufficiency and cardiac tamponade may be in severe cardiogenic shock. In this instance, the patient may tolerate only small amounts of amnestics and narcotics in addition to muscle relaxants to facilitate intubation. If a patient is severely hypotensive (systolic blood pressure of more than 50 mm Hg), muscle relaxants alone may be all that can be given as the patient is resuscitated. As is always the case, management of the airway remains the anesthesiologist's first concern. Once the patient is successfully intubated and ventilated, additional

Table 13-1. Anesthetic Requirements for Acute Aortic Dissection

1. Two large 14-gauge peripheral intravenous lines equipped with blood warmers
2. Arterial line monitor placed after bilateral pulses are confirmed, preferably placed in the left radial artery in the event that the innominate artery is clamped at the time of repair
3. Pulmonary arterial pressure monitoring
4. Transesophageal echocardiography to assess aortic valve competency and coronary ostial patency (if possible)
5. Careful attention to the patient's NPO status before anesthetic induction

narcotics, amnestics, and muscle relaxants may be given as tolerated. Once the patient is effectively placed on cardiopulmonary bypass, other anesthetic agents may be given as well. Table 13-1 presents the anesthesia requirements for management of an acute aortic dissection.

Intraoperative Management

The peri-induction period for patients such as Mr. AA may be quite difficult. Ventricular dysfunction as a consequence of aortic insufficiency or myocardial ischemia secondary to occlusion of the coronary ostia, pericardial tamponade, and hypovolemia may make the prebypass time an ongoing round of resuscitation. Avoidance of hypertension in acute dissection is intuitively obvious. Likewise, the need to preserve systemic perfusion for a patient in cardiogenic shock is also straightforward. Of course, rarely is management so simple. The hemodynamic roller coaster tends to be operative in this particular emergency situation because wide degrees of hemodynamic lability complicate patient management. Quick actions and reactions by the anesthesia staff offer the patient the best chance at maintaining organ viability before institution of cardiopulmonary bypass. Generally, the femoral artery is cannulated by the surgeon as the chest is opened. The arterial cannula is placed in the femoral artery along with bicaval venous cannula. Bypass is instituted after a suitable activated clotting time has been achieved. Once the patient is paralyzed, anesthetized, and placed on cardiopulmonary bypass, a graft can be placed into the ascending aorta in the area of the dissection (Figure 13-2). Should the aortic valve prove incompetent, a

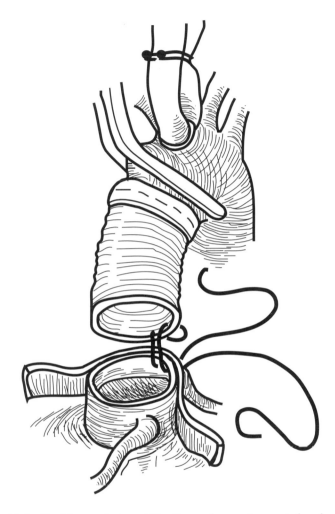

Figure 13-2. *Excision technique. The diseased aorta is resected and replaced with a graft. (Modified from JA Waldhausen, WS Pierce. Johnson's Surgery of the Chest [5th ed]. St. Louis: Mosby, 1985.)*

composite graft, including an aortic valve replacement, can substitute both the native valve and the ascending aorta. Reimplantation of the coronary ostia into the graft is necessary to preserve coronary blood flow. If the native coronary vessels are diseased, coronary bypass grafts can be performed at this time.

Careful administration of cardioplegia is necessary during the repair to ensure myocardial viability after restoration of coronary blood flow. After the surgeon has sewn the aortic graft into place, the patient is weaned from cardiopulmonary bypass. The heart may be injured as a consequence of ischemia during the prebypass period. Aortic dissection may lead to an intimal flap, occluding the coronary ostia and resulting in ischemia. Likewise, acute aortic insufficiency and ventricular distention can lead to myocardial ischemia prebypass. These factors may make it difficult to wean the patient from cardiopulmonary bypass after emergency repair of an aortic dissection. Multiple drug regimens as described in Chapter 8 will be necessary to successfully wean the patient with a poor ventricular function following cardiopulmonary bypass.

Coagulopathy and surgical bleeding also frequently complicate anesthetic management once an aortic dissection has been repaired. Hypertension is scrupulously avoided, and blood products are administered as necessary. Patients are heavily sedated and paralyzed after surgery to secure the airway in the immediate postoperative period and to prevent postoperative hypertension.

Aortic Arch Surgery

If patient AA's dissection had involved vessels of the aortic arch (the innominate artery, the left internal carotid artery, and the subclavian artery), those vessels would need to be isolated and reattached to a graft, replacing the aortic arch as well as the ascending aorta. Naturally, by occluding blood flow to the aortic arch, the brain is potentially rendered ischemic.

Anesthetic management of operations involving the aortic arch is similar to surgery involving the ascending aorta but excluding surgery on the great vessels of the aortic arch. Cardiopulmonary bypass management, however, is very different in patients undergoing arch surgery. Varying approaches are available to prevent cerebral ischemia from developing during the period of aortic arch repair. Most frequently, profound hypothermia and circulatory arrest are employed during aortic arch surgery. In this setting, the perfusionist cools the patient until a temperature of approximately 15–18°C is reached. In elective situations in which electroencephalographic (EEG) monitoring may be readily obtained, such hypothermia leads to EEG isoelectricity, indicating minimal consumption of oxygen by the central nervous system. Once the patient is appropriately cooled to the point of electrical science, cerebral protection has probably been maximized. Obviously, in an acute situation, the EEG may not be immediately available. Nonetheless, aggressive cooling remains an essential practice in those patients undergoing deep hypothermic circulatory arrest (DHCA) for repair of the aortic arch. Anesthesiologists may also provide surface cooling to the head by wrapping the patient in various ice bags. The protective effects of anesthetics (e.g., barbiturates and so forth) have been explored previously in numerous papers and monographs. Most likely there is little opportunity to improve on EEG isoelectricity once it has been attained through hypothermia. Because of the potential to exacerbate cellular ischemia, calcium and glucose administration should be avoided during performance of arch surgery with circulatory arrest.

Retrograde cerebral perfusion during profound hypothermia has been used to increase the time available for surgical repair of the aortic arch during circulatory arrest. In this modality, oxygenated blood is delivered via the superior vena cava cannula in a retrograde manner to the brain. Fortunately, the technical management of retrograde cerebral perfusion remains the responsibility of the perfusionist and surgeon. Retrograde perfusion allows the surgeon to spend an increased amount of time in completing the graft (more than 30 minutes).

Profound hypothermia may be associated with the development of coagulopathy following the bypass run. Blood product replacement as described in Chapter 16 will most certainly be necessary. Aprotinin use has been associated with increased incidences of both renal failure and mortality in patients requiring deep hypothermic circulatory arrest; however, additional studies should be forthcoming regarding its use in arch surgery requiring DHCA. If a protracted bypass run is expected or if the patient has developed an ischemic injury to the myocardium, weaning from cardiopulmonary bypass may be difficult. Weaning from bypass flow is accomplished with drug regimens described in the previous chapters. Postoperatively, patients operated on for acute aortic dissection are not only likely to have injuries to the myocardium but potential impairments in neural and renal function as well. Postoperative bleeding is quite common, both as a consequence of coagulopathy and from surgical sites due to an inadequately sewn aortic graft. Patients such as Mr. AA can exhaust a surgery and anesthesia team as well as hospital resources of blood products and materials. Nonetheless, because ascending aortic dissections remain a surgical disease, it is likely that an acute aortic dissection will be encountered by an anesthesiologist relatively early in the course of his or her experience in cardiac anesthesia practice. Because many of these surgeries are emergencies, the anesthesiologist often spends more effort on resuscitation than on providing elegant anesthesia. Nonetheless, it is important to provide tight hemodynamic control to avoid exacerbating the aortic dissection and to optimize organ perfusion until cardiopulmonary bypass can be initiated. Once the patient is placed on cardiopulmonary bypass, management of the bypass run is little different than that required in any other patient requiring cardiopulmonary bypass. However, should circulatory arrest or retrograde cerebral perfusion be required, we must be prepared for a potentially adverse neurologic outcome, the development of coagulopathy, renal dysfunction, hyperglycemia, and possible liver injury.

Anesthetic Management of Patients with Ascending Aortic Aneurysms

Unlike the acute aortic dissection, which occurs unexpectedly, many patients may be brought to the operating room for elective repair of an ascending aortic aneurysm. Unlike the patient with an acute dissection, the patient being evaluated for repair of an ascending aortic aneurysm should undergo coronary angiography to demonstrate any abnormalities in the coronary vasculature that might benefit from bypass grafting. Aneurysms of the ascending aorta may require a simple tube graft, a composite aortic valve graft, or an arch repair with circulatory arrest as in the case of acute aortic dissections. The degree to which surgical intervention is undertaken depends on the extent of the aneurysm. Common causes of ascending aortic aneurysm include Marfan's syndrome, granulomatous aortitis, syphilis, and atherosclerosis. The extent of the surgical repair depends largely on the aneurysm size and the surgeon's ability. Obviously, if deep hypothermic circulatory arrest is planned, EEG monitoring may be arranged electively to ensure that hypothermic cerebral protection is maximized. Although an elective ascending aortic aneurysm repair should avoid the problems of an acute aortic dissection or aneurysm rupture, elective ascending aortic aneurysm surgery may become complicated as well. Anesthetic management is similar to that for any patient needing tight blood pressure control prebypass. After surgical repair, the patient is weaned from bypass using protocols previously described.

Patients for Descending Thoracic Aortic Aneurysm Repairs

Repair of descending thoracic aortic aneurysms may be considered to be primarily in the field of vascular surgery. The reader is referred to any number of manuals and texts that describe management of the descending thoracic aorta in greater detail.

Briefly, descending thoracic aortic aneurysms occur distal to the left subclavian artery. Generally approached via a left thoracotomy, the surgeon routinely places an aortic cross clamp just distal to the subclavian artery to isolate the descending aortic aneurysm. Once a cross clamp is applied to the aorta, blood flow to various visceral organs, including the abdomen, kidneys, and spinal cord, is reduced. A varying number of bypass circuits and shunts have been used to deliver blood in the aorta distal to the cross clamp. Reimplantation of intercostal arteries, maintenance of mild hypothermia during the aneurysm repair, and cerebral spinal fluid drainage all improve the oxygen supply to demand ratio in the spinal cord at the time when descending aortic blood flow is interrupted.

Anesthetic management requires the careful use of pressors and vasodilators to effectively control blood pressure at the time of application of the aortic cross clamp. As descending aneurysm repair has the grave consequence of paralysis as a consequence of impaired spinal cord blood flow, patients undergoing descending thoracic aneurysms are often referred to those centers that perform the procedure with great frequency. Certainly, these cases are not ideal for the trainee in cardiac or vascular anesthesia. As always, the exact choice of anesthetic drugs employed in the management of these cases, including the methods of postoperative analgesia, remain at the discretion of the anesthesiologists themselves. Tight control of hemodynamics to prevent hypertension during aortic cross clamp and hypotension after cross-clamp release can make these cases most challenging. Likewise, the need for one-lung ventilation can be difficult as well. Maintenance of viability of the kidneys, spinal cord, and viscera is an essential task for the surgeon undertaking descending thoracic artery aneurysm repair. Whether shunts or partial bypass circuits are employed or not to provide blood flow distal to the area of cross-clamped aorta remains a surgical decision.

14

Patients with Valvular Heart Disease

So far, we have not discussed patients undergoing valvular surgery. If this gives the impression that there is some special knowledge (*gnōsis*) to understanding anesthesia for valvular surgery, we have seriously misled you. However, anesthesia for correction of valvular pathology can be among the most difficult to safely deliver (as we discuss). This is particularly true for patients requiring correction of mitral and aortic stenosis. Nevertheless, once we have managed the patient for routine coronary artery bypass grafting (such as Mr. XY) and patients with poor ventricular function, anesthesia for valvular replacement is not that much more difficult once we understand a few simple points.

First, it is the surgeon who has to replace the valve, not the anesthesiologist. If we keep focused on our actual duties in valvular surgery, we should be able to simplify patient management. Whereas the surgeon is responsible for choosing the right-sized valve and sewing the valve into place, all we need to keep focused on are things that we would routinely do in the management of any patient undergoing routine bypass surgery. In that regard, we have two principal responsibilities in managing the patient with valvular disease. We must maintain some degree of hemodynamic stability until the patient is successfully placed on cardiopulmonary bypass. This sounds significantly easier than it sometimes is. Patients with pulmonary hypertension (e.g., as a consequence of mitral stenosis or mitral insufficiency) can often develop right ventricular failure intraoperatively as a consequence of hypercarbia or hypoxemia. Patients with aortic stenosis and large aortic valvular pressure gradients (i.e., of more than 50 mm Hg) may develop significant hypotension during anesthetic induction as a consequence of vasodilation. Thus, maintaining hemodynamic stability until the initiation of cardiopulmonary bypass may be difficult indeed. Right ventricular failure, pulmonary hypertension, systemic hypotension, and myocardial ischemia can all present in the valvular surgical patient. But, what else is new? Such difficulties can happen in the routine bypass case, too. Finally, it is important to remember that cardiopulmonary bypass is available should we need to rescue the patient from any hemodynamic problems that we, despite our best efforts, are unable to correct. All we must remember is that we need to keep the patient hemodynamically stable until he or she can be placed on cardiopulmonary bypass.

Our second challenge is also not remarkably unusual. Namely, we must successfully wean the patient from bypass support. Often patients with long-standing valvular disease have significant ventricular dysfunction. Left ventricular volume overload (characteristic of mitral regurgitation and aortic insufficiency), left ventricular hypertrophy (associated with aortic stenosis), and left ventricular underloading (as occurs in mitral stenosis) can leave patients with significantly impaired left ventricular function even after valvular repair or replacement. Likewise, patients with long-standing pulmonary hypertension may be at considerable risk for developing right ventricular failure at the time of weaning from cardiopulmonary bypass.

Although left and right ventricular failure may occur with greater frequency in the valvular surgical patient as compared with the bypass population, poor left ventricular function or pulmonary hypertension can occur after coronary artery bypass in even the healthiest patients. Therefore, if poor ventricular function is encountered after valvular surgery, we may follow our approach to weaning as described in Chapter 8. Similarly, should right-sided heart dysfunction develop, we can approach the patient according to those protocols available for the improvement of right ventricular contractility.

Consequently, we have two concerns regarding the patient undergoing valvular surgery. Well, three, if we count the safe conduct of anesthesia, which we naturally assume. These concerns are to maintain hemodynamic stability until the patient is placed on bypass and to successfully wean the patient from cardiopulmonary bypass. Although the particulars of the surgical repair—for example, whether a mechanical or a porcine valve is placed—are of interest to the anesthesiologist, we need not be concerned to any great degree. After all, the surgeon is not going to ask our opinion as to whether he or she should place a mechanical valve or not. On the other hand, in the case of valvular repair, the surgeon may well ask and most likely will need our assessment of the adequacy of the valve repair as determined by transesophageal echocardiography (TEE). Likewise, the surgeon may ask for TEE assessment of mechanical valve function once the heart resumes beating. Again, this depends on our ability to interpret information provided by TEE. As we shall see, if we do not feel comfortable in this role due to a lack of training or experience with TEE, it is incumbent on us to confer with a cardiologist or anesthesiologist who can provide the surgeon with that information. But that does not mean that we should be unable to safely conduct anesthetic management of the patient.

This chapter briefly examines some of the features of valvular lesions that we will routinely encounter in our role as clinical anesthesiologists. The chapter focuses on putting the patient on the bypass machine, and as important, if not more so, separating the patient from cardiopulmonary bypass. Details of the surgical repair or surgical techniques are left to surgical texts for those who are interested.

Stenotic Lesions

Aortic Stenosis

The tricuspid aortic valve has a normal valvular orifice of 2.5–3.5 cm^2. A critical stenosis occurs when the orifice is reduced to 0.5 cm^2. As valvular obstruction worsens, a systolic pressure grading develops across the aortic valve. As that gradient increases beyond 50 mm Hg, surgical replacement is considered. Patients may develop ischemia, ventricular failure, and syncope in the course of stenosis of the aortic valve.

In response to the obstruction to ventricular outflow, the left ventricle develops an increased systolic pressure and increased stress in the ventricular wall. As a compensatory mechanism, the heart undergoes concentric hypertrophy, resulting in increased myocardial oxygen demand and decreased diastolic relaxation.

With the cardiac output fixed by an obstructive lesion, vasodilation can lead to syncope and myocardial ischemia. Patients are at risk for sudden death. Right ventricular failure may develop as a consequence of end-stage disease with left ventricular failure.

To examine the perioperative management of the aortic stenosis patient, we will discuss the case of patient AS.

Patient AS is a 63-year-old man with a bicuspid aortic valve. He has increased angina pectoris. Catheterization reveals a 70% occlusion of the left anterior descending coronary artery as well as a 60 mm Hg systolic grading across the aortic valve. The valvular orifice is estimated at 0.7 cm². Ventricular function appears unimpaired.

From an anesthesia standpoint, Mr. AS is perhaps the most straightforward valvular patient that we might encounter. His ventricular function is preserved. He has a one-vessel coronary disease that requires bypass in addition to replacement of his aortic valve.

Our first task is how to get Mr. AS safely on cardiopulmonary bypass. From the time we induce anesthesia (even before that if we routinely use heavy premedication), we must be cautious of anesthetic effects in the patient with obstruction of ventricular outflow. We need to consider the following:

1. *Anesthetic selection.* Fentanyl and sufentanil with or without midazolam may provide a suitable anesthetic that minimally affects cardiac function. However, vasodilation may lead to profound hypotension. Remember that blood pressure is equal to cardiac output multiplied by the systemic vascular resistance. Since cardiac output is limited by stenosis of the aortic valve, systemic blood pressure is routinely maintained through an increase in vascular tone. By reducing the vascular tone (and anesthetics certainly do), we can produce significant hypotension. In patients such as Mr. AS with a left anterior descending artery occlusion, this can easily lead to myocardial ischemia and the hemodynamic spiral toward ventricular failure. Of course, we should not be too concerned about this either. It is easy enough to restore vascular tone, as we have previously discussed. Phenylephrine, administered by small bolus, can augment peripheral tone without producing tachycardia. By restoring vascular tone and avoiding tachycardia, anesthesia can be safely induced using a narcotic, muscle relaxant, and amnestic technique as might be employed in any routine bypass case.

2. *Avoidance of tachycardia and bradycardia.* Tachycardia can lead to decreased myocardial oxygen supply with increased myocardial oxygen demand in patients with the concentric ventricular hypertrophy characteristic of aortic stenosis. Bradycardia can likewise reduce cardiac output, leading to hypotension.

3. *Maintenance of sinus rhythm.* Atrial contraction is essential to help fill the often noncompliant left ventricle in patients with ventricular hypertrophy secondary to aortic stenosis. Atrial fibrillation and junctional rhythms may reduce cardiac output, leading to hypotension and hemodynamic compromise.

Thus, for patients such as Mr. AS, a successful anesthetic must avoid rhythm disturbances, tachycardia, and vasodilation. This sounds familiar, doesn't it? In essence, the patient with aortic stenosis needs an anesthetic that offers maximum hemodynamic stability, if such a thing exists. Mr. AS needs the same meticulous care as does any other patient at risk for ventricular failure. The principal difference is that the degree of leeway in hemodynamic fluctuations is much reduced. Whereas the routine coronary artery bypass patient may permit transient tachycardia or transient hypotension, the patient with a fixed obstruction to ventricular ejection coupled with concentric ventricular hypertrophy may be far less adaptable should our anesthetic lead to those disturbances that result in ventricular dysfunction. A narcotic-based anesthetic that we routinely administer generally achieves this goal. As always, how carefully we provide anesthesia has far more to do with our skills in responding to changes in patient performance and predicting patient performance than it does with the particular drugs or agents that we employ. For patients such as Mr. AS, the time until the initiation of bypass can be difficult. Arrhythmias and hypotension as a consequence of vasodilation or ventricular failure need aggressive responses. Cardioversion may be necessary should atrial fibrillation or other arrhythmias develop that compromise ventricular function. As always, should we encounter a situation in which we are unable to restore hemodynamic stability, it is incumbent on us to inform the surgeon so that we may speed up the process and "crash" onto bypass.

Once the patient is successfully placed on cardiopulmonary bypass, the surgical repair proceeds through an incision in the aorta. The diseased valve is resected and the new valve sewn into place. There is little the anesthesiologist can do at this time. During the course of the surgical repair, it is important that the surgeon be confident that adequate myocardial protection has been achieved. The coronary ostia may be directly cannulated after aortotomy to deliver anterograde cardioplegia. Retrograde administration of cardioplegia should also be used to ensure adequate cardioplegia delivery in the setting of a hypertrophied left ventricle. Retrograde cardioplegia is also useful toward the end of the surgical repair to expel air from the myocardial capillary bed that may have developed as a consequence of opening the aorta. With a little luck, the surgeon expeditiously replaces the diseased aortic valve. Still, we need to be aware of the possible problems that surgeons can encounter as they attempt an aortic valve replacement. These include (1) aortic dissections, in which case the surgeon has to replace the entire aortic root; (2) sewing the valve over a coronary ostium, leading to myocardial ischemic dysfunction; and (3) inadequate removal of air in the heart, leading to air embolism of the coronary vasculature and possibly the cerebral vessels.

TEE can be useful in managing the patient undergoing aortic valvular replacement. In addition to assessing ventricular function before cardiopulmonary bypass, it can be used to assess the adequacy of air removal after completion of the surgical repair. TEE likewise can be used to ascertain that the new valve is functioning correctly. TEE can assist in visualizing the coronary arteries and potentially identifying an obstructed coronary ostia if the replacement valve is in any way occluding the coronary ostia. As TEE is useful in this population, it may be necessary to consult with either a cardiologist familiar with its use or an anesthesia colleague if one is not fully comfortable with the interpretation of TEE images.

Once the valve has been sewn into place, we must address our second issue—weaning from cardiopulmonary bypass. Before weaning from cardiopulmonary bypass, the surgeon asks the anesthesiologist to resume ventilation. At that time, the surgeon attempts to vent any air that may have collected in the heart as a consequence of opening the aorta. TEE can be used to visually inspect the adequacy of air removal. Fortunately, in patients who have relatively preserved ventricular function prior to undertaking valvular repair, it is relatively easy to wean from cardiopulmonary bypass. Often patients such as Mr. AS can be weaned from bypass support with minimal use of inotropes. Indeed, patients frequently require significant vasodilators such as nitroglycerin or nitroprusside to prevent the profound hypertension that can develop in the immediate postbypass period. In general, the surgeons want the systemic blood pressure to remain relatively low from the time of weaning from cardiopulmonary bypass through to delivery in the intensive care unit. Any degree of systemic hypertension often elicits complaints from the surgeon about the dangers of hypertension for the patient after aortotomy.

Thus, we must be prepared to provide control of hypertension when weaning from bypass by the use of vasodilators that need to be continued postoperatively. An infusion of propofol or other sedatives is useful to avoid hypertension as the patient starts to emerge from anesthesia in the intensive care unit. By using a propofol infusion, it is possible to maintain relative sedation until the patient is stable in the intensive care unit, at which point the patient can be awakened and weaned from ventilatory support. As with so many anesthetics, the exact dosage of propofol by infusion needs to be titrated to effect. Sterile technique is essential if propofol is used because of its ability to support bacteria growth.

On the other hand, not all patients with aortic valvular disease have well-preserved ventricular function. Many patients have significant ventricular hypertrophy as a consequence of long-standing aortic stenosis. Ventricular dysfunction is not uncommon in these patients. Inadequate cardioplegia delivery during the surgical repair can lead to the development of left ventricular failure at weaning from cardiopulmonary bypass. In this instance, pharmacotherapy, mechanical assistance, or both may be needed to effectively wean from bypass support. Once again, an approach as described in Chapter 8 can be applied. A combination of inotropes, vasodilators, and mechanical assistance devices, as would be used in the patient with poor ventricular function, can be employed in the patient with poor ventricular function following valvular replacement. Fortunately, in any patient undergoing correction of aortic stenosis, the principal cause of decreased cardiac output, namely the diseased aortic valve, will have been corrected. This leads to increased ventricular ejection. Many patients need control of systemic hypertension more than they need any particular augmentation in cardiac output. Nevertheless, those with end-stage aortic stenosis require the full range of inotropic support to effectively wean from cardiopulmonary bypass. Mechanical support may be necessary as well in patients who simply are unable to generate a cardiac output capable of sustaining adequate tissue perfusion.

In other words, many patients such as Mr. AS are easy to take care of if ventricular function has been preserved perioperatively. All that is often necessary postoperatively is vigorous control of postoperative hypertension. The management of the patient with aortic stenosis is relatively easy when compared with those patients with greater degrees of ventricular dysfunction.

Mitral Stenosis

The second obstructive lesion that we discuss involves stenosis of the mitral valve. Mitral stenosis frequently occurs in female patients, most often as a consequence of rheumatic valvular heart disease. The normal mitral valve orifice is 4–6 cm^2. When valvular area declines to less than 1 cm^2, mitral stenosis becomes critical. Pressure gradients of 25 mm Hg or higher may exist between the left atrial pressure and the left ventricular end-diastolic pressure. This increase in left atrial pressure is transmitted to the pulmonary vasculature, resulting in pulmonary edema, tricuspid regurgitation, and ultimately right ventricular failure. On the other hand, the obstruction to left ventricular filling often results in a relatively low left ventricular end-diastolic pressure and the underloading of the left ventricle. With the left ventricle poorly loaded, the stroke volume is reduced, resulting in diminished cardiac output. The development of tachycardia can further reduce the time available for left ventricular filling, further diminishing stroke volume and cardiac output. Atrial fibrillation, common in the mitral stenosis patient, may further reduce left ventricular filling by eliminating the atrial component of the loading of the ventricle. Both pulmonary hypertension and right ventricular failure may characterize severe mitral stenosis. As such, both left and right ventricular failure may ensue. As a consequence of decreased cardiac output, systemic vascular resistance may be elevated to preserve systemic blood pressure.

In addition to the development of pulmonary edema, right ventricular failure, pulmonary hypertension, and decreased left ventricular output, mitral stenosis patients are at risk for emboli from the mitral valve into the arterial circulation, leading to cerebral, myocardial, and mesenteric infarctions. Finally, even though the left ventricle remains underloaded as a consequence of obstruction to ventricular filling, this does not mean that left ventricular function is by any means normal. Often, left ventricular function is impaired in the patient with mitral stenosis for any number of reasons. Consequently, after valvular replacement, left ventricular function may be significantly compromised. Therefore, in the mitral stenosis patient we are once again brought to the same two questions—that is, how can we support the patient until we are safely on cardiopulmonary bypass and then how do we wean the patient from bypass support?

The answer to the first question is rather obvious. The underloaded left ventricle needs time to fill and requires us to preserve a sinus rhythm so that the atrial contribution to ventricular filling is not eliminated. Naturally, anesthetic delivery can present any number of difficulties in maintaining an adequate left ventricular volume. Anesthetics can produce profound vasodilation resulting in decreased venous return to the heart, thereby impairing volume loading of the left ventricle. Rhythm disturbances (e.g., atrial ventricular dissociation, tachycardias, atrial fibrillation) that might occur at the time of anesthesia can further reduce the volume load delivered to the left ventricle. In patients with significant pulmonary hypertension, any hypoxemia or hypercarbia that might occur at the time of anesthetic induction can result in right ventricular failure, leading to underloading of the left ventricle as well. Institution of positive pressure ventilation in patients with right ventricular hypertrophy can alter the left ventricular geometry and further diminish left ventricular filling. The administration of vasoconstrictors to restore systemic pressure as a consequence of anesthesia-induced vasodilation can result in elevation of pulmonary arterial pressures further, potentially leading to right ventricular failure. Pancuronium or inotropes (i.e., ephedrine, dobutamine) can produce tachycardia that may reduce the time needed to adequately load the left ventricle through the stenotic mitral valve. Thus, to manage the patient to cardiopulmonary bypass can be exceptionally difficult because valvular obstruction prevents adequate loading of the left ventricle.

As usual, the specific agents chosen for anesthetic management are far less important than providing for adequate loading of the left ventricle. Synthetic narcotics (e.g., fentanyl) provide the basis of routine anesthetic management. Amnestics and muscle relaxants are likewise employed. Once the patient is asleep, we may have to correct any number of rhythm abnormalities and restore vascular tone to provide hemodynamic stability until cannulation for cardiopulmonary bypass. Close monitoring of the cardiac index by the pulmonary artery flotation catheter can assist us in finding the optimal volume load, heart rate, and vascular tone for adequate perfusion until bypass is initiated. Until bypass is initiated, the anesthetic management of the patient with mitral stenosis is partially performed by trial and error. For example, if phenylephrine is given to restore systemic vascular tone to augment blood pressure, alpha-agonist effects may increase pulmonary artery pressure, leading to impaired right ventricular function, further reducing cardiac performance. Similarly, vasodilators may reduce pulmonary hypertension to a degree, but likewise may reduce venous return to the heart, further diminishing left ventricular volume loading. In general, anesthetics that retard myocardial performance are avoided. With that one caveat, those agents available to the cardiac anesthesiologist must be used with the understanding that in the patient with mitral stenosis, hemodynamic compromise may occur for any number of reasons. The anesthesiologist must be able to adjust volume loading, myocardial contractility, and vascular tone as quickly as necessary to optimize the patient's performance. Last, in spite of all of our best efforts to provide hemodynamic stability, sometimes patients

Table 14-1. Procedure for Crashing onto Bypass

1. Administer heparin centrally.
2. Begin activated coagulation time and heparin analysis.
3. Surgeon places cannulas.
4. Bypass is initiated as per routine.
5. Confirm adequacy of flow with perfusionist.
6. Manage per bypass routine.

with mitral stenosis simply do not perform well. In this instance, we have no choice but to crash onto bypass. Although hardly elegant, restoration of perfusion via cardiopulmonary bypass does end a hemodynamic emergency (Table 14-1).

Should an arrhythmia contribute to the patient's deterioration, cardioversion must be performed quickly. A pulmonary artery catheter with atrial and ventricular pacing capability (i.e., a pacing pulmonary artery catheter) can be useful to ensure atrial contractility should the patient lose atrial contraction after anesthetic induction.

Once the patient is safely on cardiopulmonary bypass, the anesthesiologist then has time to catch his or her breath. This little rest is often necessary because the time to cardiopulmonary bypass in the patient with mitral stenosis can be quite challenging. Once cardioplegia is delivered, the valve is excised and a new mitral valve sewn into place.

This operation can take a variable amount of time after which we must again try to wean the patient from cardiopulmonary bypass (see Chapter 8). Often patients have poor ventricular function after mitral valve replacement secondary to mitral stenosis. This occurs for two reasons: (1) poor left ventricular function, and (2) pulmonary hypertension and right ventricular failure.

Poor left ventricular function can occur for any number of reasons: Inadequate cardioplegia delivery and air embolism in the coronary vasculature can be sources of perioperative ventricular dysfunction. The mitral stenosis patient also has chronic underloading of the left ventricle. The left ventricle may be unable to handle the increased volume load delivered once a new mitral valve is sewn into place. In this setting, the left ventricle may become distended, with the resulting increase in myocardial oxygen demand leading to subsequent left ventricular failure. Inotropic support, mechanical support, or both to wean from cardiopulmonary bypass may be necessary as described in Chapter 8.

Right ventricular failure can be difficult to correct after bypass. Pulmonary hypertension and right ventricular failure may be long-standing in patients with mitral stenosis. Even after the valvular obstruction has been relieved, patients who have developed significant pulmonary hypertension (e.g., pulmonary artery pressure is more than half systemic pressure) continue to be affected by elevated pulmonary artery pressures. Right ventricular dysfunction may occur as well and remain after correction of the mitral valve. Development of right ventricular failure can result in underloading of the left ventricle, resulting in systemic hypotension and biventricular heart failure. Likewise, any distension of the left ventricle secondary to poor ventricular function can further increase pulmonary artery pressures, leading to acute right ventricular failure. In either scenario, right ventricular dysfunction ensues and requires support. Should pulmonary hypertension and right ventricular failure develop, weaning from cardiopulmonary bypass will require varying agents including dobutamine, phosphodiesterase inhibitors, and vasodilators. Nitric oxide, as it becomes more routinely available in operating rooms across the country, may be used to lower pulmonary artery pressures and, it is hoped, improve right ventricular ejection. It may be necessary to call the pulmonologist or intensivist to assist in the delivery of nitric oxide. In many institutions, nitric oxide has found its way into the hospital through intensive care and pulmonary medicine rather than through the efforts of the anesthesiologist. This provides a good opportunity for shared management and an opportunity to demonstrate the skills that are necessary to be an effective cardiac anesthesiologist.

Vasodilators and inotropes are carefully titrated to optimize cardiac index. Again, using a trial and error approach, inotropes and vasodilators are adjusted to find the best combination at which right ventricular function is augmented, pulmonary artery pressures are reduced, and left ventricular function provides suitable hemodynamic stability. This is not easy. Indeed, it can be quite frustrating to manage the patient with right ventricular failure that occurs after mitral valve replacement. As always, retreat to cardiopulmonary bypass is available while new agents are loaded and plans made. Should all efforts fail and if the patient may survive, mechanical assistance with ventricular assist devices may be necessary.

It would be wonderful to identify a simple formula for managing this complex scenario of pulmonary hypertension, right ventricular failure, and left ventricular dysfunction. In reality, we can simply adjust the limited agents with which we work—namely catecholamines, phosphodiesterase inhibitors, and vasodilators—in such a way that we maximize cardiac index while reducing pulmonary arterial pressures. In our practice, we begin with a phosphodiesterase inhibitor (e.g., milrinone or amrinone) with an infusion of nitroglycerin. Other agents are added as necessary once we see how the patient progresses. If biventricular failure is present, an aggressive approach to patient management is needed. Isolated right ventricular failure may necessitate placement of a right ventricular assist device if the surgery is considered survivable. In the event left ventricular function is impaired as well, intra-aortic balloon counterpulsation may be useful. However, intra-aortic balloon counterpulsation may be of limited value if the patient's principal problem is elevated pulmonary arterial pressures and right ventricular dysfunction. Once a polypharmacy approach has been exhausted, including the use of a phosphodiesterase inhibitor (milrinone), a vasodilator (nitroglycerin), a vasoconstrictor (norepinephrine), and a beta agonist (dobutamine), there is little choice but to attempt some form of mechanical assistance.

TEE can be useful in assessing ventricular function after mitral valve replacement. Not only can TEE confirm that the valve is functioning correctly, but it also can assist in identifying both left and right ventricular dysfunction. Should ventricular assist devices be placed, TEE is necessary to rule out the presence of intraventricular shunts that could lead to right-to-left shunting if left ventricular assist device placement is required.

Regurgitant Lesions

Whereas stenotic lesions require maintenance of vascular tone and reduced heart rate to optimize ventricular filling and ventricular ejection, regurgitant lesions necessitate reduced diastolic time (i.e., increasing heart rate) and lowered vascular tone to improve ventricular ejection. Mild tachycardia and systemic vasodilation become the goals of prebypass management for the patient with a regurgitant lesion. Fortunately, this is easy to achieve. Often, patients undergoing anesthesia end up both vasodilated and tachycardic. Maintaining vasodilation and tachycardia is significantly easier to achieve than is slowing the heart rate and preserving vascular tone as is desirable in the care of patients with stenotic lesions. Mild tachycardia can be a consequence of anesthetic management. Likewise, vasodilation is so common following anesthesia induction that it is routinely corrected by the use of small amounts of vasopressors (e.g., phenylephrine). What is important in dealing with regurgitant lesions is that unlike stenotic lesions, which generally progress over time, regurgitant lesions can develop either acutely or as a consequence of chronic valvular insufficiency. Patient management is often dependent on the time course of the valvular pathology.

Aortic Insufficiency

Aortic insufficiency may occur for any number of reasons: Infectious endocarditis or rheumatic heart disease, dilation of the aortic root as a consequence of connective tissue disease, Marfan's syndrome, vasculitis, and syphilis can all result in the patient developing chronic aortic insufficiency. From an anesthesia standpoint, the principal issue is not how aortic insufficiency develops but rather the time course and acuity of that insufficiency. Gradually developing aortic insufficiency is generally compensated for by the heart. Acute aortic insufficiency, however, can lead to cardiogenic shock and a high risk of imminent patient death. Thus, how we manage the patient often depends on the amount of time over which aortic insufficiency has developed.

Patients with chronic aortic insufficiency generally become dyspneic as a consequence of volume overload of the left ventricle. Incompetency of the aortic valve leads to ventricular dysfunction and pulmonary hypertension. Acute aortic insufficiency places a huge volume load on a left ventricle potentially unable to compensate for the increase in volume. Without the ventricular dilation that compensates for chronic aortic insufficiency, patients with acute aortic insufficiency develop rapid increases in left ventricular end-diastolic pressure. An elevated left ventricular end-diastolic pressure is transmitted to the pulmonary vasculature. Pulmonary edema ensues and the patient frequently presents to surgery in cardiogenic shock. Thus, patients with aortic insufficiency are seen by anesthesiologists under two very different circumstances. In one sense, the patient with chronic aortic insufficiency is taken for elective surgical repair, whereas the patient with an acute decompensation is frequently in cardiogenic shock, requiring all the hemodynamic supports available for patient management. Whether acute or chronic, the principal issues in addressing the patient with valvular surgery remain: (1) How do we place the patient on cardiopulmonary bypass, and (2) how do we get the patient off of it once the valve has been replaced?

For patients undergoing elective repair, anesthetic induction often can improve the forward flow of blood from the left ventricle. Vasodilation occurring as a consequence of anesthesia induction may improve left ventricular ejection. Mild tachycardia that similarly may result from anesthetic agents lowers diastolic time, thereby reducing the time for regurgitant flow. Thus, the routine effects of some anesthetics, mainly tachycardia and vasodilation, may assist in improving myocardial performance. Drugs that increase vascular tone, such as phenylephrine, may increase regurgitant blood flow. Nonetheless, we must be careful not to allow the patient too great a degree of vasodilation. The diastolic pressure may become dangerously low. Because left coronary artery perfusion occurs during diastole, too great a reduction in diastolic pressure may lead to myocardial ischemia. Therefore, we must attempt to reduce vascular tone without necessarily lowering left ventricular coronary perfusion pressure to the point of ischemia. Generally, a cocktail of narcotics, muscle relaxants, and amnestics serves adequately for induction. Inhalational anesthetics may be added as necessary.

Patients with acute aortic insufficiency, on the other hand, often present in the setting of an acute aortic dissection. These patients frequently present in cardiogenic shock. Many are already intubated and receiving various degrees of pharmacologic support. In this setting, anesthetic management may involve simply the administration of muscle relaxants (if blood pressure is significantly reduced, e.g., less than 50 mm Hg systolic) or the titration of the anesthetics in small amounts (e.g., amnestics, narcotics) in addition to muscle relaxants as the patient tolerates. If a patient with acute aortic insufficiency and aortic dissection presents unintubated but in cardiogenic shock, the airway must be carefully secured and anesthesia safely induced. A rapid sequence induction and intubation is necessary because many patients will not have been on NPO orders. Small amounts of amnestics, narcotics, etomidate, and muscle relaxants may be administered to facilitate intubation. If the patient is profoundly hypotensive (i.e., systolic pressure is less than 50 mm Hg), the patient may simply require muscle relaxants followed by intubation. Narcotics may then be administered as tolerated. Certainly, the patient presenting in cardiogenic shock will tolerate the administration of vasodilators and myocardial depressants poorly. In this regard, until cardiopulmonary bypass is instituted, the anesthetist's time may principally be spent on ongoing resuscitation. Open chest cardiac massage may be necessary to provide blood flow until cardiopulmonary bypass can be initiated. Because the patient with acute aortic insufficiency most likely also suffers from acute aortic dissection, surgical repair frequently involves replacement of the aortic root and possibly the aortic arch. Aortic arch surgery requires periods of circulatory arrest and profound hypothermia. This kind of patient management is both time and resource consuming. The surgeon should be certain that at least some potential for survival exists before bringing the patient with acute pathology to the operating room. Unfortunately, it is often not known whether the patient can survive and as a consequence many patients are taken through hours of surgery only to have profound cardiac or neurologic injuries (see Chapter 13).

Whether the patient presents with acute aortic insufficiency or as a consequence of a chronically regurgitant valve, these patients often have poor ventricular function postbypass. Prolonged bypass runs can be expected, particularly if the aortic root needs to be replaced in addition to the valve. Patients who have presented for repair after acute insufficiency and cardiogenic shock may be expected to have multisystem organ dysfunction, renal failure, respiratory embarrassment, and coagulopathy, all of which may complicate weaning from cardiopulmonary bypass. In either event, we may assume that ventricular function is impaired. Left and right ventricular failure may occur in this setting as a consequence of either long-standing ventricular volume overload (as in chronic aortic insufficiency) or as a consequence of myocardial ischemia potentially developing at the time of aortic dissection. TEE not only assesses the adequacy of the valvular repair, but also provides some insight into the patient's left and right ventricular function. A combination of vasodilators, inotropes, vasoconstrictors, and mechanical assist devices, as previously described, needs to be employed to wean following valvular replacement. Weaning the patient from bypass support proceeds as with any patient with impaired ventricular function (see Chapter 8).

Mitral Valve Regurgitation

Aortic insufficiency can occur as a consequence of many etiologies. So too can a number of pathologies affect the mitral apparatus. These include endocarditis, ruptured chordae tendineae, dysfunctional papillary muscles, and rheumatic heart disease. Degeneration of the mitral apparatus can likewise lead to mitral regurgitation. As with aortic insufficiency, mitral regurgitation may develop clinically as either an acute or a chronic event. Acute mitral regurgitation secondary to ischemic injury often leads to rapid decompensation and cardiogenic shock. As with aortic insufficiency, chronic mitral regurgitation is better tolerated. The left atrium enlarges to accept flow from the left ventricle. Eventually, in the chronic mitral regurgitation patient, pulmonary hypertension and right ventricular failure may ensue. In the patient experiencing acute mitral regurgitation secondary to ischemia or infarction, the left atrium cannot dilate to the degree needed to accept the volume delivered through the regurgitant mitral valve, leading to acute pulmonary edema and right ventricular failure. Biventricular failure occurs, and the patient frequently presents in cardiogenic shock.

Like aortic insufficiency, management until bypass is initially directed at minimizing regurgitant flow and improving forward left ventricular ejection. Mild tachycardia and vasodilation may help to improve left ventricular output and minimize mitral regurgitation. In chronic mitral insufficiency, a narcotic, amnestic, and muscle relaxant anesthetic generally provides suitable conditions to safely manage the patient until cardiopulmonary bypass is initiated. Those patients presenting to the operating room with acute mitral insufficiency often are in cardiogenic shock. They are frequently intubated and routinely require multiple inotropes and vasodilators. Anesthetic management is directed at maintaining systemic perfusion until cardiopulmonary bypass can be expeditiously initiated. Anesthetic management in this instance consists of muscle relaxants and those anesthetics that can be hemodynamically tolerated by the patient at any particular moment. Should the patient be awake and responsive but remain in cardiogenic shock, a rapid induction with a muscle relaxant and small amounts of etomidate, midazolam, or sufentanil may provide suitable hemodynamic stability to facilitate intubation. Resuscitative efforts may be ongoing until bypass is initiated. Should the patient acutely decompensate, it will be necessary to crash onto bypass.

Once bypass has been initiated, the regurgitant mitral valve may be repaired rather than replaced. In patients undergoing mitral valve repair, facility with TEE is essential to assess the adequacy of repair (i.e., to be sure that mitral regurgitation has been minimized or eliminated) after completion of the surgeon's work. It is not unusual for a mitral repair to be ineffective, leaving a significant mitral regurgitant flow even after the surgeon has attempted to repair the mitral valve.

At this point, facility with TEE becomes essential in making definitive clinical decisions. If TEE is incorrectly interpreted, it is possible that patients may receive an inadequate repair, leaving them with continued mitral regurgitation after surgery. Frequently, this necessitates a return trip to the operating room for eventual mitral valve replacement. Often, it is in the anesthesiologist's interest to have the interpretation of the adequacy of the mitral valve repair confirmed not only by the cardiac surgeon, but also by a second anesthesiologist or cardiologist. Such duplication can help to eliminate any subjective variability in TEE interpretation. TEE also helps to confirm air removal from the heart following mitral replacement or repair.

Once the mitral valve has been replaced or repaired, the patient needs to be weaned from cardiopulmonary bypass. Again, the ease with which the patient is weaned from bypass support is often dependent on his or her preoperative condition. Patients presenting with acute mitral regurgitation and cardiogenic shock frequently have significant injury to other organ systems, in particular, the kidneys, potentially complicating postoperative management. As the patient with acute mitral regurgitation is likely to have experienced significant myocardial ischemia, it is probable that ventricular dysfunction will be likely secondary to recent myocardial infarction. Arrhythmias may further complicate separation from cardiopulmonary bypass. In patients who have undergone repair or replacement for chronic mitral insufficiency, the regurgitant pathway for low impedance ventricular ejection (into the left atrium) is eliminated. As a consequence, this can result in an increase in left ventricular end-diastolic pressure, ventricular distension, myocardial ischemia, and difficulty weaning from cardiopulmonary bypass. In both instances, inotropes, vasodilators, and mechanical assist devices as previously described may well be necessary to effect separation from cardiopulmonary bypass (see Chapter 8).

Tricuspid Disease

The tricuspid valve separates the right atrium from the right ventricle. Although the right ventricle was once thought to be a passive conduit, the right ventricle actively loads the left heart and as such is a critical component in generating cardiac index. Right ventricular failure can lead to circulatory collapse. Proper functioning of the tricuspid valve is critical to everyone's well-being. Tricuspid stenosis results in a pressure gradient developing between the right atrium and the right ventricle. Patients present signs of right ventricular failure characterized by development of ascites and hepatomegaly. Tricuspid stenosis is associated with rheumatic disease. Anesthetic management is directed at maintaining an adequate venous return to the heart. Certainly, positive pressure ventilation can result in reduced venous return, potentially leading to circulatory embarrassment in an underloaded right ventricle secondary to tricuspid stenosis. Anesthetics producing significant vasodilation may likewise impair venous return to the heart, further decreasing right ventricular output. Once the stenosis has been relieved, patients may develop both right-sided and left-sided heart failure as a consequence of volume overload in chronically underloaded ventricles. Pharmacologic and mechanical support as previously described may be necessary to effectively manage the patient.

Tricuspid regurgitation often occurs secondary to other valvular lesions such as mitral stenosis or pathologies that result in pulmonary hypertension. Intravenous drug abuse may lead to the development of endocarditis in which the tricuspid valve becomes the source of infectious vegetations. Generally, management of the patient with tricuspid regurgitation is principally directed toward the primary lesion, namely, correction of mitral or other valvular heart disease. Anesthetic techniques are chosen to correct the principal valvular lesion. Nonetheless, the presence of tricuspid regurgitation can impair right ventricular function, which in pulmonary hypertension may lead to ineffective right ventricular performance, resulting in not only right ventricular failure but also the underloading of the left ventricle and cardiogenic shock. As usual, pharmacologic and mechanical support may be necessary to effectively wean the patient following correction of tricuspid regurgitation as with any other valvular pathology that may exist.

Hypertrophic Cardiomyopathy

Idiopathic hypertrophic subaortic stenosis leads to obstruction of the aortic outflow tract. Unlike the fixed obstruction of aortic stenosis, idiopathic hypertrophic subaortic stenosis presents a dynamic obstruction that occurs as the ventricle contracts, leading to a reduction in ventricular outflow. Maneuvers that increase ventricular size (i.e., increased afterload, increased preload, and decreased myocardial contractility) decrease the obstruction and improve the forward flow of blood.

Inotropic agents, decreased ventricular volumes, and vasodilators all tend to exacerbate outflow obstruction. In patients with hypertrophic cardiomyopathy, the hypertrophied ventricular septum contacts the anterior leaflet of the mitral valve, leading to a narrowed ventricular outflow path. Medical therapy is aimed at reducing ventricular contractility (i.e., beta blockade). If this is ineffective, the patient is taken to surgery for septal myomectomy, mitral valve replacement, or both. Management of the patient is aimed at reducing outflow obstruction until cardiopulmonary bypass is initiated by providing a suitable volume to the left ventricle and an elevated vascular resistance. Phenylephrine is employed to preserve vascular tone after anesthesia induction with a variety of agents. The patient's preoperative medical regimen may be continued to prevent an increase in myocardial contractility secondary to preoperative anxiety and its associated increase in sympathetic outflow. Adequate volume replacement is essential once positive pressure ventilation is initiated to be certain that the heart is adequately loaded. Inhalational anesthetics may be given to decrease myocardial contractility, along with beta-blockers. Short-acting beta-blockers such as esmolol can be useful in providing transient reductions in myocardial contractility until bypass flow is initiated. Systemic vascular tone can be maintained with phenylephrine, which may be administered by either bolus or infusion. Once cardiopulmonary bypass is initiated, the surgeon performs either valvular replacement to relieve obstruction from the anterior leaflet of the mitral valve, septal myomectomy, or both. TEE is useful to be certain that the obstruction has been relieved after completion of the myomectomy or valvular replacement. Distortions in ventricular anatomy as a consequence of the resection may impair myocardial performance when weaning from cardiopulmonary bypass. Heart block and the development of ventricular septal defects are of particular concern. Competency of an unreplaced mitral valve needs to be assessed also. Development of a perioperative ventricular septal defect and mitral regurgitation must be ruled out before the patient leaves the operating room. Weaning from cardiopulmonary bypass may be initiated using protocols described in Chapter 8.

15

The Cardiac Anesthesiologist and Postoperative Care

After having spent a variable amount of time caring for patients such as Mr. XY, we can look forward to safely delivering them to the intensive care unit (ICU). Once this is done (and indeed transport to ICU can be quite difficult), we must come to an understanding of what the anesthesiologist's role is in the ICU.

As we face numerous reductions in reimbursement, a movement has taken hold to transform anesthesia into a specialty called perioperative medicine. Although our involvement in total patient management appears to be a valid and worthy goal, we must nevertheless be prepared to commit our resources to undertake this endeavor successfully. Management of patients such as Mr. XY and others in the ICU provides us with an opportunity to demonstrate successfully our ability as perioperative physicians or to fail miserably as the "gas passers of bygone days." How we are perceived largely depends on how effectively we do what we say we will do. On the one hand, if we are gifted with a quality ICU nursing staff, it is possible for the busy clinical anesthesiologist to assist in patient management while simultaneously practicing operating room anesthesia—that is, ventilatory adjustments, titration of vasoactive infusions, diabetes control, and so forth can be accomplished through communication with an experienced nursing staff. If this kind of "housekeeping" management is expected of the operating room anesthesiologist, these goals can be readily attained by the operating room practitioner. In other words, if being a perioperative physician means only to make those adjustments that can be made while already involved with another patient, we can easily practice perioperative medicine.

Of course, this is hardly the ideal role for the cardiac anesthesiologist in caring for the cardiac patient in the ICU. Ideally, a dedicated anesthesiologist should be available to provide for an immediate response to patient's needs in the ICU. A sudden fibrillatory arrest is difficult to treat when the perioperative anesthesiologist is already occupied in the operating room with a "to follow" patient. In this event, claiming to be a total perioperative physician can only lead the anesthesiologist into great difficulty if he or she is unable to respond to a patient emergency. Thus, anesthesiologists have only a few options in dealing with postoperative intensive care, including the following:

1.   The patient is managed by the surgeon after delivery in the ICU by the anesthesiologist. This is a frequent method of practice in community care. Once the patient is delivered to the ICU, all medical orders are at the discretion of the surgeon. From the anesthesiologist's standpoint, this allows the anesthesiologist to concentrate on the next patient undergoing anesthesia without responsibility for postoperative care. Unfortunately, this also denies the patient the potentially valuable insights of the anesthesiologist in assisting in postoperative management. Although this method may be most common in community care, it is certainly true that in many of the large university settings with strong cardiac surgery programs and weak anesthesia departments, there is little influence of the anesthesiologist in postoperative management at all. Indeed, even if anesthesiology intensivists are present, the surgeons often continue to dominate postoperative care.

2.   The anesthesiologist assumes full responsibility for ICU management. In this model, the anesthesiologist provides the primary perioperative ICU services. The attending surgeon addresses surgical concerns (e.g., wound healing, chest tubes, and so forth), whereas medical management is left to an intensive care team under the anesthesiologist's direction. This approach provides both the surgeon and the operating room anesthesiologist the opportunity to devote attention to their follow-up patients. Of course, such a model requires a dedicated ICU anesthesia team with 24-hour attending coverage and the authority from the surgeon to make critical decisions. None of these things are readily achieved. In a few university centers, anesthesiologists have assumed responsibility for postoperative care. In general, these institutions are supplied with an inexpensive source of resident and fellow labor to staff these units on a 24-hour basis, 365 days per year. Such a deployment is often difficult to maintain in community cardiac practice.

3. The anesthesiologist, surgeon, pulmonologist, and others contribute to patient management. In this approach, the surgeon remains responsible for the ICU care of the patient. Medical intensivists and pulmonologists, along with the cardiac anesthesiologist, assist the surgeon with management as necessary. This approach continues anesthesia involvement with the patient following surgery and allows the patient the opportunity to possibly benefit from the anesthesiologist's input in postoperative management. Ideally, this provides the most collegial management scheme by which various practitioners recognize and appreciate the abilities and skills of one another.

If we are to be the practitioners of perioperative medicine that ultimately we may hope to be, we must aim toward eventually supplying complete perioperative care, including ICU management. Still, economic questions and "turf battles" between the surgery and anesthesiology and pulmonary and anesthesiology fields make this worthy ideal difficult to achieve in both the university and community settings. Because many university departments have not yet achieved the status of providing complete perioperative medicine, it is unlikely that in community practice cardiac anesthesiology practitioners will more easily deliver total perioperative care. Nevertheless, physician anesthesiologists, if they are to continue to exist, must continually emphasize their abilities both in and out of the operating room. Ultimately, it is the patient such as our friend Mr. XY who will benefit most from anesthesia involvement in perioperative intensive care.

Having completed this editorial gloss, it is now time to focus on those areas that we need to address in dealing with postoperative care of the cardiac surgery patient. Because practice model 3 (i.e., the cooperative model) remains the one most easily achieved in the community setting, we address the management of those issues that can be attended to by a cardiac anesthesiologist with responsibilities for operating room care. We emphasize those areas in which the anesthesiologist might be primarily responsible (i.e., respiratory care and pain management) and where he or she may assist with consultation (i.e., managing renal dysfunction, neurologic injury, and so forth). To facilitate our discussion, we take a collegial approach in addressing our sample patient, Mr. XY, who now suffers innumerable complications from surgery.

Pulmonary Complications

As previously mentioned, patients presenting for cardiac surgery often have coexisting pulmonary disease. Both chronic obstructive pulmonary disease (e.g., emphysema, chronic bronchitis, and so forth) and restrictive lung disease (e.g., pulmonary fibrosis, external chest wall restrictions such as obesity) may complicate perioperative management of the cardiac surgical patient. Additionally, many patients without preexisting pulmonary disease may develop postoperative atelectasis and pulmonary edema that can impair respiratory gas exchange.

The combination of chronic pulmonary disease coupled with the effects of cardiac surgery can make pulmonary management in the ICU quite difficult. Because anesthesiologists generally have significant experience in dealing with management of the airway and the use of mechanical ventilators, postoperative pulmonary function ideally should be addressed by the operating room anesthesiologist.

Patients such as Mr. XY, whom you may recall was relatively free of pulmonary disease before undergoing coronary artery bypass (CAB), require mechanical ventilation for brief periods after routine CAB. Some patients can be routinely extubated in the operating room after minimally invasive CAB; however, the many effects of cardiopulmonary bypass and the potential for coagulopathy when cardiopulmonary bypass is employed may leave patients somewhat unstable at the conclusion of surgery. To ensure a patent airway and to facilitate other management, patients are often routinely anesthetized, paralyzed, and ventilated at the conclusion of cardiac surgery.

Although there are many timetables available by which the routine CAB patient may be awakened and extubated after surgery, there is no one universal rule. Many patients can be awakened and extubated in the surgical suite after CAB with cardiopulmonary bypass. Nevertheless, rapid deterioration can occur in the immediate postoperative period (e.g., from arrhythmias, pericardial tamponade, and so forth). It is prudent to keep the patient ventilated for some time postoperatively. Additional doses of muscle relaxants, narcotics, and amnestics may be needed so that the patient can tolerate endotracheal intubation during elective postoperative ventilation. Administration of propofol by continuous infusion can provide patients with adequate sedation so that they can tolerate mechanical ventilation in the immediate postoperative period. They can be readily awakened on discontinuation of the propofol infusion. Should sedation with propofol be planned, nursing staff must be made aware of the potential infective risks of propofol due to its ability to support bacterial growth. Strict adherence to aseptic techniques by the anesthesiology and nursing staffs alike will prevent the development of septicemia.

Patients managed with a narcotic-based anesthetic may be relatively anesthetized at the conclusion of the procedure from residual anesthetic medications. In this instance, it may not be necessary to supplement the anesthetics postoperatively. Nevertheless, many patients find themselves in the ICU intubated, partially paralyzed, and relatively awake in considerable discomfort. Tachycardia and hypertension not only can lead to the potential for myocardial ischemia (although we hope this has been corrected), but also will panic the surgeon concerned about bleeding from an anastomotic site. To avoid both immediate postoperative hypertension and a panicked surgeon, it is far better to ensure that the patient remains relatively asleep and hemodynamically stable immediately after surgery. Propofol allows us to achieve this end without necessarily having to maintain prolonged intubation. Propofol administration is titrated to effect by intravenous infusion. The dose must be titrated to the individual patient. Sedation with propofol and other agents should be commenced before transporting the patient from the operating room to the ICU. Obviously, the addition of anesthetic drugs may lead to decreased cardiac output and vasodilation. Thus, the anesthesiologist must be certain that a stable hemodynamic profile remains after the administration of additional amnestics and narcotics. At the time of transport from the operating room the patient should be easily ventilated by hand and monitored per the hospital routine. Because motion may impair the electrocardiographic signal on the travel monitor, it is often best to follow the arterial pressure tracing to provide a reliable monitor not only of electrical activity and rhythm of the heart, but also of the adequacy of systemic perfusion pressure. Even if the electrocardiographic trace is less than clear, an arterial trace that appears to be more or less regular ensures both an effective rhythm and an adequate blood pressure.

If infusions of vasoactive drugs are continued throughout transport, care is taken to avoid the loss of intravenous lines and monitors during mobilization. Of course, most experienced anesthesiologists at one time or another have lost an occasional intravenous line at the time of transport.

As hospitals reduce staffing in response to managed care, the number of assistants available to help transport patients decreases precipitously. It is important to have a suitable number of staff available to assist in patient movement. Often the loss of monitors and intravenous lines can be attributed to an inadequate number of individuals available to free the anesthesiologist to concentrate on patient monitoring and the safe transport of intravenous lines.

Routine Ventilatory Management

On arriving in the ICU, the patient is placed on mechanical ventilation. If the patient has been extubated in the operating room as is common

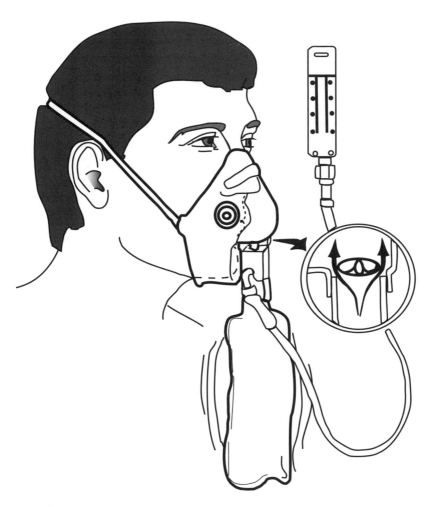

Figure 15-1. *A nonrebreathing mask. (Modified from WJ Hoffman, JD Was-nick. Postoperative Critical Care of the Massachusetts General Hospital. Boston: Little, Brown, 1992;41.)*

in minimally invasive surgery, the patient should be transported with sup-plemental oxygen administered via a nonrebreathing mask (Figure 15-1).

If the patient is at risk for ventilatory failure secondary to the elim-ination of hypoxic respiratory drive, that patient should remain venti-lated postoperatively even after minimally invasive surgery. Patients are placed on a mechanical ventilator with a volume cycle ventilator after

Table 15-1. Modes of Mechanical Ventilation

Mode	Description
Intermittent mandatory ventilation (IMV)	Ventilator delivers a preset tidal volume and respiratory rate. Patient can spontaneously breathe between IMV breaths.
Assist control ventilation (AC)	Ventilator delivers a preset tidal volume and a backup respiratory rate. Patient triggers full mechanical breaths through his or her own respiratory efforts.
Control mandatory ventilation (CMV)	Ventilator delivers a preset tidal volume and respiratory rate.
Pressure support ventilation (PSV)	Ventilator delivers a gas volume to a preset airway pressure. Patient's respiratory effort determines the respiratory rate. The tidal volume is determined by pulmonary compliance. The more compliant, the greater the tidal volume for a given amount of pressure support.
Inverse ratio ventilation (IRV)	Ventilator delivers a breath in which the inspiratory time is greater than the expiratory times. IRV recruits alveoli in noncompliant lungs (e.g., patients with adult respiratory distress syndrome).
Positive end-expiratory pressure (PEEP)	Ventilator recruits alveoli to increase the functional residual capacity of the lung, improving oxygenation. PEEP maintains a positive airway pressure at the end of a ventilation cycle.

cardiac surgery. The ventilator delivers a given gas volume during inspiration. A number of ventilatory modes are currently available on modern ventilators with which the CAB patient may be managed. In routine circumstances, however, intermittent mandatory ventilation (IMV) can be easily used. Table 15-1 describes a number of modes of ventilation.

When patients arrive from the operating room to the ICU, ventilator orders are given as described in Table 15-2. Common ventilatory settings are listed here:

   1.   *The mode.* IMV is generally chosen for routine cases. Assist control or control mandatory ventilation may be employed if pro-

tracted ventilation is envisioned. Generally the inspired oxygen concentration (FIO_2) is started at 60% but may be increased depending on how adequate the oxygen saturation has been in the operating room. Pulse oximetry is useful to immediately assess the adequacy of the FIO_2 to meet the patient's oxygen needs.

2.   *Minute ventilation = body weight (kg) × 100.* A tidal volume of 10–15 cc per kg is set along with a respiratory rate of 8–12 breaths per minute to generate the appropriate minute ventilation. In patients with left or right internal mammary artery grafts, expansion of the lungs can lead to disruption of the anastomosis. Most surgeons test lung expansion in the operating room to be certain that there is sufficient room for the lungs to expand without producing stretch or tearing the bypass grafts. In setting the postoperative tidal volume, it is important that the lungs be expanded no more than that which was tested in the operating room. In the case that the graft should fall apart, the surgeon most certainly will blame the venti-

Table 15-2. Ventilatory Orders in the Intensive Care Unit

Ventilator orders on arrival to the intensive care unit*

Mode	IMV
FIO_2	60–100% initially
Rate	8–12 breaths/min
Tidal volume	10–15 cc/kg
PEEP	2–5 cm H_2O
I:E ratio	1:2–1:3

Adjunctive orders

CPT

    Types of CPT: turning, postural drainage, vibration, percussion, etc.

    Frequency

    Cautions to therapist or nurse

Aerosol medications

    Device (nebulizer, USN, hydrosphere)

    Dose

    Dilution and diluent

    Frequency

    When to withhold

Weaning orders

All types of weaning

FiO$_2$

PEEP

Timing of measurements: arterial blood gas levels, VC, IF

When to call physician (e.g., systolic blood pressure of >200, respiratory rate of >35, diaphoresis)

IMV weaning

IMV respiratory rate

Conventional weaning

T piece or CPAP

How long off ventilator

How often off ventilator

Earliest and latest time of day for weaning

IMV = intermittent mandatory ventilation; FiO$_2$ = inspired oxygen concentration; PEEP = positive end-expiratory pressure; I:E = ratio of inspirations to expirations; CPT = chest physiotherapy; USN = ultrasonic nebulizer; VC = vital capacity; IF = inspiratory force; CPAP = continuous positive airway pressure.
*These are ventilator settings commonly used in the usual postoperative anesthetized adult patient on arrival in the intensive care unit. Exceptions certainly occur.
Source: Modified with permission from WJ Hoffman, JD Wasnick. Postoperative Critical Care of the Massachusetts General Hospital. Boston: Little, Brown, 1992;47.

latory management for the problem if a tidal volume larger than what has been tested in the operating room has been delivered.

3. *Inspiratory to expiratory ratio.* Generally, the respiratory therapist adjusts the inspiratory to expiratory ratio. An inspiratory to expiratory ratio of 1 to 2 is suitable for most patients. Individuals with obstructive pulmonary disease require a longer expiratory time. Inverse ratio ventilation lengthens the inspiratory time to improve oxygenation in patients with respiratory failure.

4. *Positive end-expiratory pressure (PEEP).* PEEP recruits collapsed alveoli, thereby increasing the functional residual capacity of the lung. After surgery, atelectasis causes a reduction in functional residual capacity that is quite common. A PEEP of 5 cm H$_2$O is routinely given so that the FiO$_2$ may be reduced. Although PEEP has been proposed as a prophylaxis against adult respiratory distress syn-

drome, this has not been shown to be the case. PEEP is not without potential complications. It can contribute to a reduced venous return to the heart, a reduced cardiac output, an increase in barotrauma, and an increase in secretion of antidiuretic hormone, leading to a decrease in urine output. In cases of severe hypoxemia in which higher levels of PEEP are employed, a PEEP of much greater than 10 cm H_2O can lead to an intraventricular septal shift, distorting the left ventricular anatomy and potentially compromising left ventricular filling and cardiac output. Often a "best PEEP" is sought, being the point at which the improvement of oxygen delivery to the tissues is greatest. This is done by examining mixed venous oxygen saturation to assess the results of improved oxygenation as a consequence of PEEP versus the potential decrease in cardiac output occurring as a result of the effect of PEEP on the venous return.

Once these ventilator orders are given, the respiratory therapist puts the patient on the ventilator. As the patient is put on the ventilator, the anesthesiologist should observe the patient to be certain that ventilation is acceptable. The rise and fall of the chest should be noted. Lungs should be auscultated. The endotracheal tube should be checked, as it may become kinked or dislodged during transport. A right main stem bronchus intubation also can occur as a consequence of transportation. Pulse oximetry and capnography should be used in the ICU as much as they are in the operating room. Fifteen to 30 minutes after the patient arrives in the ICU and after institution of mechanical ventilation, an arterial blood gas is obtained.

Problems with Mechanical Ventilation

Several common occurrences can complicate patient management:

1. The endotracheal tube becomes dislodged. The airway should be reestablished.

2. Mucus plugs the endotracheal tube. The endotracheal tube should be suctioned.

3. Bronchospasm may occur, especially in chronic obstructive pulmonary disease. Albuterol (beta$_2$-agonist), 0.2–0.3 ml of 0.5% solution in 2–3 ml normal saline via nebulizer, should be begun. Severe bronchospasm may require intravenous epinephrine.

4. A pneumothorax or hemothorax may develop. A chest tube should be placed.

5. Respiratory failure in the postoperative cardiac patient may complicate recovery and lead to patient death in spite of a successful surgical procedure. The inability to successfully oxygenate the postoperative cardiac patient can fundamentally occur because of only three etiologies: hypoventilation, ventilation perfusion mismatch, and shunting.

Decreased ventilation with increasing carbon dioxide tension leads to hypoxemia. Therapy is directed at improving ventilation by adjusting tidal volume and respiratory rate.

Ventilation-perfusion mismatch represents the primary source of arterial hypoxemia in any number of pulmonary diseases. Atelectasis, pneumonia, and adult respiratory distress syndrome all produce hypoxemia because of the inability of the lung to effectively match ventilation with perfusion.

Right-to-left shunting does occur in the cardiac surgical patient. Patients with a patent foramen ovale or atrial septal defect can produce right-to-left shunting in the event that left atrial pressure decreases below right atrial pressure. Left ventricular assist device placement may be complicated by shunting across a patent foramen ovale or atrial septal defect because of right to left shunting in the setting of the drainage of the blood volume from the left ventricle. Transesophageal echocardiography must rule out any intra-atrial defects prior to using a left ventricular assist device on the failing ventricle.

Problems with ventilation can complicate the postoperative recovery of the cardiac surgical patient. Elevation of arterial carbon dioxide tension ($PaCO_2$) can occur for only two primary reasons: increased carbon dioxide (CO_2) production (i.e., malignant hyperthermia, shivering) or decreased ventilation. Increased CO_2 production is not uncommon after surgery because hypothermic patients shiver secondary to thermogenesis. Severely hypothermic patients should be paralyzed with nondepolarizing muscle relaxants and warmed to prevent the increase in oxygen consumption and CO_2 production that accompanies shivering. Inadequate ventilation may contribute to an increase in CO_2 tension for a number of reasons, including bronchospasm and chronic obstructive pulmonary disease.

Should the patient develop hypoxemia in the immediate postoperative period he or she should be evaluated as described in Figure 15-2.

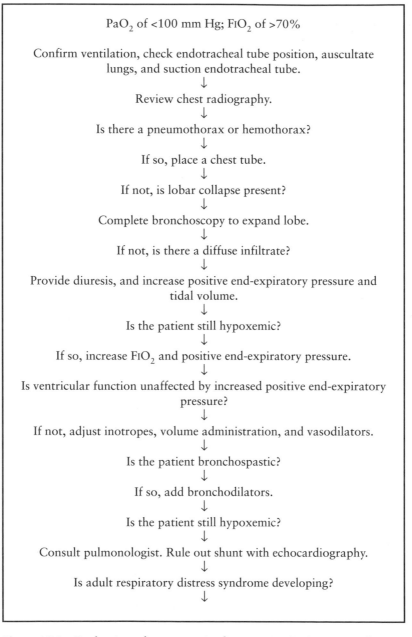

Figure 15-2. *Evaluation of postoperative hypoxemia. (PaO$_2$ = arterial oxygen saturation; FiO$_2$ = inspired oxygen concentration.)*

Continue supportive care, continue invasive monitoring, treat pneumonia, renal dysfunction, pulmonary hypertension, and so forth. Paralyze and sedate patient. Begin inverse ratio ventilation and attempt to improve oxygenation.
↓
Continue supportive ventilatory care. Watch for barotrauma. Provide nutritional support.
↓
Await respiratory improvement.

There are a number of calculations that are helpful in assessing the critically ill patient with postoperative pulmonary disease (Table 15-3).

Whether patients will develop pulmonary embarrassment postoperatively is difficult to predict. Heart surgery remains a traumatic event that can be complicated with significant blood loss and blood product replacement. Alveolar capillary leakage associated with adult respiratory distress syndrome can present in the postoperative period to the point of the development of pulmonary fibrosis, pulmonary hypertension, right ventricular failure, and subsequent patient death. Consultation with a pulmonologist or anesthesia intensivist early in the course of the patient's ICU course may be helpful to provide adequate support. Sepsis and renal dysfunction should be addressed as well. Nutritional support must be provided if the patient requires prolonged ventilation. Careful attention to patient positioning must be made if the patient is at bed rest for a prolonged period. Although numerous experimental therapies have been tried to treat adult respiratory distress syndrome the essence of therapy for the patient with respiratory failure remains aggressive support through ventilatory management and correction of underlying disease processes in the hope that pulmonary function will improve.

Should the postoperative cardiac surgery patient develop adult respiratory distress syndrome (ARDS), care must be taken to avoid lung trauma from overdistension of the few functional alveoli that might participate in the patient's gas exchange. Inverse ratio ventilation is used to attempt to improve oxygenation. High-frequency oscillatory ventilation employs less than dead space tidal volumes in an effort to

Table 15-3. Evaluating Respiratory Failure

1. Obtain arterial blood gas/SaO_2
2. Obtain mixed venous blood gas/SvO_2
3. Calculate alveolar gas equation:

$$PAO_2 = FIO_2 \times (P_B - 47) - \frac{PaCO_2}{RQ}$$

   PAO_2 = alveolar oxygen tension
   PaO_2 = arterial oxygen tension
   FIO_2 = inspired oxygen tension
   P_B = barometric pressure
   47 = partial pressure of water vapor
   $PaCO_2$ = arterial CO_2 gas tension
   RQ = respiratory quotient
   Normal PaO_2 on 100% FIO_2 = 600–500 mm Hg
4. Calculate A-a gradient. Increases in A-a gradient signify $\dot{V}/\dot{Q}$ mismatch
   $[PAO_2 - PaO_2]$.

recruit additional lung volume to participate in gas exchange with a reduction in lung trauma. As additional studies become available, high-frequency oscillatory ventilation may prove to be useful in the management of adult ARDS patients.

Weaning the Postoperative Cardiac Surgical Patient from Ventilatory Support

The patient who has tolerated surgery and has little preoperative history of pulmonary or other systemic disease should be able to waken and be weaned from ventilatory support relatively quickly postoperatively. There is no reason to provide prophylactic ventilation in an otherwise awake, stable patient in the belief that mechanical ventilation is somehow protective to the patient. If the patient is awake, hemodynamically stable, and not bleeding, the patient can be weaned from mechanical ventilation quite readily. On the other hand, if a patient has active bleeding, reduced cardiac output, requires multiple drugs and mechanical supports, or is oliguric, weaning from ventilatory support should not be immediately considered. In this setting it is far better to control the airway and provide for ventilatory support in the event that the patient deteriorates.

After routine surgery patients should be quickly extubated in the ICU. Although the occasional patient can be extubated in the operating room, there is little need for this in the patient operated on with cardiopulmonary bypass. The risk of coagulopathy, arrhythmias, or other instability in the immediate perioperative period would seem to warrant keeping the patient intubated for 2–4 hours postoperatively. Nonetheless, if the patient is doing well without evidence of instability, is not bleeding, and is awake, he or she can be extubated within a shorter period if breathing adequately.

Generally, an IMV weaning program is quickly commenced as soon as the patient is sufficiently awake and is otherwise stable. Because a patient in pain does not breathe adequately, intravenous narcotics (e.g., morphine sulfate) should be given as necessary. Similarly, anxiolysis (e.g., with midazolam) may be given to patients who become agitated on emerging from anesthesia. Although the administration of systemic narcotics and anxiolysis may render a patient somewhat more somnolent, the judicious administration of such drugs generally provides a suitable level of comfort to effectively wean from ventilatory support.

If an average-sized patient presents with a spontaneous tidal volume of less than 300 ml during weaning from IMV ventilation, pressure support ventilation may be employed to augment tidal volume while IMV breathing is reduced. Once the patient is spontaneously breathing with the assistance of pressure support only, pressure support itself can be gradually reduced and the patient extubated. Before extubation, respiratory mechanics are performed by the respiratory therapist. Generally, to extubate, appropriate mechanics include an inspiratory force of more than (–) 20 cm of H_2O pressure, a vital capacity of more than 15 ml per kg, and a spontaneously ventilating patient. An acceptable arterial blood gas measurement on 40–50% FIO_2 and a respiratory rate of less than 30 should also be considered necessary before extubating. Obviously, nothing is absolute, and each patient must be examined individually. Patients who breathe fast, more than 30 breaths per minute, are generally sick. This is a handy rule to remember when assessing a patient before extubation. Even if respiratory mechanics and blood gas measurements are acceptable, the tachypneic patient should always be viewed suspiciously because tachypnea may indicate an excessive work of breathing. Likewise, the use of accessory muscles of respiration or paradoxical breathing should be considered a warning against extubation. In these situations, the experienced anesthesiologist can simply tell when a patient is or is not capable of "flying off the ventilator."

Occasionally, correction of inadequate analgesia, diuresis, treatment of metabolic alkalosis with acetazolamide, and endotracheal suction are necessary before attempting an IMV wean. If IMV weaning is initiated and the patient becomes tachypneic, tachycardic, or hemodynamically unstable, the patient should be restored to full ventilatory support. Once fully ventilated, the source for failure to wean may be sought.

If patients become dependent on ventilation, it is best for the cardiac anesthesiologist to turn over ventilatory management to either a medical or anesthesia intensivist. In this instance, it is most prudent for the physician responsible for weaning to be immediately available in the ICU. Continuous positive airway pressure weaning trials and the use of pressure support ventilation may assist the ventilatory-dependent patient in weaning from mechanical support. A continuous positive airway pressure wean involves placing the patient on continuous positive airway pressure for increasingly longer periods of time during the day over a protracted period. Early performance of a tracheostomy (within a few days of surgery) makes weaning management easier for both patient and nursing staff. Nutritional support must always be initiated to prevent loss of muscle mass.

Neurologic Complications

Nothing is more distressing for a surgical team than to successfully take a patient through cardiopulmonary bypass and cardiac surgery uneventfully, only to find the patient awakens with a severe neurologic deficit or fails to awaken at all. The risks in cardiac surgery to the central nervous system occur as a consequence of the altered hemodynamics of cardiopulmonary bypass, the possibility of severe hypotension and reduced cardiac output, and various particulate and air emboli that may develop secondary to vascular manipulations. Fortunately, most perioperative deficits improve with time. Nevertheless, the prospect of stroke after cardiac surgery remains one of the complications most feared by the patient, family members, and surgical team alike. Efforts to prevent stroke by careful intraoperative management is perhaps the best approach to perioperative stroke. Transesophageal echocardiographic assessment of the ascending aorta may assist the surgeon in placing the arterial cannula away from potential sources of embolic material. The surgeon's palpation of the aorta may also be useful in guiding him or her away from areas of calcification likely to produce a shower of emboli. Although the anesthesiologist generally does not have the ability to prevent embolic stroke, the anesthesiologist does need to be certain that an adequate perfusion pressure and oxygenation are maintained to avoid stroke as a consequence of hypotension. In certain instances, particularly patients presenting emergently in great distress, stroke may occur as a result of prolonged hypoperfusion in the setting of cardiopulmonary resuscitation. The internist's warnings to avoid hypoxemia and hypotension naturally are the best guides by which the anesthesiologist can avoid neurologic injury. Hypothermia can be helpful in preventing neurologic injury by reducing oxygen requirements during the bypass period. Although various pharmacologic aids have been used (e.g., barbiturates, propofol, and so forth) to produce brain electrical silence and cerebral protection, hypothermia provides the greatest degree of protection to neural tissues with reduced oxygen delivery. As mentioned in Chapter 13, if circulatory arrest is necessary to facilitate surgical repair, deep hypothermia is perhaps the best protection against neurologic injury. Retrograde cerebral perfusion may also be helpful when circulatory arrest is necessary.

If a neurologic deficit is noted, there is little that the anesthesiologist can do but offer supportive care. Seizures may be treated with diazepam, phenytoin, or both. Computed tomography and magnetic resonance imaging may be completed over a period of days to localize areas of brain injury, as well as to rule out any intracranial hemorrhage that might require evacuation. Electroencephalographic studies, as conducted by neurologists, may be necessary to confirm brain death should that be a concern. Because hyperglycemia is considered to contribute to cellular injury, it should be scrupulously avoided in patients at risk for neurologic ischemia.

Anesthesiologists should have a basic sense of the patient's neurologic functioning preoperatively to facilitate a postoperative comparison. The following tests may be easily reproduced:

1.   Motor and cranial nerves are assessed.

2.   Mental status and orientation to person, place, and time are checked.

3.   Memory recall, specifically short-term memory, is tested.

4.   Speech and identification of objects are tested.

5.   Visual fields and pupil symmetry are tested.

Patients recover from anesthesia for heart surgery at varying speeds. Elderly patients may be particularly prone to somnolence after surgery. Analgesics and muscle relaxants may render the patient with hepatic or renal impairment unresponsive for many hours after surgery. Similarly, patients with a previous history of neurologic injury may show transient neurologic dysfunction after anesthesia and surgery. Over time, patients who are slow to awaken as a consequence of the poor metabolism of anesthetic drugs as well as those who suffer a reappearance of a previous neurologic deficit will improve. Reversal of narcotics, muscle relaxants, and amnestics may be attempted if there is concern that a neurologic injury has occurred. Of course, this may lead to hypertension, tachycardia, and great pain for the patient, potentially leading to other complications as well. A comatose patient should have blood sugar levels checked to rule out any hypoglycemia. Patients with a history of parkinsonism may be unresponsive as a consequence of dopamine receptor antagonists (droperidol, haloperidol) encountered during the perioperative period. Time will tell whether a patient successfully awakens or not. If the anesthesiologist is concerned about a possible neurologic injury, neurologic consultation should be obtained. If patients develop seizures, neurologic deficits (Todd's phenomenon) may complicate diagnosis. Unfortunately, as dreaded as neurologic injury may be, there is little that the anesthesiologist can do to improve patient functioning after a perioperative neurologic injury other than to assist in providing supportive care.

Renal Dysfunction

As with neurologic injuries, a small population of patients taken for cardiac surgery develop renal dysfunction perioperatively. Many patients who are taken to surgery as a consequence of widespread vascular disease or diabetes mellitus already have impaired renal function as measured by the serum creatinine (i.e., creatinine of more than 1.6–1.7 mg per dl). Altered blood flow associated with cardiopulmonary bypass, the potential for hypotension, decreased cardiac output, the use of vasoconstrictors, and embolic phenomenon can all contribute to the development of acute renal failure perioperatively (Table 15-4).

Renal dysfunction in the cardiac surgery patient should be approached as with any patient developing a transient renal embarrassment. Prerenal, postrenal, and renal sources of injury can contribute to a low urine output in both the cardiac surgical patient as well as any other patient who develops renal dysfunction perioperatively. Prerenal causes

Table 15-4. Causes of Acute Renal Failure

Prerenal	Intrinsic Renal Disease	Postrenal
Hypovolemia	Acute tubular disease	Ureteral obstruction
Volume redistribution	ischemia (postshock)	Intrinsic
Impaired cardiac	Sepsis (postoperative)	Extrinsic
function	Toxins	Bladder, outlet
Renovascular disease	Contrast dye	obstruction
Hepatorenal syndrome	Drugs, heavy metal	Urethral obstruction
	pigment	
	Calcium, urate	
	Acute glomerulonephritis	
	Interstitial nephritis	
	Vascular disease	
	Emboli (arterial)	
	Vasculitis	
	Intrarenal thrombosis	
	Thrombotic thrombocyto-	
	penic purpura	

Source: Modified from DH Ellison, MJ Bia. Acute renal failure in critically ill patients. J Intern Care Med 1987;2:8.

of renal dysfunction likely to be encountered in the cardiac patient include hypotension, reduced cardiac output, and vascular constriction. Renal sources include embolic and ischemic injuries to the kidney, and contrast dye–mediated injuries in patients who have had recent cardiac catheterization. Postrenal causes include an occluded bladder catheter (Table 15-5).

Therapy for acute renal dysfunction is aimed at correcting the source responsible for the acute renal failure. In patients with postrenal obstruction, a patent bladder catheter can often relieve an obstructive uropathy. Those patients afflicted with prerenal causes often benefit from improved cardiac output and reduced use of vasoconstrictors. Those patients suffering renal injury as a consequence of ischemia are best treated with supportive measures as necessary to improve renal blood flow. Low-dose dopamine, 1–3 μg per kg per minute, may questionably improve urine output in renal injury. However, tachycardia and arrhythmias may develop, potentially complicating cardiac management. Diuretics (e.g., bumetanide) given by infusion may improve urine output, making fluid management easier in the patient who develops acute renal failure. Fluid retention may lead to pulmonary edema and myocar-

Table 15-5. Diagnostic Tests of Renal Dysfunction

	Prerenal	Renal
Urine (sodium)	<10 mEq/liter	>20 mEq/liter
Urine (chloride)	<10 mEq/liter	>20 mEq/liter
FE_{na}[a]	<1%	>2%
Urine osmolarity (mOsm/liter)	>500	<350
Urine/serum (creatinine)	>40	<20
Renal failure index (RFI)[b]	<1%	>2%
Urine/serum (urea)	>8	<3
Serum (BUN)/creatinine	>20	≈10

FE_{na} = fraction excretion of sodium; BUN = blood urea nitrogen.
[a] $FE_{na} = (U_{na}/P_{na}) \div (U_{cr}/P_{cr}) \times 100$, where U_{na} is the urine concentration of sodium; P_{na} is the plasma concentration of sodium; U_{cr} is the urine concentration of creatinine; and Pcr is the plasma concentration of creatinine.
[b] Renal failure index = $U_{na} \div (U_{cr}/P_{cr})$, where U_{na} is the urine concentration of sodium; U_{cr} is the urine concentration of creatinine; and P_{cr} is the plasma concentration of creatinine.
Source: Modified with permission from WJ Hoffman, JD Wasnick. Postoperative Critical Care of the Massachusetts General Hospital. Boston: Little, Brown, 1992;363.

dial ischemia in the patient who develops oliguric acute renal dysfunction. Diuretics may help prevent fluid retention; however, they will not improve renal function per se. The accumulation of acids and potassium may potentially complicate electrolyte management. Dialysis or ultrafiltration may ultimately be needed to correct fluid and electrolyte balance in the patient perioperatively. Consultation with a nephrologist is encouraged early if acute renal failure appears likely. Patients at risk for fluid retention should remain intubated and sedated until an effective mechanism for diuresis has been secured. The development of pulmonary edema as a consequence of impaired renal function can lead to significant respiratory embarrassment and patient injury perioperatively.

Postoperative Rhythm Disturbances

It is hoped that the heart's function will have been improved by the time the patient arrives in the ICU. Much of the ICU care directed toward the cardiovascular system is an extension of that therapy commenced in the operating room to successfully wean the patient from cardiopulmonary bypass. Treatment of ventricular failure in the intensive care unit follows those protocols to wean the failing heart from bypass support (see Chapter 8). As hemodynamics improve in the ICU, inotropes, vasopressors, and vasodilators can be withdrawn as the patient's cardiac function permits. On awakening, the patient may commence an oral regimen for blood pressure control, arrhythmia prophylaxis, and diuresis (e.g., beta blockers, furosemide).

Should patients develop rhythm disturbances (e.g., atrial fibrillation), they will need aggressive therapy. Atrial fibrillation is among the greatest causes of postoperative morbidity and increased hospital stay after coronary artery bypass. Beta$_1$ selective beta blockers and amiodarone may provide prophylaxis against postoperative atrial fibrillation. Digoxin, procainamide, verapamil, and beta blockers may be used to control the ventricular response to atrial fibrillation, to attempt a chemical conversion to normal sinus rhythm, or both. Should a patient become unstable secondary to the new onset of atrial fibrillation, synchronized direct-current cardioversion should be attempted.

In the event that ventricular arrhythmias appear in the postoperative patient, electrolyte levels, including magnesium concentrations, should be checked. Hypokalemia and hypomagnesemia need to be corrected if present, because they may contribute to the development of ventricular ectopy. Should the patient have a pulmonary arterial catheter, the catheter's position in the pulmonary artery should be confirmed by chest x-ray, examination of the pulmonary arterial waveform, or both. Should the pulmonary catheter be found to be in the right ventricle, it can be advanced into the correct position or removed, depending on the patient's condition.

Should sustained ventricular tachycardia present, it can be treated with a variety of agents. Lidocaine, procainamide, and bretylium can all suppress ventricular tachycardia. Amiodarone (IV) may also be given in the postoperative period to suppress refractory sustained ventricular tachycardia. Close cooperation with the patient's cardiologist and electrophysiologist should ensure a unified approach to postoperative dysrhythmia management.

Other Issues in the Intensive Care Unit

Other issues that complicate ICU management of the cardiac surgical patient include perioperative hemorrhage (see Chapter 16). If acute deterioration occurs, leading to cardiac arrest, re-exploration of the chest in the ICU may be necessary to relieve tamponade and attempt salvage. If the surgeon is unavailable, the anesthesiologist must be prepared on rare occasions to open the chest if the patient is in full arrest. The ICU must be equipped with the necessary equipment to facilitate opening the chest postoperatively to relieve tamponade. Cardiopulmonary resuscitation will need to be initiated and maintained in the event of an arrest. Once the chest is open, often patients are transported, with ongoing open chest massage, back to surgery to be placed on cardiopulmonary bypass to resuscitate the patient and repair any bypass grafts that may be contributing to the patient's deterioration. Bleeding sites must be corrected and pericardial tamponade relieved. Patients returned to the operating room from the ICU in this setting have a particularly poor prognosis, with the likelihood of both neurologic and renal injury being quite high. Prognosis in this setting is grim.

Postoperative analgesia consists of intravenous narcotics (e.g., morphine sulphate, meperidine, etc.). Anxiety can be treated with intravenous midazolam. Should sedation be desired, propofol by infusion (IV) can likewise be administered. Once the patient is extubated and taking liquids by mouth, oral analgesics may be used for pain control. Regional techniques (e.g., thoracic epidural analgesia) and intravenous patient controlled analgesia may likewise be used.

Management of stress ulcers, diabetes, nosocomial infections, pneumonias, pressure sores, as well as patient comfort issues must also be addressed in patients requiring ICU stays. There are any number of texts available on intensive care medicine ranging from exhaustive tomes to handy manuals. The individual returning to cardiac anesthesia practice is advised to have one available to assist in dealing with these postoperative care issues.

16

Bleeding Patients

So far, we have encountered several patients in the course of this introduction to cardiac anesthesia practice. Fortunately, even the sickest patients presented thus far have recovered, even those with left ventricular assist devices. Of course, things are rarely so certain in actual cardiac anesthesia practice. Complications frequently challenge both patients and physicians. In Chapter 15, we focused briefly on the many renal, pulmonary, and neurologic complications that can make cardiac surgery a frustrating experience for all concerned. As difficult and life-threatening as these problems may be, patients with postoperative bleeding leading to an acute deterioration in the intensive care unit (ICU) present most frequently. Often, such postoperative bleeding necessitates a return trip to the operating room for surgical re-exploration. Table 16-1 lists the number of possible ramifications of postoperative hemorrhage in the cardiac surgical patient.

The development of postoperative bleeding (more than 300 ml per hour of chest tube drainage), whether as a consequence of a surgical bleeding site (e.g., from suture deficiency) or as a consequence of coagulopathy, can place the patient at risk for development of pericardial tamponade, hemodynamic embarrassment, and organ injury. Whether correction by surgical intervention, blood-product administration, or both, postoperative bleeding needs to be aggressively treated by both anesthesiologist and surgeon as a shared responsibility. This chapter briefly reviews the coagulation system, discusses how it is affected by cardiac surgery, and reviews some strategies for managing blood component therapy.

In this age of potentially lethal blood-borne pathogens, administration of blood products must not be approached casually. Blood prod-

Table 16-1. Complications of Postoperative Hemorrhage
in the Cardiac Surgical Patient

Hypovolemia

Anemia

Hypotension

Decreased cardiac output

Decreased renal perfusion

Decreased oxygen delivery

Need for blood product replacement

Pericardial tamponade

---

uct replacement must be given for a reason. Gone are the days when the surgeon (generally a surgical resident) would yell over the drapes to the anesthesiologist, "I don't want to see anything not yellow hanging." In other words, the surgeon wished to use fresh frozen plasma (FFP) as a volume expander for some mythologic prophylactic need. Today, such a request (or demand) would be readily dismissed. Careful administration of blood products is essential to the survival of the cardiac patient as in any patient at risk for postoperative bleeding.

Coagulation System

Before we can even begin to explore how the typical patient such as Mr. XY would develop postoperative hemorrhage, we briefly review (and I do mean briefly) the coagulation cascade. We have all had to memorize those factors at one time or another, so let's not do it this time. You will never need to reproduce the coagulation cascade in the operating room. Still, the process by which a clot forms or fails to form, as is more likely the case, remains relevant in our diagnosis and treatment of postoperative hemorrhage. Figure 16-1 provides us a schematic of the coagulation cascade.

Although Figure 16-1 is a sketchy diagram, it does provide the essential information needed by the clinical anesthesiologist to understand the coagulation system. The requirements for clot formation are relatively obvious, as is the fact that clot formation is limited by the presence of antithrombin III, protein C, and protein S. Fibrinolysis also serves to limit the extent of clot formation. It is clear that various components are necessary to initiate coagulation. Absence of those components can impair the body's ability to successfully form a clot after tissue injury.

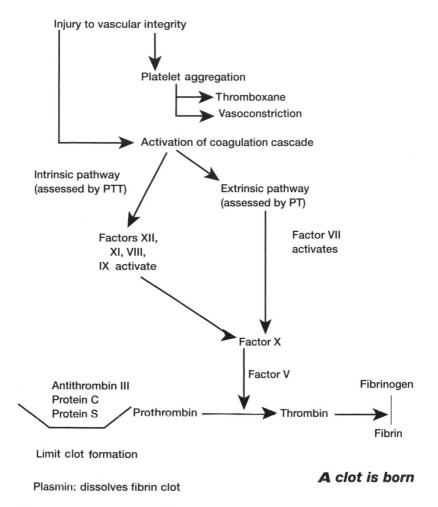

Figure 16-1. *The making of a clot. (PTT = partial thromboplastin time; PT = prothrombin time.)*

Causes of Coagulopathy

In the cardiac patient, assuming a surgical cause of bleeding has been excluded, there are a number of potential sources that could render the patient coagulopathic. These sources, like the clotting system itself, reflect the balance between clot formation and clot degradation. Inadequate clot formation is a consequence of platelet dysfunction, platelet insufficiency, and dilution of coagulation factors (such as fibrinogen). Activation of the fibrinolytic system as a consequence of cardiopulmonary bypass can all lead to clot degradation, requiring aggressive therapy to restore hemostasis.

Tissue Injury

It is certainly an understatement that tissue injury can be a source of bleeding. There is never a shortage of potential bleeding sites as a consequence of heart surgery. Repeat cardiac surgery, in particular, can leave countless sites requiring clot formation to prevent bleeding. Of course, any bleeding site that requires surgical correction must be attended to. No amount of clot will correct an arterial bleed from a high-pressure vessel such as a torn mammary artery or bypass graft.

Platelet Consumption and Dilution

Platelets are necessary to produce the platelet plug to initiate the process of clot formation. Platelet consumption and dilution as a consequence of cardiopulmonary bypass may be a common cause of postoperative bleeding. Antiplatelet therapy, such as aspirin, is so common in antianginal regimens that many patients' platelets are ineffective even with a normal preoperative platelet count.

Dilution of Coagulation Factors

Dilution of coagulation factors, although less likely than platelet dilution, may also account for coagulopathy after heart surgery. Preoperative hepatic disease, not uncommon in the cardiac patient, may further contribute to the patient's inability to form suitable clots after surgery. Potentiation of antithrombin III by residual heparin may also impair the formation of clot after the administration of protamine if heparin reversal has been inadequate.

Fibrinolysis

Although not a process of clot formation per se, activation of the fibrinolytic system during cardiopulmonary bypass does occur, potentially leading to fibrinolysis. In particular, if a patient is inadequately heparinized during cardiopulmonary bypass, activation of the fibrinolytic system can lead to significant perioperative coagulopathy and patient hemorrhage.

Assessing and Responding to Postoperative Bleeding

With this basic review, let's now look at a bleeding patient postoperatively and see how we might assess and respond to the patient who hemorrhages after cardiopulmonary bypass. Although bleeding may be a particular problem postoperatively, attaining acceptable hemostasis should be a concern for the surgical team from the minute surgery is commenced. From the onset, the surgeon must be careful to coagulate or suture possible bleeding sites as he or she proceeds with the operation. Anastomotic sites must be checked and rechecked to ensure vascular integrity. Vein bypass grafts and arterial conduits need to be inspected by the surgical team to be certain that no obvious sources of bleeding are present. Cannulation sites in particular should be checked to ensure that they are securely sutured. Sudden hemorrhage and quick development of tamponade can occur if atrial or aortic cannula sutures become dislodged postoperatively. The anesthesiologist should be concerned with the patient's propensity for bleeding from the onset of surgery. If the preoperative platelet count and coagulation study results are abnormal, one can expect bleeding postoperatively. Hepatic disease or renal dysfunction can lead to both reduced production of coagulation factors or platelet impairment, respectively. Patients treated with heparin for a prolonged period before surgery may develop a heparin-induced thrombocytopenia.

Nonetheless, assuming an uneventful surgical course, protamine is administered as our first attempt to restore coagulation to where effective hemostasis may be obtained.

As with so many things in cardiac anesthesia, visual inspection is often a reliable first test of the adequacy of the coagulation system or platelet function. Namely, if the patient oozes blood from every operative surface and around intravenous insertion sites, we suspect that clot formation is inadequate.

The failure to develop a clot in the chest after protamine administration may mean that the patient's ability to achieve effective hemostasis is impaired. Once we have come to this conclusion, even before we measure activated clotting time (ACT) and perform a heparin concentration analysis, we should begin to think about why hemostasis is abnormal and what we might do about it.

Before we do that, however, a word to the individual returning to cardiac anesthesia practice or beginning cardiac anesthesia is in order. After prolonged surgery, there is often the tendency on the part of the surgeon and the anesthesiologist alike to hurriedly close the chest. Be very careful in undertaking this course of action. Should a patient appear "wet" after administration of protamine, too quickly closing the chest can lead to pericardial tamponade and the need for surgical re-exploration. Generally, it is wise to search for the cause of bleeding before leaving the operating room, if possible. If coagulopathy is suspected, a quick laboratory assessment can provide a great deal of assistance in effectively diagnosing abnormalities in hemostatic function.

We may ask, why is the patient bleeding? Unfortunately, the answer at times is obfuscated. Immediately, we tend to suspect a surgical source of bleeding. In this regard, we must assume that the surgeon has thoroughly examined potential sites for bleeding so that a surgical cause may be readily eliminated. Occasionally, a discrete bleeding site can be identified such as a tear in the right atrium at the site of the venous cannula or an inadequately sewn bypass graft. During the inspection for bleeding sites, it is not uncommon for the surgeon to lift the beating heart in an effort to locate the potential trouble spot. Lifting the heart can frequently lead to hypotension, ventricular dysfunction, and arrhythmias. We must be prepared to tell the surgeon at this point to stop the search while the heart is manipulated so that we may have the opportunity to restore hemodynamic stability. That stability may be short-lived, as no doubt the surgeon will lift the heart again and again. Clearly, it is the surgeon's duty to complete a full inspection of the pericardial cavity. Our role as anesthesiologists is to support the circulation as best we can while this is done after separation from cardiopulmonary bypass. If, however, the patient cannot hemodynamically tolerate manipulation by the surgeon and prolonged repairs are necessary after separation from bypass, it may be necessary to recannulate, reheparinize, and resume cardiopulmonary bypass to complete the surgical repair. So, assuming that there are no obvious surgical sources of bleeding, again we must ask, why is the patient bleeding?

Preexisting Conditions that Predispose to Bleeding

Hemophilias and von Willebrand's Disease
Presumably, we will be well aware of preexisting causes of bleeding. Such causes include the hemophilias and von Willebrand's disease.

Both hemophilia A and von Willebrand's disease affect different parts of factor VIII. In von Willebrand's disease, there is a deficiency of factor VIII (von Willebrand's factor). Factor VIII V.W. is that part of the factor complex that interacts with platelets. An elevated bleeding time often serves as a sign of von Willebrand's disease. Hemophilia A is a sex-linked deficiency of Factor VIII procoagulant. An elevated activated partial thromboplastin time (aPTT) is associated with hemophilia A. Obviously, patients with either hemophilia A or von Willebrand's disease or any other bleeding disorder should come to heart surgery only after close consultation with a hematologist. The hematologist is an asset in providing for perioperative factor replacement.

Liver Disease

Patients with hepatic disease may have both decreased production of clotting factors and hypersplenism leading to platelet sequestration. If patients are taken to surgery with significant hepatic disease, it may be necessary to provide an aggressive transfusion of FFP, platelets, and cryoprecipitate to restore hemostatic integrity. Vitamin K administration may be given preoperatively over a period of time to improve coagulation. The patient with significant hepatic disease and impaired coagulation should be reviewed with the hematologist prior to coming for surgery. Additionally, in a patient with a grossly diseased liver, we must be concerned for the development of perioperative hepatitis as a consequence of hypoperfusion during cardiopulmonary bypass or periods of reduced cardiac output.

Platelet Dysfunction

Preoperative thrombocytopenia can lead to obvious bleeding postoperatively. Various causes of thrombocytopenia or platelet dysfunction do occur in the cardiac surgery patient population, making platelet deficiency a common source of postoperative bleeding. Impaired platelet production may occur as a consequence of bone marrow disease. Platelet destruction as mediated through autoimmune phenomena may similarly reduce platelet numbers. Heparin, as previously mentioned, can produce a thrombocytopenia in patients coming to surgery. Because patients are frequently treated with heparin as part of an anti-ischemia regimen for some days before surgery, it is possible that patients will have dramatically reduced platelet counts perioperatively. Uremia and aspirin and other drug use may also result in significant perioperative platelet dysfunction.

Nonetheless, assuming that no preoperative abnormalities of hematologic function are noted (normal prothrombin time [PT], aPTT, bleeding time, platelet count), the patient is considered ready for surgery. However, even if perioperative measures of hemostatic function are normal, this does not preclude the development of significant coagulopathy postbypass.

Assessing Hemostasis Postbypass

After administration of protamine, a heparin analysis and ACT are completed. The ACT is used routinely to monitor the effects of heparin anticoagulation before the initiation of cardiopulmonary bypass. Blood is mixed with diatomaceous earth, which activates the intrinsic coagulation system. The normal ACT is 90–120 seconds. Kaolin-based ACTs are necessary if aprotinin is used. As you may recall, aprotinin is employed in some patients to inhibit fibrinolysis associated with cardiopulmonary bypass. Aprotinin can prolong non–Kaolin-based ACTs, giving a falsely elevated measurement. After cardiopulmonary bypass and the administration of protamine, it is hoped that the ACT will return to baseline. In so doing, we assume that the effects of heparin have been neutralized. A heparin concentration determination also serves to confirm that protamine has effectively neutralized heparin. However, even if the ACT is normal, the patient may experience significant nonsurgically correctable bleeding as a consequence of inadequate platelet function. Thus, if a normal ACT is present after administration of protamine and a heparin analysis confirms the lack of heparin should the patient appear "oozy," then platelet dilution or dysfunction must be suspected. An abnormally elevated ACT after the administration of protamine reflects either inadequate protamine administration or impairment of the intrinsic and common coagulation pathways. Often, dilution of clotting factors may be suspected in this setting.

Assuming that a heparin concentration assay has been completed, residual heparin or inadequate protamine administration may be ruled out as a possible cause of the patient's clotting difficulty. The ACT, in and of itself, tells nothing about platelet function, whether normal or abnormal. If the ACT is elevated, not only must we suspect impairment of the clotting cascade, but we must also consider the possibility that platelet function and number may be inadequate. With a patient bleeding and an elevated ACT, there may be the desire on the part of the sur-

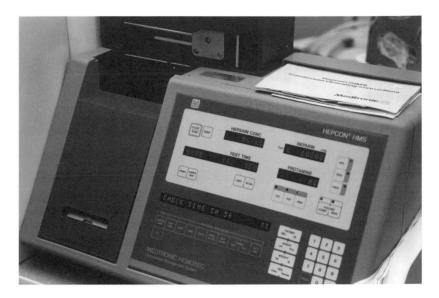

Figure 16-2. *Hepcon Heparin Analysis (Hepcon HMS, Medtronic, Minneapolis) and activated clotting time machine.*

geon to administer ever increasing amounts of protamine to eliminate residual heparin. Be cautious if this occurs. Excessive protamine administration can lead to coagulopathy itself. Once a heparin assay has been determined, there is little need to administer additional protamine unless heparinized blood is administered to the patient after being drained from the bypass circuit (Figure 16-2).

Thus, if we encounter an ACT that is normal and the patient is bleeding, we must first suspect platelet dysfunction or platelet dilution. Pooled platelets will need to be administered to restore either the platelet count or to provide functioning platelets to the patient. Generally, if a platelet count obtained during cardiopulmonary bypass is significantly less than 100,000 platelets per μl, we may expect platelet-mediated bleeding postbypass. If a low platelet count is obtained and the patient does not appear to be bleeding, the patient does not need a platelet transfusion. Generally, 5–10 U of platelets will be administered to an average-sized individual to augment the platelet count.

If on the other hand, the ACT is abnormally high, several additional tests of coagulation need to be performed as quickly as possible to diagnosis the deficiency in hemostatic functioning:

- Thrombin time. Thrombin time measures the conversion of fibrinogen to fibrin (normal thrombin time is 15 seconds). The thrombin time is elevated in hypofibrinogenemia or in the presence of excessive fibrin split products as might be expected during fibrinolysis.

- Fibrinogen concentration. Fibrinogen concentration normally is 200–400 mg per dl. Fibrinogen concentration is reduced by either consumption or hemodilution.

- Prothrombin time (PT). PT is prolonged by reductions in fibrinogen as well as factors V, VII, and X. The normal PT is 11–12 seconds.

- Activated partial thromboplastin time. It is prolonged by deficiencies in the intrinsic and common pathways.

- Fibrin split products. They are present in consumptive coagulopathies such as disseminated intravascular coagulation and fibrinolysis. The D-dimer portion of fibrin is produced during fibrinolysis and can be detected by the laboratory's indicating fibrin degradation.

With the assistance of a speedy laboratory, these tests can rapidly help to determine which additional blood products need to be administered to the patient in the form of FFP, cryoprecipitate, platelet concentrates, or packed red blood cells.

Other tests such as thromboelastography provide an assessment of both clot formation and fibrinolysis by measuring the viscoelasticity of blood clot. Thromboelastography provides a relatively rapid assessment of clot formation that can be useful to guide therapy. The availability of thromboelastography is dependent on institutional preference. In reality, if the laboratory and blood bank function well, it should be possible to diagnose and treat the coagulopathic patient using specific tests of coagulation.

Diagnosis and Treatment of the Bleeding Patient Postoperatively

Low platelet count before weaning from cardiopulmonary bypass should obviously alert the anesthesiologist to a possible source of bleeding after heparin reversal. It is important to remember that as patients bleed postoperatively and are given additional volume in the form of either crystalloid, packed cells, or other volume expanders, further dilution of both platelets and possibly other factors may occur, leading to further decreases in clotting factors, platelets, and fibrinogen. Thus, even if just the platelet count is initially low and is the cause of bleeding, it is possible that volume replacement while awaiting the delivery of pooled platelets from the blood bank may further dilute other components of the coagulation system. This may impair clot formation even after the platelet number and function have been corrected. This can lead to a coagulopathic spiral in which control of hemostasis is difficult because varying factors become diluted while awaiting platelets. If a low platelet count is noted, certainly fewer than 50,000 platelets per µl, then it would be prudent to order platelets before separation from bypass in the high likelihood that a platelet transfusion will be necessary. In addition to platelets, there are other blood products available to help individualize correction of postoperative coagulopathy.

Packed Red Blood Cells

Patients undergoing cardiopulmonary bypass are hemodiluted. A hematocrit of between 22% and 25% is routine after the termination of cardiopulmonary bypass. Diuresis frequently leads to increases in hematocrit postoperatively. Nonetheless, if the hematocrit decreases significantly below 20%, packed red blood cells may be needed if postoperative bleeding develops. If patients remain hemodynamically stable and oxygen delivery to the tissues is adequate as assessed by blood gas determination and mixed venous oxygen saturation, patients may be able to tolerate significantly reduced hematocrits in the immediate postoperative period. Patient performance must guide the administration of packed red blood cells rather than the establishment of any arbitrary hematocrit. Each unit of packed cells has a hematocrit of approximately 70–80%. Therefore, these highly concentrated units have the ability to augment the patient's hematocrit and improve the oxygen-carrying capacity of the blood. If a patient is diagnosed as being coagulopathic and requires multiple transfusions of FFP, platelet transfusions, or both, in addition to crystalloid, further hemodilution may be expected, reducing the hematocrit. In this instance, the addition of packed red blood cells (PRBCs) may be needed to provide adequate oxygen-carrying capacity.

Fresh Frozen Plasma

FFP preserves much of the coagulant activity of whole blood. FFP may be administered to restore factor activity if clotting is reduced after cardiopulmonary bypass. Although dilution of clotting factors is a less likely cause of postoperative hemorrhage when compared with thrombocytopenia, it can lead to postoperative hemorrhage. As such, FFP may be needed to correct obvious postoperative coagulopathy. FFP should never be given solely as a volume expander.

Cryoprecipitate

Cryoprecipitate is a concentrated source of fibrinogen and factor VIII. When the fibrinogen concentration is reduced as a consequence of dilution or consumption, cryoprecipitate provides a ready supply of fibrinogen to the patient.

Platelet Concentrates

Platelet concentrates are given to correct thrombocytopenia. One unit of platelets improves the platelet count by approximately 7,000 in an average-sized 70-kg individual.

Naturally, whenever blood products are administered there remains a risk for the transmission of infectious disease. Additionally, whenever blood products are administered there is the risk of potentially transfusing a unit of the wrong type, leading to a transfusion reaction. It is important that all protocols be followed closely to ensure that each transfused unit is correctly identified. FFP, PRBCs, and cryoprecipitate should never be given prophylactically for any reason. The only reason to administer blood products is to correct coagulopathy or to increase oxygen-carrying capacity.

An Approach to the "Wet" Patient

So how then should we approach a bleeding patient after cardiopulmonary bypass? Let's take Mr. XY again, our routine coronary artery bypass patient. In this instance, he has undergone an uneventful course and has had protamine administered. After this, the surgeon looks at

Table 16-2. An Approach to the Bleeding Patient

1. Surgeon confirms there is no active surgical bleeding. Note: Lifting the heart to inspect for bleeding sites may cause hemodynamic compromise.

2. Recheck ACT and heparin analysis.

   a. If ACT is elevated and heparin is present, administer protamine.

   b. If ACT is elevated and heparin is absent, consider factor deficiencies: Quickly obtain PT, aPTT, thrombin time, CBC, fibrinogen, and FSP.

   c. If ACT is normal and no heparin is detected but patient appears "wet," assess platelet count and administer platelets.

3. Review laboratory data as they become available.

   a. If decreased platelet count and bleeding, administer platelets.

   b. If PT, aPTT, and thrombin time are increased and fibrinogen level is decreased, consider dilution of clotting factors, and administer FFP and cryoprecipitate.

   c. If FSP is increased or if D-dimers are increased, consider fibrinolysis. Administer fresh frozen plasma, cryoprecipitate, and additional ε-aminocaproic acid (ε-aminocaproic acid is routinely administered as an antifibrinolytic perioperatively).*

   d. Administer packed red cells as necessary to restore hematocrit based on individual patient assessment.

   e. After administration of blood products, repeat CBC, PT, PTT, thrombin time, FSP, and fibrinogen tests.

   f. If patient continues to bleed, repeat search for surgical site of bleeding and if none are found, consult with hematologist.

FFP = fresh frozen plasma; ACT = activated clotting time; PT = prothrombin time; aPTT = activated partial thromboplastin time; CBC = complete blood count; FSP = fibrin split products.
*Never administer aminocaproic acid in the setting of intravascular thrombosis.

the anesthesiologist and says, "Hey, doctor, the patient looks wet." What are we to do? See Table 16-2.

As with many things in cardiac anesthesia, providing rules may be helpful but can also become overly rigid. Such is often the case with postoperative bleeding. Although it is true that thrombocytopenia is often the principal cause of nonsurgical bleeding perioperatively, the administration of pooled platelets as well as the volume to keep up with blood loss can soon lead to dilutions of other factors as well. This sometimes necessitates an inelegant but nonetheless effective "shotgun" approach to coagulopathy. In coagulopathic spiral, continued hemo-dilution and continued bleeding lead to the consumption of factors and platelets alike. In this instance, varying blood components, including PRBCs, platelets, FFP, and cryoprecipitate may need to be administered to the patient. Once coagulopathy is diagnosed, expeditious delivery of appropriate blood products to the patient minimizes the overall extent of postoperative blood loss. Additionally, specific blood component therapy can prevent patients from requiring multiple blood component transfusions because therapy is directed toward replacing what is specifically needed to restore hemostasis. Should blood components be unavailable to the operating room, other factors become diluted, requiring still more component transfusions. In addition to the hemo-dynamic effects of hypovolemia, protracted blood loss and blood replacement can lead to pulmonary embarrassment postoperatively. In this regard, it is important that nonsurgical bleeding, like surgical bleeding, be controlled as quickly as possible by specific blood product replacement to prevent the ramifications of prolonged hemorrhage and massive blood transfusion with its associated potential hepatic, pul-monary, renal, and electrolyte abnormalities.

The best prophylaxis against blood-borne disease is not to require any blood component transfusion. Unfortunately, anesthesiologists have little control over whether nonsurgical bleeding will develop or not. Certainly, careful anticoagulation before the initiation of car-diopulmonary bypass will help to prevent fibrinolysis, especially if cou-pled with prophylactic administration of ε-aminocaproic acid or aprotinin. Beyond this maneuver, however, there is little the anesthesi-ologist can do to prevent coagulopathy from developing. Prolonged bypass runs with excessive amounts of cardioplegia can readily lead to hemodilution and thrombocytopenia in spite of efforts by the per-fusionist to hemoconcentrate the patient's blood volume while on car-diopulmonary bypass. The ability of the blood bank and laboratory to provide quick information and blood component therapy as neces-sary will prevent nonsurgical bleeding from producing further hemod-ilution as a consequence of the need for continued volume replacement secondary to ongoing blood loss. Through careful cooperation between the surgeon, anesthesiologist, perfusionist, laboratory staff, and blood bank staff, it is nonetheless possible to quickly identify with simple tests the basic types of postoperative hemorrhage likely to be encountered. Because both platelet deficiencies and hemodilution of other factors often coexist, it becomes necessary to provide blood component ther-apy aimed at restoring platelets and clotting factors. As a consequence

Table 16-3. ABO Blood Groups

Blood Group	Antigen on Red Blood Cell	Antibody in Serum	Selection of Red Blood Cells for Transfusion	Selection of Plasma for Transfusion
O	None	Anti-A, anti-B	O	O, A, B, or AB
A	A	Anti-B	A or O	A or AB
B	B	Anti-A	B or O	B or AB
AB	AB	None	AB, A, B, or O	AB

Source: Modified with permission from WJ Hoffman, JD Wasnick. Postoperative Critical Care of the Massachusetts General Hospital. Boston: Little, Brown, 1992;318.

of these volume administrations, additional units of packed red blood cells may be needed to provide for a suitable oxygen-carrying capacity. Nonetheless, at no time should blood products be given frivolously. Remember that they harbor the potential to transmit significant infectious agents, in spite of modern screening procedures.

Bleeding in the Intensive Care Unit

Although we hope to control postoperative hemorrhage in the operating room before bringing the patient to the ICU, this is not always possible. In the event that the wet patient has had his or her sternum closed, chest tube drainage will be our guide as to the adequacy of coagulation. Generally, chest tube drainage in excess of 300 ml per hour must be considered significant bleeding, possibly necessitating surgical re-exploration. On the other hand, if massive amounts of blood quickly wells into the chest tubes postoperatively, then we must assume that a cannulation site has become disrupted, requiring an emergency re-exploration. It may, in fact, be necessary to open the chest in the ICU in an effort to control the hemorrhagic site or to release pericardial tamponade. In the event of massive bleeding, blood transfusions of components including PRBCs, cryoprecipitate, FFP, and platelets may be necessary as dictated by clinical instinct and laboratory examination. Table 16-3 provides a guide to ABO blood types for appropriate transfusion should large amounts of packed red cells become necessary either in the operating room or the ICU.

Should transfusion of multiple units of cells, FFP, platelets, and cryoprecipitate be needed postoperatively, complications can include electrolyte abnormalities, hypokalemia, metabolic alkalosis, hypothermia, hypocalcemia, further clotting and platelet dilution, respiratory distress syndrome, and peripheral edema. These complications can certainly add to the postoperative ICU course and delay recovery from anesthesia and surgery.

Conclusion

Although much effort is spent in attempting to control postoperative hemorrhage, it is clear that with a few simple tests and a little clinical experience, it is possible to troubleshoot nonsurgical bleeding with the judicious administration of blood products. Careful preoperative screening and bypass management should allow a rapid response to coagulopathy after administration of protamine. Patients have a tendency to bleed sometimes following cardiopulmonary bypass. If the surgeon can rule out a distinct bleeding site, we must accept that the patient has coagulopathy either as a consequence of platelet dilution, factor deficiency, or fibrinolysis. The use of simple laboratory tests generally can determine which particular cause is principally responsible for the bleeding problem. This should allow for specific therapies to be administered. However, bleeding as a consequence of one etiology can quickly lead to impairment in other components of the coagulation cascade. It is often not possible to titrate specific therapy unless experience has guided the anesthesiologist to be ready to respond briskly to potential bleeding after the conclusion of cardiopulmonary bypass. Although this is not always possible, anesthesiologists should be suspicious of thrombocytopenia while on pump. If the platelet count is significantly reduced on bypass, even with hemodilution and hypothermia, we must be prepared for the quick administration of platelets postbypass. Rapidly addressing the needs of the patient can prevent the transfusion of multiple units of blood components, leading to a variety of complications including the risk of blood-borne pathogens.

17

Anesthesia for Heart Transplantation

Patients with chronic ventricular failure and those supported by mechanical assist devices may present for heart transplantation. Because heart transplantation is generally limited to certain institutions, it is not always a component of routine adult practice. Even within those institutions where heart transplants are performed, often a transplant anesthesia team is selected in order to provide consistency in the management approach. Because much media attention is focused on patient outcomes after transplantation, it is highly unlikely and unusual that the initiate in cardiac anesthesia practice would be given the opportunity to undertake such high-profile anesthesia. Nevertheless, the principles of caring for a patient undergoing transplantation are similar to those of any patient with poor ventricular function coming to cardiac surgery. Patients may be found in a variety of conditions as they are listed for transplantation. Patients requiring inotropic or mechanical support who are free of other disease states are generally placed on the transplant list.

Anesthetic Management of the Donor

As the recipient patient is prepared for surgery, a harvest team is sent to secure any organs necessary for transplantation. Although the anesthesiologist for the recipient is often a part of a select team, the donor anesthesiologist is chosen with considerably less care. After all, the patient is already dead. Still, the anesthesiologist must preserve organ function until any organs are harvested. Dopamine is frequently used to support the blood pressure, along with volume resuscitation. In providing donor anesthesia, the anesthesiologist needs to control hypertension by administering nitroprusside; prevent hypotension by giving volume, dopamine, or both; eliminate movement by administering nondepolarizing muscle relaxants; and correct any electrolyte abnormalities. Most transplant organizations have a form to be completed by the anesthesiologist, who records the various arterial blood gases and drugs employed in the donor prior to organ harvest. Once the various transplant surgeons—and they often travel in large packs—have isolated the vessels of the organs to be harvested (liver, kidneys, and so forth), the heart is arrested through the administration of cardioplegia. Ventilation is discontinued, and the anesthesiologist withdraws from the operating room.

Providing donor anesthesia is often the first task as an anesthesia trainee. On the other hand, the recipient's anesthesiologist is often part of a team of individuals with some experience in managing cardiac surgical patients. These patients can obviously be challenging both in the prebypass period as well as after cardiopulmonary bypass. However, anesthesia for cardiac transplantation is not terribly different from any other case in which the patient has remarkably poor ventricular function. The anesthesiologist must keep the patient stable enough until bypass is initiated and then wean the patient from cardiopulmonary bypass after placement of the new heart.

Since the donor heart may have been arrested for up to several hours before the restoration of perfusion, poor ventricular function may require the anesthesiologist to employ aggressive therapy to successfully wean the recipient from cardiopulmonary bypass.

Anesthetic Management of the Recipient

As can be expected, patients presenting for heart transplant generally have poor ventricular function. Pulmonary hypertension with right ventricular failure may also complicate the prebypass patient. Monitoring is as expected for patients with poor ventricular performance. Using strict sterile techniques, central access is achieved and a pulmonary artery catheter advanced in its sleeve into the central circulation. The pulmonary artery catheter then can be advanced into the new heart after discontinuation of cardiopulmonary bypass. Transesophageal echocardiography is employed to assess ventricular function. Anesthesia may be induced with a combination of narcotics, amnestics, and muscle relaxants, as is the routine for any patient with poor ventricular function being taken for heart transplant surgery. Because many patients may have eaten before being alerted that a heart has become available and may have taken oral medications, care must be taken to prevent aspiration in those patients who have not been on nothing by mouth orders. Once induction is complete, the anesthesiologist needs to provide whatever inotropic support is necessary and relieve pulmonary hypertension as best as he or she can until bypass is initiated. If the patient deteriorates as a consequence of ventricular dysfunction or if life-threatening arrhythmias develop, the patient can be heparinized and bypass initiated as in any other surgery. Once the patient is placed on bypass, the donor heart is sewn into position. When completed, the surgeon removes air in the new heart and the patient is weaned from cardiopulmonary bypass support. Again, this is not that different from other patients with poor ventricular function. However, the transplanted heart is free of autonomic innervation. This means that only direct-acting agents (e.g., isoproterenol) have effects on the heart's function. Indirect-acting agents, which depend on an intact autonomic nervous system, are ineffective. With this understanding, we can attempt to wean the patient from cardiopulmonary bypass as tolerated. Isoproterenol, dobutamine, and other inotropes are administered as necessary to optimize myocardial performance. Using pulmonary artery pressures, monitoring cardiac output assessment, and viewing transesophageal echocardiography as guides, additional inotropic drugs, vasodilators, or both may be administered as needed.

Should right ventricular failure occur as a consequence of the recipient patient having long-standing pulmonary hypertension, therapy as previously described for right-sided heart failure is administered. Inotropes, vasodilators, inhaled nitric oxide, and prostaglandin E_1 all have been used to one degree or the other to improve pulmonary blood flow and relieve right ventricular failure.

Once weaned from cardiopulmonary bypass, the patient is transferred to the intensive care unit, where he or she is weaned from ventilatory and pharmacologic support as tolerated over a period of hours as in any other patient. Obviously, two differences in the care of the transplant patient are the increased risk of infection and donor heart rejection. In this regard, it is incumbent on the operating room anesthesiologist to take special care to employ sterile techniques. Whatever immunosuppressive agents the surgeon may request are administered in a timely fashion. Cyclosporine, azathioprine, and methylprednisolone are routinely administered perioperatively.

18

Transesophageal Echocardiography and the Cardiac Anesthesiologist

It would be foolhardy to attempt to summarize the principles and practice of transesophageal echocardiography (TEE) in a brief chapter in a brief introductory text. Nevertheless, it is critically important that any individual attempting to practice cardiac anesthesia either as a trainee or an individual returning to cardiac anesthesia practice have an understanding of this helpful diagnostic tool. This may seem like an onerous task for many anesthesiologists, especially those returning to cardiac anesthesia practice only to find that technology not available to them during their training is now considered a routine skill to one degree or another for the practice of cardiac anesthesia. Since the 1990s, many graduates of residency programs have had formal training in TEE so that to them it is no more involved than placing Swan-Ganz catheters was to anesthesiologists who trained in the 1970s and 1980s. It is important to remember, however, that in both instances the faculty who taught those residents probably had to learn the techniques themselves without the benefit of training during their own residencies. Many established cardiac anesthesia practitioners have had to turn to various books and courses to learn TEE.

Whereas videotapes and text coupled with review courses may contribute much to learning TEE, established practitioners now have the opportunity to turn to their home computer and CD-ROM technology to access TEE educational materials that provide a sense of real-time performance. It is important that the anesthesia practitioner make a definitive effort to acquire these valuable skills.

Although anesthesiologists have contributed much to the use of intraoperative TEE, it is likely that many anesthesiologists who have some facility with this technology have done so in collaboration with noninvasive cardiologists. Ideally, a noninvasive cardiologist should always be available to both the surgeon and the anesthesiologist should a TEE diagnosis be uncertain. If the anesthesiologist, whatever his or her level of TEE training, is uncertain of a TEE image, it is far better to seek the counsel of either a cardiologist or another anesthesiologist to assist in clinical decision making, rather than make clinical judgments based on potentially flawed TEE interpretations. Because TEE can have specific ramifications on patient care (e.g., in mitral valvular repair), it is important that we be as comfortable as possible with this technology. If the surgeon and anesthesiologist are uncertain about a TEE image, it is imperative that additional opinions be sought before taking any particular action when possible.

What Transesophageal Echocardiography Reveals

Through this text we have frequently mentioned the use of TEE in guiding one aspect of therapy or another. The perioperative uses for it include (1) assessing valvular function and integrity; (2) estimating left and right ventricular function; (3) examining intraventricular and intra-atrial shunting; (4) detecting intracavitary masses (e.g., atrial myxomas); (5) examining the aorta for dissections, atheromas, and intra-aortic balloon pump placement; (6) ruling out atrial septal defects in patients with left ventricular assist devices; (7) assessing the adequacy of mitral valvular repair; (8) examining the coronary ostia after aortic valvular replacement; (9) confirming coronary sinus catheter placement for retrograde delivery of cardioplegia; (10) identifying pericardial effusion; and (11) examining for intracavitary air. A knowledge of any of these issues could be very helpful in patient management. That is what is important about TEE. It can help us to manage patients with a variety of disease states.

It is important that each individual develop a unified TEE examination that covers all the structures that TEE allows us to view—not only the valves or ventricular function, but also the intraventricular and intra-atrial septa, as well as the aorta. Through a guided examination, the anesthesiologist, even with limited experience, should be able to identify if something is wrong.

TEE employs a piezoelectric crystal that generates ultrasonic waves that are reflected at various surfaces depending on acoustic densities. This permits us to obtain a real-time visualization of the heart. Greater detail on the technology underlying the workings of echocardiography can be found in any number of the fine texts and videotapes. Rather than focusing on the science behind TEE, it is far more important at this stage to determine how it can assist us in the operating room. Obviously, to use TEE, the first thing we must be aware of is that it must be placed in the esophagus. Generally, this is done after induction of anesthesia, at which point the lubricated TEE probe is placed into the esophagus. Care must be taken not to force the probe or cause substantial injury to the pharynx or the esophagus. Because esophageal tears can lead to mediastinitis, it is important that the probe not be forcibly placed. Additionally, patients with varying esophageal pathologies (tumors, strictures, and so forth) should not undergo TEE examination.

Figure 18-1 shows the various views that can be obtained by placing the TEE probe in the esophagus. Using these different views, the anesthesiologist can note the various pathologies outlined previously. Color flow Doppler allows for the detection of an abnormal flow of blood in the heart, which can help in identifying both valvular pathologies and shunts. Before we attempt to diagnose the dysfunctional heart, however, it is important to know exactly what we are looking for in these images. Figure 18-2 provides a schematic view of the blood supply to the heart in the principal views obtained through TEE. The four-chamber view (Figure 18-3) shows the atria as well as the mitral and occasionally the tricuspid valve. The three-chamber view (Figure 18-4) shows the aortic valve and left ventricular outflow. The short-axis view helps to assess ventricular function (Figure 18-5). Using these views we can begin to comment on the questions that we would like TEE to help us answer.

Namely, how well do the ventricles contract? Does the valve leak? Is the mitral valve repair complete? These questions are not going to be answered by reading a book or even looking at static pictures in a text specifically devoted to TEE. Rather, time must be spent with the TEE machine gaining experience during real-time TEE examinations. Videotapes and CD-ROMs also help to educate the practitioner in interpreting TEE images. Once educated, the anesthesiologist becomes familiar with the routine structures that can be revealed through TEE examination. Next, the anesthesiologist can begin to appreciate the various pathologies demonstrated through TEE. Even though we may have a specific purpose in mind when using TEE (e.g., does a mitral valve

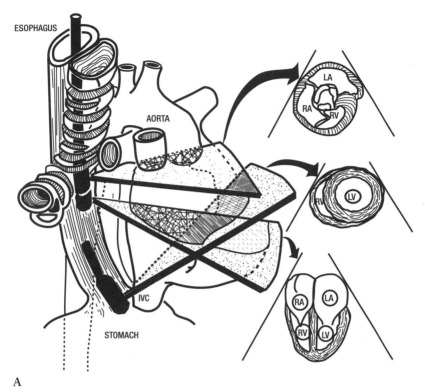

A

Figure 18-1. *Transesophageal echocardiographic views (A,B). (LA = left atrium; RA = right atrium; RV = right ventricle; LV = left ventricle; RPA = right pulmonary artery; IVC = inferior vena cava; SVC = superior vena cava; Ao = aorta; LAA = left atrial appendage.) (Modified from TE Oh. Intensive Care Manual [4th ed]. Oxford: Butterworth–Heinemann, 1997.)*

repair leak?), we should examine all aspects of the heart when performing an examination.

We must be careful in using TEE as well. At times, TEE imagery can distract us from our other duties to the patient. We must keep an eye on hemodynamic performance as well as the surgical field while we attempt to perform a TEE examination. In many regards TEE is but one part of a complete patient management approach by which we direct vasodilator and inotropic therapy in response to information provided through TEE images, direct visualization of the heart, and hemodynamic monitoring. Thus, when TEE is used in combination with other modalities it helps to ensure a safely delivered anesthetic.

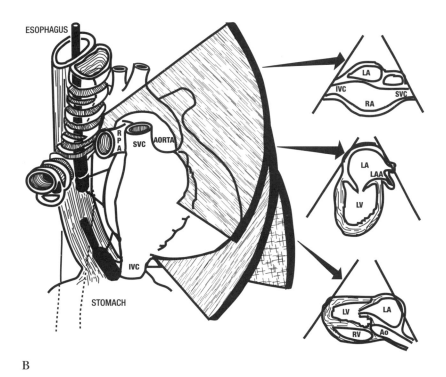

B

How Transesophageal Echocardiography Is Used

Assessing Valvular Function

Observation of the valves can determine the integrity of the valvular apparatus, vegetations, myxomatous degeneration, and ruptured chordae tendineae (Figures 18-6 and 18-7). Stenotic lesions are also readily identified by TEE examination. Color flow Doppler helps to detect abnormalities in blood flow in the heart, often revealing the extent of the valvular pathology (Figure 18-8). TEE assessment of valves after valvular repair and replacement can be used to confirm that the underlying pathology has been corrected.

Assessing Ventricular Function

Although the precise quantification of left ventricular function using TEE requires some experience, even the novitiate can readily determine

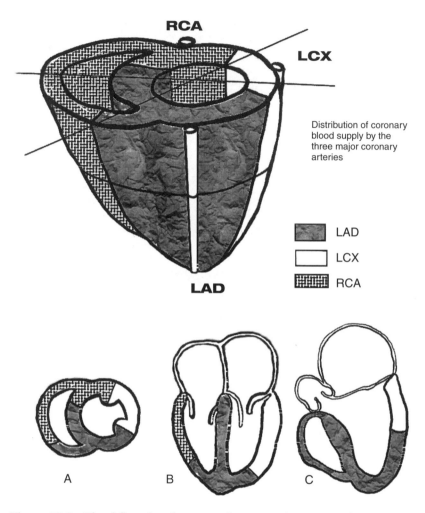

Figure 18-2. *Blood flow distribution to the myocardium in (A) the ventricular short-axis view, (B) the four-chamber view, and (C) the three-chamber view. (LAD = left anterior descending artery; LCX = left circumflex artery; RCA = right coronary artery.) (Modified from Y Oka, P Goldiner. Transesophageal Echocardiography. Philadelphia: Lippincott, 1992.)*

whether the ventricle is contracting or not. The distended noncontractile heart characteristic of a failing ventricle is readily observed through a TEE examination using the short-axis view. Right ventricle dysfunction can similarly be noted on TEE as well. Although in the surgical

Figure 18-3. *The four-chamber view (A,B). The atria and ventricles are easily seen. The tricuspid valve and mitral valve are visualized as well.*

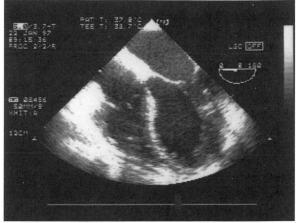

A

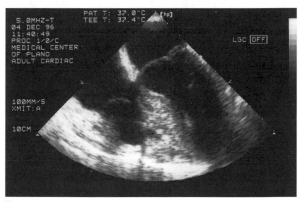

B

candidate, direct observation of the heart over the sterile drape generally provides the first inkling of a patient with a failing pump, TEE is useful to confirm that impression. Naturally, measures of cardiac output and pulmonary artery pressures also serve to help guide therapy for ventricular failure. By using the short-axis view and by being knowledgeable about the various arterial blood vessels supplying the walls of the heart, it is possible to determine which vessels are providing inadequate blood flow, resulting in ventricular decompensation. Using such an approach it is possible to occasionally identify a kinked bypass graft after myocardial revascularization.

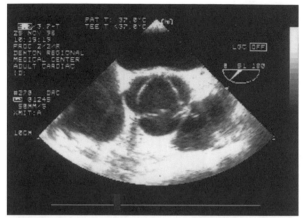

Figure 18-4.
(A) The aortic valve and (B) left ventricular out-flow.

A

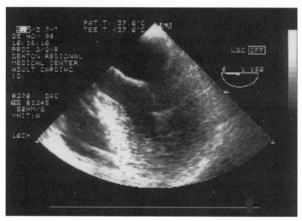

B

Detecting Shunts, Masses, Effusions, and Unexpected Pathologies

A quick survey of all the views obtainable through a TEE examination may reveal unexpected pathology at the time of surgery. Various shunts, ventricular aneurysms, pericardial effusions, and unexpected valvular pathologies can be detected during the course of a routine examination. Should an unusual pathology be noted by the anesthesiologist, this

Figure 18-5. *The short-axis view showing the right and left ventricles.*

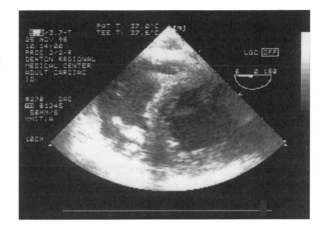

Figure 18-6. *Vegetation on the mitral valve.*

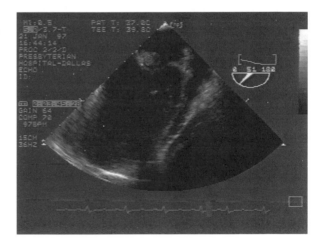

needs to be discussed with the surgeon to determine the significance of the finding. If necessary, a cardiologist or more experienced anesthesia echocardiographer may need to determine whether any newly discovered pathology warrants immediate surgical treatment. This is particularly true should significant mitral valvular disease be found in a patient scheduled for simple coronary artery bypass grafting.

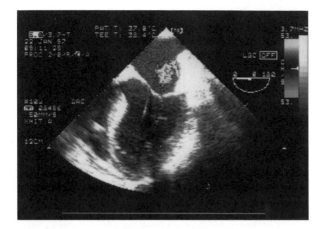

Figure 18-7.
Minimal mitral regurgitation.

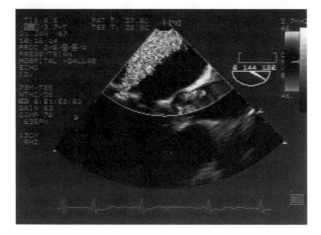

Figure 18-8.
Doppler color flow showing severe mitral regurgitation.

Guiding Therapy

TEE assessment of the aorta can assist the surgeon in detecting atheromas that could lead to embolization on aortic cannulation (Figure 18-9). Using TEE and surface echocardiography, it is possible for the surgeon to direct aortic cannula placement away from areas more likely to promote systemic embolization.

Figure 18-9.
Transesophageal
echocardio-
graphic view of
the aorta and aor-
tic valve (A,B).

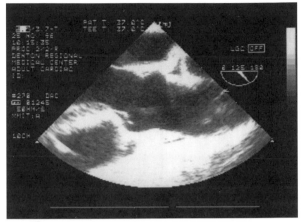

A

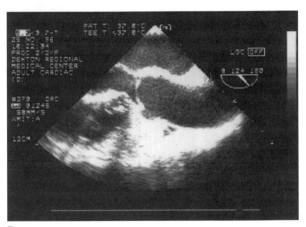

B

   Ultimately, only by working with the TEE machine and reviewing live images will the anesthesiologist become comfortable with this important technology. It is important that any anesthesiologist returning to cardiac anesthesia practice make a considerable effort to become as familiar as possible with the diagnostic modality. Most important, anesthesiologists, if uncertain as to the interpretation of TEE imagery, should seek appropriate assistance from cardiology or anesthesiology colleagues when necessary.

19

Anesthesia for Minimally Invasive Cardiac Surgery*

The anesthetic management of patients undergoing minimally invasive cardiac surgery represents nothing uniquely innovative with regard to anesthesia. Nevertheless, this evolving surgical technique presents a number of challenges to the anesthesiologist that must be quickly addressed to ensure successful minimally invasive surgery. Although the techniques, agents, and methods employed in caring for the minimally invasive cardiac patient should be well known to any experienced anesthesiologist, the unique circumstances and combinations of required skills can make minimally invasive cardiac surgery among the most challenging anesthetics to safely deliver.

This chapter reviews those techniques and procedures necessary to provide a satisfactory operating environment and the patient's quick recovery from minimally invasive cardiac surgery. Although it is beyond the scope of this chapter to provide a complete review of the various nuances of cardiac anesthesia practice, the unique synthesis of mechanical skills, pharmacologic manipulations, and communication abilities necessary to successfully anesthetize these challenging patients are reviewed.

In undertaking any discussion of anesthesia for this patient population, it is best to consider how these patients are similar to and dif-

---

*Modified with permission from J Wasnick. Anesthesia for Minimally Invasive Cardiac Surgery. In M Mack, et al. (eds), Minimally Invasive Cardiac Surgery. St. Louis: Quality Medical Publishers, (in press).

ferent from other candidates for cardiac revascularization. As with any patient scheduled for bypass surgery, it is implicitly understood that there is a potential risk for myocardial ischemia, infarction, and dysrhythmia in the perioperative period. Although the patient presenting for minimally invasive surgery is more than likely not afflicted with diffuse multivessel disease, it is also true that such patients frequently have significant left anterior descending artery stenosis with a varying amount of clinical symptomatology. Thus, simply because a patient may have single-vessel disease does not in any way permit any decrease in perioperative vigilance. The anesthesiologist should not assume a false sense of security by thinking that the minimally invasive cardiac patient is somehow less sick than any other patient scheduled for coronary revascularization.

So what is fundamentally different about anesthetic management in this setting? In essence, there are three critical points of difference in anesthetic management between patients revascularized via sternotomy with cardiopulmonary bypass and those operated on using minimally invasive techniques.

First, patients undergoing minimally invasive surgery will for varying amounts of time have blood flow occluded in the operated vessel, usually the left anterior descending artery. Whereas anesthetic management generally aims to preserve coronary blood flow until application of the aortic cross clamp in patients revascularized with the assistance of cardiopulmonary bypass, the anesthesiologist must be prepared to respond to the development of myocardial ischemia at the time of completion of the arterial anastomosis in the minimally invasive patient. Generally, the successful surgical team produces a trial occlusion of the vessel to be bypassed before performing the arteriotomy. This maneuver allows time to assess the adequacy of collateral blood flow by noting preservation of myocardial function through measurements of cardiac output or transesophageal echocardiography (TEE). Additionally, trial occlusion of the artery to be bypassed may provide for ischemic preconditioning to better protect the myocardium during the actual performance of the anastomosis.

Thus, first and foremost, patients operated via the minimally invasive approach without cardiopulmonary bypass present a challenge in that a coronary artery is intermittently occluded, leading to the potential for the development of myocardial ischemia. As any experienced cardiac surgery team knows, myocardial ischemia is not an infrequent occurrence in patients taken for revascularization. Inadequate myocardial oxygen supply to meet the myocardial oxygen demand invariably leads to the development of ischemia and potentially ventricular dysfunction. The treatment of both ischemia and ventricular failure should be nothing new to any anesthesiologist attempting to care for the patient undergoing minimally invasive surgery. Nevertheless, whereas the cardiopulmonary bypass machine has long provided a ready escape for the anesthesiologist faced with circulatory collapse secondary to myocardial ischemia, the patient operated via the minimally invasive approach will most likely not be cannulated to permit immediate institution of bypass. Thus, both the surgeon and anesthesiologist should be confident of the patient's ability to tolerate vascular occlusion before completion of the arteriotomy. Obviously, if deterioration occurs beyond which pharmacologic manipulations can relieve ischemia and restore ventricular function, the patient needs to be placed emergently on either femoral bypass or the have the surgical excision extended and atrial and aortic cannulations completed in the usual fashion.

The second obvious area of difference between the patient operated via the minimally invasive technique and those patients revascularized employing routine sternotomy centers on access and visualization of the heart. As many experienced anesthesiologists may readily admit, perhaps the best monitor of the heart is direct observation, which assists in patient management. Without ever looking on any other measurement or number, most anesthesiologists can tell how the patient is doing simply by watching the brisk right ventricle contract in the open chest. This valued monitor is lost in patients operated via the minimally invasive technique. Extra attention must be paid to electrocardiography, hemodynamic monitors, and TEE for careful surveillance for myocardial ischemia in the minimally invasive patient.

More important, because direct access to the heart is limited, certain precautions should be taken to provide appropriate substitutes for those frequently employed modalities that require direct epicardial contact. First and foremost among these concerns is the need for a quick, sterile mechanism for defibrillation and cardioversion. Minimally invasive approaches do not permit application of epicardial paddles to the heart. Additionally, patient draping and positioning may prevent application of cutaneous defibrillation paddles in a timely fashion should a life-threatening rhythm develop. As such, transcutaneous defibrillation pads must be placed on the patient and connected to the cardioverter defibrillator before preparing the surgical field.

Additionally, epicardial pacing is not immediately possible in the minimally invasive approach. As heart rate reductions are frequently requested by the surgical team to facilitate completion of the anastomosis, it is prudent to establish an alternative pacing capability should heart block and sinus bradycardia require emergent treatment. Although transesophageal atrial pacing may be employed, atrioventricular pacing is necessary should heart block ensue. Transvenous pacing is, therefore, established before surgical incision. Generally, either a pace port or pacing Swan-Ganz pulmonary artery flotation catheter can provide the necessary pacing capabilities as well as the standard hemodynamic information useful in managing any critically ill patient.

Third, the minimally invasive cardiac patient differs from the patient operated via sternotomy with cardiopulmonary bypass in the amount of communication required between the anesthesiologist and surgical team. Whereas the essential part of the surgery of the patient with cardiopulmonary bypass is done on an arrested heart, the minimally invasive patient's heart remains beating. This reality represents a significant difference in the role of the anesthesiologist in the operating room. In the patient undergoing coronary revascularization via sternotomy with cardiopulmonary bypass, the anesthesiologist's primary role in the procedure comes during induction and weaning from the cardiopulmonary bypass machine. Assuming a relatively autonomous perfusionist, the anesthesiologist has little to do during the actual performance of the bypass grafts.

In minimally invasive surgery, the anesthesiologist has the ability either to advance or hinder completion of the anastomosis. Additionally, the anesthesiologist must ensure adequate delivery of oxygen to the tissues while simultaneously securing a suitable operating environment for the surgical team. Often these goals are not readily attainable. Because cardiac output is dependent on stroke volume and heart rate, it is clear how minimally invasive surgery can impair delivery of oxygenated blood to the body.

Frequently, to gain access to the anastomotic site, the shape of the heart must be slightly distorted by flat, malleable retractors and immobilizers. Such retraction can reduce stroke volume, lowering cardiac output. Additionally, frank ischemia, should it develop, obviously can impair myocardial contractility with a resultant reduction in stroke volume and cardiac output. More frequently, however, the surgeon requests a slowing of the heart rate during the period of vascular occlusion. This serves two purposes. First, a reduced heart rate may decrease myocardial oxygen demand and lengthen diastolic time to improve the balance between myocardial oxygen supply and demand in the left ventricle. Second, and perhaps more importantly, heart rate reduction provides a slowly beating heart that facilitates completion of the vascular anastomosis.

Obviously, communication between the anesthesiologist and surgeon is essential at this time to facilitate completion of the bypass graft. Both the anesthesiologist and surgeon must be certain that an adequate cardiac output and systemic pressure are maintained to secure organ viability. The information exchanged between the anesthesiologist and surgeon is much closer to that which is needed in pulmonary surgery where manipulation of one-lung ventilation is necessary to facilitate pulmonary excision. Because it is often necessary to provide one-lung ventilation during minimally invasive surgery as well, this analogy has a practical implication. Although one-lung ventilation may not be essential to minimally invasive direct vision cardiac surgery, it does facilitate mammary artery harvesting in patients in which thoracoscopic or video assistance is to be employed. Various modalities can provide single-lung ventilation. Double-lumen endotracheal tubes, bronchial blockers, and the Univent tube (Fuji Systems, Tokyo) can successfully achieve one-lung ventilation depending on the preferences of the individuals involved.

Thus, when compared with routine bypass, the minimally invasive technique presents specific concerns relating to myocardial ischemia, myocardial access, and intraoperative communications. How these concerns are addressed are now explored by reviewing the anesthetic management of a typical minimally invasive thoracoscopically assisted coronary artery bypass patient.

Mr. X is a 37-year-old man scheduled for minimally invasive thoracoscopically assisted coronary artery bypass. He has had a previous subendocardial myocardial infarction and a prior angioplasty. He has had recurrent angina of increasing severity and has become refractory to medical therapy. Cardiac catheterization revealed a 95% stenosis of the left anterior descending artery, with an ejection fraction of approximately 50%. His history is also noteworthy for a 90–packs-a-year smoking history and significant ethanolism. Physical examination reveals a slightly overweight, hypertensive man with decreased breath sounds bilaterally. Preoperative laboratory is within normal limits except for a room air arterial oxygen tension (PaO_2) of 60 mm Hg.

From this history, it is clear to see that a number of anesthesia-related difficulties can occur in bringing the typical minimally invasive cardiac surgery patient to the operating room. These difficulties are no different than those that might well be encountered in any other patient taken for bypass surgery. The constellation of smoking, hypertension, and obesity must be addressed in this patient as with any other patient presenting for coronary revascularization. Careful preoperative anesthesia assessment should minimize any particular problems in this patient population.

Preoperative Assessment

A brief history and physical examination should assist in identifying any particular problems that might complicate anesthetic management. In addition to eliciting any history of increased angina pain or respiratory difficulty before surgery, it is especially prudent in this population to identify any past difficulties in airway management. Because double-lumen endotracheal intubation will most likely be requested, it is useful to determine if the patient has had any particular difficulty with any type of airway management in the past. Because double-lumen intubation is generally more difficult than single-lumen tube placement, it is prudent to recognize that double-lumen endotracheal intubation may prove most difficult in patients with a previous history of airway difficulty. In this instance, should lung isolation be deemed essential, the single-lumen Univent tube may be employed to provide bronchial blockade. If it does not appear that the patient can be intubated, either awake intubation or fiberoptic intubation should be considered. As always, failure to secure the airway can lead to significant intraoperative morbidity and mortality. Even in that patient with myocardial ischemia, safe airway management remains the cornerstone of cardiac anesthesia practice. Additionally, attention should be given to the patient's smoking history. Lung disease may make one-lung ventilation difficult to manage intraoperatively. Pulmonary disease may lead to significant ventilation-perfusion mismatch during one-lung ventilation, resulting in significant hypoxemia. Intraoperative bronchospasm can further complicate patient management during periods of one-lung ventilation.

Physical examination for the minimally invasive cardiac patient should especially focus on the ease of airway management and considerations for double-lumen endotracheal tube placement if a thoracoscopic approach is planned. Equivalence of bilateral radial arterial pulses should be confirmed to determine the site of arterial line placement. Additionally, a reduced left radial arterial pulse may signify subclavian stenosis, potentially retarding flow through the left internal mammary artery. Although the surgeon most likely will have noted this already, if unequal pulses are detected, it is prudent to remind the surgical team that flow in the left arm is impaired. The laboratory data and electrocardiogram results are reviewed and, assuming they are in order, the patient is considered ready for bypass.

As with any other bypass patient, antihypertensive and anti-ischemic medications are continued up through the time of surgery. Premedication may be given at the discretion of the anesthesiologist, but it is hardly essential for successful and safe patient management.

Anesthesia Induction

On arriving in the operating room suite, the patient is monitored in the usual fashion. A 14-gauge intravenous line is begun, and a radial arterial catheter is placed. Five-lead electrocardiography (leads V_5 and 2) is applied to provide surveillance for myocardial ischemia. Assuming normal airway anatomy is present, anesthesia induction may be undertaken with any number of anesthetics currently available. As is always the case in cardiac anesthesia and is so frequently misunderstood by many anesthesia practitioners, no one combination of drugs offers a magical formula for successful anesthetic management. Any number of induction agents (thiopental [Pentothal], propofol, midazolam, etomidate) can be used in the management of these patients depending on individual preference. Generally, the combination of amnestics (e.g., propofol), a narcotic (e.g., sufentanil), and a muscle relaxant (e.g., rocuronium) may be administered to achieve anesthetic induction and acceptable conditions for intubation. As always, the anesthesiologist must be both actor and reactor. Quick reactions and thoughtful actions should prevent hemodynamic embarrassment.

Peri-induction hypertension and tachycardia most likely reflect inadequate anesthesia and as such, supplemental boluses of narcotics and inhalational agents (e.g., desflurane) may be given. Bradycardia accompanied by hypotension may reflect decreased sympathetic tone accompanying anesthesia induction. Judicious administration of ephedrine should readily correct induction-related hypotension. Obviously, both peri-induction hypotension and hypertension can lead to myocardial ischemia and cardiovascular collapse. Rapid correction of either hypertension or hypotension and ischemia should prevent hemodynamic instability that results in significant ventricular dysfunction.

Once anesthetized, a pacing pulmonary artery flotation catheter is placed via the right internal jugular vein. Ability to pace both the atrium and ventricle is confirmed. Baseline hemodynamic measurements are obtained.

A TEE probe and assessment may next be undertaken. Although TEE is hardly essential in the management of every bypass patient, it does provide an additional source of information regarding ventricular performance. It is potentially worthwhile in this patient population. Although ventricular wall motion abnormalities may have many causes, the development of ventricular dysfunction after occlusion of the coronary artery by vascular snares more than likely indicates true ischemic dysfunction. Finally, defibrillation pads are applied before preparation of the surgical field.

The patient is placed in a modified right lateral decubitus position with the left arm secured. This position allows the surgeon to access the left internal mammary artery. Careful positioning prevents peripheral nerve injury.

Anesthesia induction should be directed toward the same hemodynamic goals as in any patient at risk for myocardial ischemia—that is, myocardial oxygen supply must be greater than myocardial oxygen demand. The patient should ideally remain normotensive without developing any relative tachycardia. The combination of propofol (100 mg), sufentanil (50 µg), and a muscle relaxant (e.g., vecuronium, 0.1 mg per kg) for the typical 70-kg individual generally achieves suitable hemodynamics. As always, induction may be complicated by ischemia and ventricular dysfunction. In that event, intravenous nitroglycerin, phenylephrine, and other inotropes (dobutamine, milrinone) may be necessary to correct ischemia, hypotension, and ventricular dysfunction as employed in any other cardiac anesthetic. The application of vasodilators and vasopressors in the peri-induction period is no different than in any other patient taken for coronary revascularization (Table 19-1).

Anesthetic Management

Maintenance of anesthesia should be with inhalational agents (desflurane, isoflurane), narcotics (sufentanil, fentanyl), and muscle relaxants (vecuronium, rocuronium, pancuronium) that permit early extubation at the conclusion of surgery and support early patient mobilization. Although a high-dose narcotic technique will successfully anesthetize these patients like any other cardiac patient, there is no need to provide a 50 µg per kg dose of intravenous fentanyl. Careful hemodynamic management should permit the use of relatively short acting anesthetics. Consequently, the goal of anesthetic induction and maintenance should be early extubation and mobilization.

Table 19-1. Specific Considerations for the Minimally Invasive Thoraco-scopically Assisted Coronary Artery Bypass Patient

1. Transvenous pacing ability
2. Transcutaneous defibrillation capability
3. Ability to provide one-lung ventilation
4. Anesthetic selection leading to early extubation and mobilization

The crucial point in anesthetic management of the minimally invasive patient such as Mr. X comes when performing the anastomosis. Before this point, anesthetic management and goals are directed toward the same hemodynamic necessities as in any other bypass patient. At the time of completion of the anastomosis, however, the anesthesiologist must provide both a slowly beating heart and provide for adequate organ perfusion in a patient experiencing the iatrogenic occlusion of a coronary artery.

Once the surgeon has harvested, either through direct vision or thoracoscopically, the left internal mammary artery, 10,000 U of heparin is given (Figure 19-1). Additional heparin is readily available to be quickly administered via a central line should cardiopulmonary bypass become necessary. The perfusionist is available in the room with a bypass machine.

With the pericardium opened and the left anterior descending artery exposed, the surgeon places proximal and distal vascular snares around the site of the anastomosis. Once in place, a trial occlusion of the vessel is instituted. Electrocardiogram, TEE, and hemodynamic monitors are quickly assessed to see if any signs of ischemia or ventricular dysfunction develop. After a brief test, flow is restored to the left anterior descending artery through relaxation of the vascular snares. Once the surgeon is confident that the patient has tolerated a trial occlusion, blood flow through the vessel to be bypassed is again interrupted. At this point the heart rate is frequently reduced to facilitate operating conditions by reducing myocardial movement and to minimize rate-related myocardial ischemia. Individual surgeons may demand varying degrees of bradycardia to comfortably complete the anastomosis. Heart rates may be slowed anywhere to 60–30 beats per minute. The beta$_1$-specific, short-acting beta blocker esmolol (bolus dosage [10–20 mg intravenously] and infusion) can slow the heart rate to provide a suitably quiet surgical field. Adenosine (6–12 mg intra-

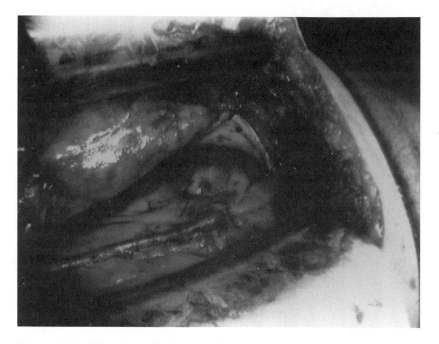

Figure 19-1. *The minimally invasive direct-vision coronary artery bypass approach.*

venous bolus) can transiently slow atrioventricular conduction, leading to brief periods of cardiac standstill.

While attempting to fulfill the surgeon's request for a slowly beating heart, the anesthesiologist must recognize that reducing the heart rate also impairs cardiac output and blood pressure. Generally, phenylephrine can be titrated to maintain systemic pressure. However, alpha agonists do not augment cardiac output. In essence, near completion of the anastomosis, systemic pressures of approximately 80–100 mm Hg systolic with a variable cardiac index are tolerated. Fortunately, the time required to complete the anastomosis is relatively short (6–10 minutes). Therefore, any reduction in cardiac index is generally transitory.

If significant myocardial ischemia is noted on the electrocardiography or TEE or through hemodynamic measurements, nitroglycerin is infused. Phenylephrine may be administered to provide pressure support. If outright cardiovascular collapse develops, additional heparin is administered and the patient placed on either femoral-femoral bypass,

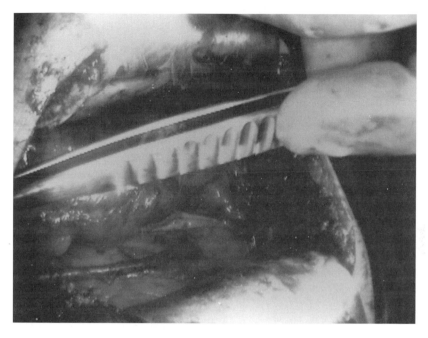

Figure 19-2. *Anastomosis of the left internal mammary artery to the left anterior descending artery.*

or the sternotomy is completed and the patient cannulated. Obviously, if the heart becomes completely dysfunctional, sternotomy and direct cardiac massage would be necessary until cardiopulmonary bypass can be initiated or the patient defibrillated.

Once the anastomosis is successfully completed, esmolol is discontinued and pacing commenced to restore a heart rate in the range of 70–80 beats per minute (Figure 19-2). Adequacy of graft patency is determined by either thermal imaging or Doppler flow. Protamine in a ratio of 1 to 1 to heparin is given to reverse anticoagulation. The surgical incision is closed. After closure, an intercostal block with 0.25% bupivacaine may be performed to lessen pain on emergence. Anesthetic agents are discontinued and reversal of muscle relaxants achieved. When the patient is awake and spontaneously breathing, the patient is extubated and transported, with appropriate monitoring, to the recovery area.

In addition to the intercostal block, other modalities of pain management may be successfully employed in this population. Epidural or subarachnoid narcotics can no doubt be successful in controlling perioperative pain. However, there is some risk of dural puncture headache and nerve injury that might affect postoperative mobilization. Intravenous morphine or meperidine administered via a patient-controlled analgesia apparatus satisfactorily controls perioperative discomfort. Ketorolac may be given as well in certain select patients. Ketorolac must be administered with caution, however, in elderly patients, those with renal dysfunction, and those with peptic ulcer disease.

Early mobilization and discontinuation of vascular monitoring should be accomplished, assuming stable hemodynamic, pulmonary, and renal function. Incentive spirometry, bronchodilator therapy, and positive pressure breathing may be particularly necessary in patients such as Mr. X who have some degree of pulmonary impairment. The staff of the intensive care unit should be cautioned not to expect the kind of large diuresis that frequently accompanies patients after revascularizations done with cardiopulmonary bypass.

Conclusion

Although the extent to which minimally invasive surgery will be employed in the future remains uncertain, it is clearly a technique in constant evolution. Although no new anesthesia maneuvers are necessary to accommodate this rapidly developing surgical approach, well-established anesthetic techniques have had to be refined and synthesized to provide for successful minimally invasive surgery.

20

Real World Concerns for the Cardiac Anesthesiologist in Community Practice

We have now spent a considerable amount of time reviewing the many aspects of community cardiac anesthesia practice. Although we have not covered every issue in great detail, we have provided the basis by which routine cardiac cases should be readily managed by the novitiate, particularly if an experienced colleague is available for consultations. As the established general anesthesia practitioner becomes more and more comfortable in managing the cardiac surgery patient, he or she will no doubt wish to seek a more detailed and comprehensive text to expand his or her knowledge of cardiac anesthesia. One area of particular importance is the many policy issues that influence both the cardiac surgery patient and the cardiac anesthesiologist. Currently, there are an increasing number of social, ethical, economic, and legal issues that influence the practice of cardiac anesthesia and cardiac care in general. As practitioners become ever more comfortable with the medical issues involved in cardiac anesthesia practice, the numerous social and ethical concerns may take on greater importance. This chapter briefly reviews a number of the social aspects of cardiac anesthesia practice.

Jehovah's Witnesses

Jehovah's Witnesses as a matter of belief refuse blood products. Their refusal of blood products presents a particularly difficult problem for the anesthesia practitioner. The refusal of blood products by a cardiac surgery patient can easily lead to patient death after cardiopulmonary bypass. Nonetheless, patients still have the right to refuse treatment, even that which we might consider life-saving therapy. Anesthesiologists must be careful to respect the view of Jehovah's Witnesses and to understand that their refusal to accept blood products is grounded in specific beliefs. At the same time, anesthesiologists must be certain of their ability to permit a patient who might otherwise survive to bleed to death after cardiac surgery. Thus, the individual physician and patient must come to an understanding in that regard. Many hospitals have prepared specific release forms by which the patient absolves the hospital for failing to provide transfusion therapy should that be necessary. In our practice, we agree to anesthetize all Jehovah's Witness patients when they desire surgery. Nonetheless, we are extremely frank in discussing the risk of death with these patients. We inform them that we will permit them to die as a consequence of withholding blood products. If they still refuse blood products, under no circumstances do we give blood products once an understanding has been made not to do so.

Patients with Human Immunodeficiency Virus Infection

With antiviral therapy becoming increasingly successful, it is possible that we may be called on to care for an ever greater number of individuals living with human immunodeficiency virus (HIV) infection. Coexisting cardiac disease is likely to present as HIV patients age. Therefore, anesthesiologists must be reminded they have an ethical duty to provide anesthesia care for all patients afflicted. Appropriate caution must be taken for all patients (i.e., universal precautions) whether they are known to be HIV positive or not.

Patients with Do Not Resuscitate Orders

The patient with do not resuscitate orders has little chance of being selected for cardiac surgery. The very nature of cardiac surgery may in and of itself be considered a resuscitative event to a degree. Still, occasionally a patient with do not resuscitate orders presents for surgery but rarely for cardiac repair. As always, living wills and patient directives need to be followed should complications develop.

Consent

Patients need to be frankly informed of the risks of anesthesia in heart surgery. We have a frank discussion regarding the risk of surgery and death with both patients and families. Generally, patients and family members do not want to participate in this discussion. Many are frightened by the frankness with which risks are discussed. Nonetheless, in today's litigious atmosphere, there is little choice but to proceed with a full and complete consent regarding all the risks in anesthesia and surgery in front of witnesses.

Although cardiac surgery is not possible without anesthesia, it remains prudent to detail the possible complications from anesthesia-related maneuvers. These things include pulmonary artery line placement, intubation-related injuries, and other complications that might be directly traced to anesthesia in addition to those things likely to occur as a consequence of cardiac surgery.

Recent media reports of the dangers of pulmonary artery line placement often need to be explained to patients. Other mass media scares regarding anesthetic practice need to be addressed at the time of informed consent (e.g., risk of awareness, and so forth).

Litigation

Cardiac surgery carries a significant mortality. Approximately 1–2% of routine patients may have a serious complication. This means that if an anesthesiologist sees 200 patients per year, he or she could be involved with up to four perioperative deaths per year. The death of a patient generally brings family anger no matter how sick the patient may have been. Strokes and other injuries also occur that enrage patients and families who are unable to appreciate the complexity or severity of illness. Although it may be true that the risks of cardiac surgery are known, patients and their families will engage in legal action against the anesthesiologist even if anesthesia has had little to do with a poor outcome. As always, truthfulness and accurate record keeping remain the best defense against litigation. The cardiac anesthesia practitioner should be certain that suitable solvent malpractice coverage has been arranged before entering into cardiac anesthesia practice.

Economic Concerns

The changing nature of medical practice may reduce the number of patients brought to heart surgery as medical therapy is ever more advocated for the treatment of life-threatening cardiovascular disease. Likewise, managed care may prevent patients from being taken for surgical revascularization. It is highly likely that reimbursement for anesthesia services will continue to decline in the years to come. Many anesthesiologists have responded to this change by forming ever larger collectives in the hope that they might preserve the value of anesthesia services through collective bargaining. At present, however, the overabundance of anesthesiologists and certified registered nurse anesthetists makes this practice only moderately successful. The ability of hospitals and insurers to marshal legal expertise to challenge anesthesiologists using antitrust laws can prevent anesthesiologists from achieving a strong negotiating position.

The dramatic decline in the popularity of anesthesiology as a specialty by medical school graduates may reduce the overabundance of practitioners. Nonetheless, it may take some time to witness a decline in physician-anesthesia supply. As the overall number of anesthesiologists decreases, specialty anesthesia practice may no longer be practical. With managed care reducing surgery volumes, the need for anesthesia specialists may decline. Therefore, subspecialty certification in cardiac anesthesia seems increasingly unnecessary. Flexible practitioners would appear to be essential for the survival of anesthesia as a specialty. Additional subspecialty certification requirements may only serve to further limit the flexibility of our practitioners, thereby weakening the position of the anesthesia clinician.

It is hoped that as anesthesiology declines as an alluring specialty those individuals attracted to it will be able to work well together in a collegial fashion so that patients receive the best possible care. Only time will tell if anesthesiologists can effectively work together to respond to medicine's new age. Ultimately, a praxis approach may provide the kind of insight that allows anesthesiologists to provide effective, cost-conscious, quality anesthesia care.

21

Where Do We Go From Here?

Having now presented a basic overview of adult community care, where do an anesthesiologist go for additional information? Obviously, there is much more to the pharmacology and physiology of adult anesthetic cardiac care that can be presented in a text, providing principally a praxis introduction to community practice. Also, the many influences of cardiology, pulmonology, and critical care medicine as they affect the ever changing delivery of cardiac care require that the anesthesiologist be vigilant to stay current and focused. Only when so prepared can the anesthesiologist provide the highest quality of cardiac anesthetic care possible in the community setting.

In this chapter we examine some of the resources that assist the anesthesiologist undertaking cardiac practice in staying informed and prepared to meet the challenge of anesthetic delivery into the next century and beyond.

Where to Find Information

Internet Sources

We live at the dawn of a new age of technology. Much as the printing press offered the cumulative knowledge of Western society to the masses, so too can the Internet serve to instantly communicate new ideas, technical developments, warnings, and advice for the anesthetic practitioner in general and the cardiac anesthesiologist in particular.

Table 21-1. Useful Web Sites for the Cardiac Anesthesiologist

Organization	Web Site
American Society of Anesthesiologists	www.asahq.org/
Wright's anesthesia and critical care resources on the Internet	www.eur.nl/fgg/anest/wright/
Gasnet	gasnet.med.yale.edu
Anesthesiology	www.anesthesiology.org/
New England Journal of Medicine	www.nejm.org
Journal of the American Medical Association	www.ama-assn.org/public/journals/ pubhome.htm
The Heart Surgery Forum	www.hsforum.com/HeartSurgery/ homeHSF.html
Society for Cardiovascular Anesthesiologists	dacc.uchicago.edu/sca/welcome.html

Whereas most books offer a series of texts and articles by which one is advised to seek additional information (and so will we), at this point perhaps it is to the Internet and computerized literature searches where the inquisitive practitioner first might turn.

Considering the delay in book publication after its writing, the reader who seeks references from a published source may perhaps be reading information that is 1–2 years old (as you may be doing now). Who can project into the next century the number of anesthesiology-related chat rooms, virtual textbooks, and other services that will be available to instantly locate information essential to clinical practice? Although at the moment, the number of Internet offerings dealing with anesthesiology may be limited, we can only expect that these will grow in the years to come. Whether one turns to Gasnet or simply employs a good search engine such as Alta Vista, it becomes possible to identify the topic of choice (with a little work). (See Table 21-1 for useful web sites for the cardiac anesthesiologist.)

University anesthesia web sites often contain links to other related anesthesia sites located on the Internet such as Gasnet or Anesthesia Web (www.anesthesiaweb.com). These can be useful to the practitioner as well. Increasingly, the journals themselves have developed web sites to complement the printed media. The *Journal of Cardiothoracic and*

Vascular Anesthesia is now in the process of developing its own web site at http://www.jcardioanesthesia.com. The *Journal of the American Medical Association* and other journals have also found their way onto the worldwide web.

The ready availability of computerized literature searches also assists the physician in seeking current or relative information by employing keywords. Of course, once a particular search is initiated, one is often astounded to find a plethora of general entries and literature relating to a given topic, some of a very esoteric character. As such, we must have both vision and discernment to sort through the vast amounts of medically related published material to be found in the various scientific journals. Naturally, new pharmaceuticals and technologies must be carefully considered before becoming a part of routine practice. As cost containment becomes a greater concern in day-to-day health care management, we must be that much more critical of journal entries that advocate improved clinical responses from the use of one new pharmaceutical or another. With due consideration, we should be able to update cardiac anesthesia practice on a year-to-year basis so that we may not only meet the standard of care but exceed it.

Texts, Journals, CD-ROMs, Videos, and Colleagues

Although anesthesiologists are well known for their love of gadgetry, we should not assume that all are computer literate enough to the point of being able to access web sites, although we hope everyone is working to this end. Certainly, we would not have spent the time and effort to create a readily accessible published text if we did not believe that books and published journals are and will remain a valuable resource into the next century. Whereas the exhaustive tomes produced on this field may give way to CD-ROM text, the trusty handbook in the back pocket for quick reading (as we hope you will use this book) will be with us for some time. Either in CD-ROM format or through print media, a certain number of texts should be a part of the clinician's library. The key anesthesia texts are so well known that it is pointless to name them. Suffice it to say that a comprehensive text of the specialty as a whole is essential as a reference. Miller's *Anesthesia* or *Clinical Anesthesia* by Barash et al. and other texts should provide an easily accessible source of basic information. Likewise, because the cardiac patient still can present with many of the same concerns as any adult patient presenting for general anesthesia, a text such as Stoelting's *Anesthesia and Co-Existing Disease* can be extremely helpful as well. Other texts useful to cardiac anesthesia include but are not limited to the following books:

Barrie PS, Shires GT. *Surgical Intensive Care.* Boston: Little, Brown, 1993.

Braunwald E. *Heart Disease: A Textbook of Cardiovascular Medicine.* Philadelphia: Saunders, 1997.

Civetta J, et al. *Critical Care.* Philadelphia, Lippincott, 1988.

Estafanous FG, et al. *Cardiac Anesthesia: Principles and Clinical Practice.* Philadelphia: Lippincott, 1994.

Oka Y, Goldiner PL. *Transesophageal Echocardiography.* Philadelphia: Lippincott, 1992.

This list is by no means exclusive, as there are many texts written each year. Basically, the cardiac anesthesia practitioner needs to have references relating to cardiac anesthesia per se, including critical care medicine, transesophageal echocardiography (TEE), and cardiology. Although we have maintained that one does not need to be a cardiologist or intensivist to safely manage the routine cardiac patient, the knowledge of these areas is essential to patient care.

TEE remains an area of uncertainty among anesthesia practitioners as to what constitutes levels of skills necessary to undertake and ensure a quality TEE examination. As mentioned earlier, if the anesthesiologist is not comfortable with his or her own TEE skills, it is incumbent on the anesthesiologist to arrange for a cardiologist or another anesthesiologist to assist in TEE evaluation. Various courses are available to assist in developing TEE skills as well. Working with cardiologists in one's own institution can also give the anesthesiologist the resources necessary to facilitate and to employ TEE effectively. Michael K. Cahalan and Churchill Livingstone have produced a very useful interactive publication titled *Intraoperative Transesophageal Echocardiography* that presents various TEE images using CD-ROM technology. Illustrative videotapes are likewise available to accompany the myriad texts that provide introductions to TEE. Many institutions already have a system for proctoring the use of TEE in the operating room to be certain that the anesthesiologist's TEE examination is completed in accordance with acceptable standards. The

anesthesiologist must be certain that he or she has met the requirements of his or her particular institution. Likewise, it is expected that
the anesthesiologist will have developed a level of sophistication necessary to safely place the TEE probe and to provide a basic interpretation of the imagery.

Journals provide yet another source of information that the anesthesiologist may find useful. Of course, many of our journals contain
information that is essential to the future of clinical practice and to the
survival of the specialty as a whole, yet that information is often too far
removed from day-to-day clinical application to be readily employed.
Nonetheless, it is important to recall that what we consider practical
today and applicable had its basis in the sciences of years ago. Therefore, we should not dismiss the basic science literature contained in the
principal specialty journals out of hand.

Obviously, *Anesthesiology* and *Anesthesia and Analgesia* focus on
the entire spectrum of anesthetic practice. The *Journal of Cardiothoracic and Vascular Anesthesia* often contains material that would not
be of interest to the noncardiac practitioner but can nonetheless offer
useful information to the cardiac anesthesiologist in particular. In addition to review articles, it contains "pro-and-con" presentations on a
variety of controversies relating to current anesthesia practice. Indeed,
a year's review of the *Journal of Cardiothoracic and Vascular Anesthesia* should provide an introduction to most of the current topics at
play in the field.

Survey of Anesthesiology provides useful summaries of noteworthy
articles found in a variety of publications and therefore can be useful
to stay abreast of various reports in the literature.

Colleagues and coworkers can often give great insight into practice
in a given individual patient. A good rapport with the person working next door often can provide a wealth of information and the essential second pair of hands should difficulties arise.

Last, we have focused on many of the issues in the course of providing a praxis approach to community care with the idea of making cardiac anesthesia as readily accessible, manageable, and
functional as possible. In these final pages, I have included lists of
reference articles that may help a person get started toward
researching a topic in greater degree if so interested. Although it
may be preferable in this day and age to do a fresh library search
rather than rely on a reference list, these are provided in the event
library computerized searches are unavailable or quick access to an
article is desired.

Cardiac Risk Factors

Braunwald E, et al. The stunned myocardium: prolonged, post-ischemic ventricular dysfunction. Circulation 1982;66:1146.
Goldman L, et al. Multifactorial index of cardiac risks in non-cardiac surgical procedures. N Engl J Med 1977;297:845.
Higgins TL, et al. Risk factors for respiratory complications after cardiac surgery. Anesthesiology 1991;75:A258.
Higgins TL, et al. Stratification of morbidity and mortality outcome by preoperative risk factors in coronary artery bypass patients. JAMA 1992;267:2344.
Lahey SJ, et al. Preoperative risk factors that predict hospital length of stay in coronary artery bypass patients greater than sixty years old. Circulation 1992;86:I-181.
Mangano DT. Perioperative cardiac morbidity. Anesthesiology 1990;72:153.
Zehender M, et al. Eligibility for and benefit of thrombolytic therapy in inferior myocardial infarction: focus on the prognostic implications of right ventricular function. J Am Coll Cardiol 1994;24:362.

Nitrates

Jugdutt BI, Warnica JW. Intravenous nitroglycerin therapy to limit myocardial infarct size, expansion and complications: effects of timing, dosage and infarct location. Circulation 1988;78:906.

Beta Blockade

Cork R, et al. The effect of esmolol given during cardiopulmonary bypass. Anesth Analg 1995;80:28.
Mangano D, et al. Effect of atenolol on mortality and cardiovascular morbidity after non-cardiac surgery. N Engl J Med 1996;335:1713.
Norwegian Multi-Center Study Group. Timolol induced reduction in mortality and reinfarction in patients surviving acute myocardial infarction. N Engl J Med 1981;304:801.

Calcium Antagonists

Kloner RA. Nifedipine in ischemic heart disease. Circulation 1995;92:1074.
Reves JG, et al. Calcium entry blockers: uses and implications for the anesthesiologist. Anesthesiology 1982;57:504.
Strauss WE, Parisi SF. Combined use of calcium channel and beta adrenergic blockers for the treatment of chronic stable angina. Ann Intern Med 1988;109:570.

Angiography and Cardiac Catheterization

Kulick DL, Rahimtoola SH. Risk stratification in survivors of acute myocardial infarction: routine cardiac catheterization and angiography is a reasonable approach in most patients. Am Heart J 1991;121:641.

Ross J, et al. Guidelines for coronary angiography. A report of the American College of Cardiology/American Heart Association Task Force on Assessment of Diagnostic and Therapeutic Cardiovascular Procedures (Subcommittee on Coronary Angiography). J Am Coll Cardiol 1987;10:935.

Schwab ST, et al. Contrast nephrotoxicity: a randomized controlled trial of a non-ionic and ionic radiographic contrast agent. N Engl J Med 1989; 320:149.

Nuclear Cardiology

Mangano DT, et al. Dipyridamole thallium 201 scintigraphy as a preoperative screening test. A re-examination of its predictive potential. Circulation 1991;84:493.

Pohost G, Henzlova M. The value of thallium 201 imaging. N Engl J Med 1990;323:190.

Schofer J, et al. Thallium-201/technetium-99m pyrophosphate overlap in patients with acute myocardial infarction after thrombolysis. Am Heart J 1986;112:291.

Varma S, et al. Qualitative comparison of thallium 201 scintigraphy after exercise and dipyridamole in coronary artery disease. Am J Cardiol 1986; 64:871.

Tests of Cardiac Function: Enzyme Studies

Antman E, et al. Evaluation of a rapid bedside assay for detection of serum cardiac troponin. JAMA 1995;273:1279.

Ellis A. Serum protein measurements and the diagnosis of acute myocardial infarction. Circulation 1991;83:1107.

Gibler W, et al. Early detection of acute myocardial infarction in patients presenting with chest pain and non-diagnostic ECGs. Serial CPKMB sampling in the emergency department. Ann Emerg Med 1990;19:1359.

Hamm C. New serum markers for acute myocardial infarction. N Engl J Med 1994;331:607.

Angioplasty and Thrombolytic Therapy

Anderson H, Willerson J. Thrombolysis in acute myocardial infarction. N Engl J Med 1993;329:703.

Braunwald E. Thrombolytic reperfusion of acute myocardial infarction: resolved and unresolved issues. J Am Coll Cardiol 1988;12:85A.

Califf R, et al. Experience with the use of TPA in the treatment of acute myocardial infarction. Ann Emerg Med 1988;17:1176.

Grines CL, et al. A comparison of immediate angioplasty with thrombolytic therapy for acute myocardial infarction. N Engl J Med 1993;328:673.

The Gusto Angiographic Investigators. The effects of tissue plasminogen activator, streptokinase, or both on coronary artery patency, ventricular function and survival after acute myocardial infarction. N Engl J Med 1993;329:1615.

The Gusto IIb Investigators. A clinical trial comparing primary coronary angioplasty with tissue plasminogen activator for acute myocardial infarction. N Engl J Med 1997;336:1621.

Landau C, Lange RA. Percutaneous transluminal coronary angioplasty [review]. N Engl J Med 1994;330:981.

Lange RA, et al. Immediate angioplasty for acute myocardial infarction. N Engl J Med 1993;328:726.

Ryan TJ, et al. ACC/AHA Task Force Report: guidelines for percutaneous transluminal coronary angioplasty. A report of the American College of Cardiology and American Heart Association Task Force on Assessment of Diagnostic and Therapeutic Cardiovascular Procedures. (Committee on Percutaneous Transluminal Angioplasty). J Am Coll Cardiol 1993;22:2033.

Surgical Procedure: Coronary Artery Bypass Grafting

Garrett HE, et al. Aortocoronary bypass with saphenous vein graft: seven year follow-up. JAMA 1973;223:792.

Loop FD, et al. Influence of internal mammary artery graft on 10-year survival and other cardiac events. N Engl J Med 1986;314:1.

Schaff HV, et al. Detrimental effects of perioperative myocardial infarction on late survival after coronary bypass. J Thorac Cardiovasc Surg 1984;88:972.

Echocardiography and Perioperative Evaluation

Buda A, et al. Comparison of two-dimensional echocardiographic wall motion and wall thickening abnormalities in relation to the myocardium at risk. Am Heart J 1986;111:587.

Marcovitz P, Armstrong W. Accuracy of dobutamine stress echocardiography in detecting coronary artery disease. Am J Cardiol 1992;69:1269.

Technical Aspects of Coronary Artery Bypass Surgery

He G, et al. Risk factors for operative mortality and sternal wound infection in bilateral mammary artery grafts. J Thorac Cardiovasc Surg 1994;107:196.

Jones E. Conduits for coronary artery bypass (key references). Ann Thorac Surg 1993;55:194.

Kirklin J, et al. Guidelines and indications for coronary artery bypass graft surgery: a Report of the American College of Cardiology/American Heart Association Task Force on Assessment of Diagnostic and Therapeutic Cardiovascular Procedures (Subcommittee on Coronary Artery Bypass Surgery). J Am Coll Cardiol 1991;17:543.

Loop F, et al. Influence of the internal mammary artery graft on 10-year survival and other cardiac events. N Engl J Med 1986;314:1.

Naumheim K, et al. The changing profile of the patient undergoing coronary artery bypass surgery. J Am Coll Cardiol 1988;11:494.

The Writing Group for the Bypass Angioplasty Revascularization Investigation (BARI) Investigators. Five-year clinical and functional outcome comparing bypass surgery and angioplasty in patients with multi-vessel coronary disease. JAMA 1997;277:715.

Risk Evaluation and the Coronary Artery Bypass Patient

Force T, et al. Perioperative myocardial infarction after coronary artery bypass surgery: clinical significance and approach to risk stratification. Circulation 1990;82:903.

Lahey J, et al. Preoperative risk factors that predict hospital length of stay in coronary artery bypass patients greater than sixty years old. Circulation 1992;86:181.

Mangano DT. Perioperative cardiac morbidity. Anesthesiology 1990;72:153.

Mangano DT. Cardiac anesthesia risk management: multi-center outcome research. J Cardiothorac Vasc Anesth 1994;8:10.

Preoperative Pulmonary Dysfunction

Shih H, et al. Frequency and significance of cardiac arrhythmias and chronic obstructive lung disease. Chest 1988;94:44.

Preoperative Renal Dysfunction

Kaul T, et al. Cardiac operations in patients with end stage renal disease. Ann Thorac Surg 1994;57:691.

Manske C, et al. Coronary revascularization in the insulin-dependent diabetic patient with chronic renal failure. Lancet 1992;340:998.

Straumann E, et al. Aortic and mitral valve disease in patients with end stage renal failure on long-term renal dialysis. Br Heart J 1992;67:236.

Endocrine Disease and Heart Surgery

Dilmann WH. Cardiac function in thyroid disease: clinical features in management considerations. Ann Thorac Surg 1993;56:S9–S15.

Pulsinelli W, et al. Increased damage after ischemic stroke in patients with hyperglycemia with and without established diabetes mellitus. Am J Med 1983;74:540.

Salomon WW, et al. Diabetes mellitus and coronary artery bypass. J Thorac Cardiovasc Surg 1983;85:264.

Savage MP, et al. Acute myocardial infarction in diabetes mellitus and significance of congestive heart failure as a prognostic factor. Am J Cardiol 1988;62:665.

Hematology and Coronary Artery Bypass

The Heparin/Aspirin Reperfusion Trial (HART) Investigators: a comparison between heparin and low dose aspirin as adjunctive therapy with tissue type plasminogen activator for acute myocardial infarction. N Engl J Med 1990;323:1434.

Hirsch J, Levine M. Low molecular weight heparin. Blood 1992;79:1.

Horrow J, Ellison N. Effective hemostasis during cardiac surgery. Can J Anaesth 1992;39:309.

Lewis H, et al. Protective effects of aspirin against acute myocardial infarction and death in men with unstable angina: results of Veterans Administration Cooperative Study. N Engl J Med 1983;309:396.

Ridker P, et al. Low dose aspirin therapy for chronic stable angina: a randomized placebo control clinical trial. Ann Intern Med 1991;114:835.

Sethi G, et al. Implications of pre-operative administration of aspirin in patients undergoing coronary artery bypass grafts. J Am Coll Cardiol 1990;15:15.

Theroux P, et al. Reactivation of unstable angina after discontinuation of heparin. N Engl J Med 1992;327:141.

Premedication

Thomson I, et al. Drug interaction with sufentanil. Hemodynamic effects of pre-medication and muscle relaxants. Anesthesiology 1992;76:921.

Anesthesia Induction and Maintenance

Buzello W, et al. Hypothermic cardiopulmonary bypass and neuromuscular blockade by pancuronium and vecuronium. Anesthesiology 1985;62:201.

Fleming N. The choice of muscle relaxants is not important in cardiac surgery. J Cardiothorac Vasc Anesth 1995;9:772.

Helman J, et al. The risk of myocardial ischemia in patients receiving desflurane versus sufentanil anesthesia for coronary bypass graft surgery. Anesthesiology 1992;77:47.

Higgins T, et al. Propofol versus midazolam for intensive care unit sedation after coronary bypass artery grafting. Crit Care Med 1994;22:1415.

Leung J, et al. Isoflurane anesthesia and myocardial ischemia: comparative risk versus sufentanil anesthesia in patients undergoing coronary artery bypass graft surgery. Anesthesiology 1991;74:838.

Lowenstein E, et al. Cardiovascular responses to large doses of intravenous morphine in man. N Engl J Med 1969;281:1389.

Lunn J, et al. High dose fentanyl anesthesia for coronary artery surgery. Anesth Analg 1979;58:390.

O'Connor J, et al. The incidence of myocardial ischemia during anesthesia for coronary bypass surgery in patients receiving pancuronium or vecuronium. Anesthesiology 1989;70:230.

Paulissian R, et al. Hemodynamic responses to pancuronium and vecuronium during high dose fentanyl anesthesia for coronary artery bypass grafting. J Cardiothorac Vasc Anesth 1991;5:120.

Philbin D, et al. Fentanyl and sufentanil anesthesia revisited: how much is enough? Anesthesiology 1990;73:5.

Priebe H. Isoflurane and coronary hemodynamics. Anesthesiology 1989; 71:960.

Ramsay J, et al. Pure opioid versus opioid-volatile anesthesia for coronary bypass graft surgery: a prospective, randomized double blind study. Anesth Analg 1994;78:867.

Rooke G, et al. The hemodynamic and renal effects of sevoflurane and isoflurane in patients with coronary artery disease and chronic hypertension. Anesth Analg 1996;82:1159.

Ruff R, Reeves J. Hemodynamic effects of a lorazepam/fentanyl anesthetic induction for coronary artery bypass surgery. J Cardiothorac Anesth 1990;4:314.

Russell G, et al. Propofol-fentanyl anesthesia for coronary artery bypass surgery and cardiopulmonary bypass. Anaesthesia 1989;44:205.

Slogoff S, Keats A. Randomized trial of primary anesthetic agents on outcome of coronary artery bypass operations. Anesthesiology 1989;70:179.

Slogoff S, et al. Steal prone coronary anatomy and myocardial ischemia associated with four primary anesthetic agents in humans. Anesth Analg 1991;72:22.

Starr N, et al. Bradycardia and asystole following the rapid administration of sufentanil with vecuronium. Anesthesiology 1986;64:521.

Thomson I, et al. A comparison of desflurane and isoflurane in patients undergoing coronary artery surgery. Anesthesiology 1991;75:776.

Thomson I, et al. Drug interactions with sufentanil. Hemodynamic effects of pre-medication and muscle relaxants. Anesthesiology 1992;76:922.

Tuman K, et al. Does choice of anesthetic agents significantly effect the outcome after coronary artery surgery? Anesthesiology 1989;70:189.

Tuman K, et al. Comparison of anesthetic techniques in patients undergoing heart valve replacement. J Cardiothorac Vasc Anesth 1990;4:159.

Arterial Line Placement

DeHert S, et al. Central to peripheral arterial pressure gradient during cardiopulmonary bypass: relation to pre- and intra-operative data and effects of vasoactive agents. Acta Anaesthesiol Scand 1994;38:479.

Gravlee G, et al. A comparison of brachial, femoral, and aortic intra-arterial pressures before and after cardiopulmonary bypass. Anaesth Intensive Care 1989;17:305.

Mangano D, Hickey P. Ischemic injury following uncomplicated radial artery catheterization. Anesth Analg 1979;58:55.

Mohr R, et al. Inaccuracy of radial artery pressure measurement after cardiac operations. J Thorac Cardiovasc Surg 1987;94:286.

Slogoff S, et al. On the safety of radial artery cannulation. Anesthesiology 1983;59:42.

Pulmonary Artery Catheterization

Connors A, et al. Effectiveness of right heart catheterization in the initial care of critically ill patients. JAMA 1996;276:889.

Dalen J, Bone R. Is it time to pull the pulmonary artery catheter? JAMA 1996;276:916.

Eidelman L, Pizov R. Pulmonary artery catheterization at the crossroads? Crit Care Med 1994;22:543.

Hardy J, et al. Patho-physiology of rupture of the pulmonary artery by pulmonary artery balloon tipped catheter. Anesth Analg 1983;62:925.

Johnston W, et al. Pulmonary artery catheter migration during cardiac surgery. Anesthesiology 1986;64:258.

Magilligan D, et al. Mixed venous oxygen saturation as a predictor of cardiac output in a post-operative cardiac surgical patient. Ann Thorac Surg 1987;44:260.

Marini J. Acute lung injury. Hemodynamic monitoring with the pulmonary artery catheter. Crit Care Clin 1986;2:551.

Pulmonary Artery Catheter Consensus Conference Participants. Pulmonary artery consensus conference: consensus statement. Crit Care Med 1997; 25:910.

Robin E. Death by pulmonary artery flow directed catheter. Chest 1987; 92:727.

Shah K, et al. A review of pulmonary artery catheterization in 6245 patients. Anesthesiology 1984;61:271.

Swan HJC, Ganz W. Hemodynamic measurements in clinical practice: a decade in review. J Am Coll Cardiol 1983;1:103.

Thomson I, et al. Right bundle branch block and complete heart block caused by the Swan-Ganz catheter. Anesthesiology 1979;51:359.

Tuman K, Roizen M. Outcome assessment and pulmonary artery catheterization: why does the debate continue? Anesth Analg 1997;84:1.

Tuman K, et al. Effect of pulmonary artery catheterization on outcome of patients undergoing coronary artery surgery. Anesthesiology 1989; 70:199.

Vedrinne C, et al. Predictive factors for usefulness of fiberoptic pulmonary artery catheter for continuous oxygen saturation in mixed venous blood monitoring in cardiac surgery. Anesth Analg 1997;85:2.

Airway Management

Benumof JL. Management of the difficult adult airway. Anesthesiology 1991;75:1087.

Benumof J. Laryngeal mask airway and the ASA difficult airway algorithm. Anesthesiology 1996;84:686.

Butler P, et al. Prediction of difficult laryngoscopy: an assessment of the thyromental distance and Mallampati predictive tests. Anaesth Intensive Care 1992;20:139.

Heath ML, et al. Intubation through the laryngeal mask: a technique for unexpected difficult intubation. Anaesthesia 1991;46:541.

Pennant JH, White PF. The laryngeal mask airway, its uses in anesthesiology. Anesthesiology 1993;79:685.

Task Force on Guidelines for Management of a Difficult Airway. Practice guidelines for the management of a difficult airway. Anesthesiology 1993; 78:597.

Perioperative Hypertension

Estafanous F, Tarazi R. Systemic arterial hypertension associated with cardiac surgery. Am J Cardiol 1980;46:685.

Flacke JW, et al. Reduced narcotic requirement by clonidine with improved hemodynamic and adrenergic stability in patients undergoing coronary bypass surgery. Anesthesiology 1987;67:11.

Girard D, et al. The safety and efficacy of esmolol during myocardial revascularization. Anesthesiology 1986;65:157.

Goldman L, Caldera D. Risk of general anesthesia in elective operation in the hypertensive patient. Ann Intern Med 1983;98:504.

Kaplan JA. Clinical considerations for the use of intravenous nicardipine in the treatment of post-operative hypertension. Am Heart J 1990;119:443.

Newsome L, et al. Esmolol attenuates hemodynamic response during fentanyl pancuronium anesthesia for aorto-coronary bypass surgery. Anesth Analg 1986;65:451.

Arrhythmia Management

Atlee JL. Perioperative cardiac dysrhythmias: diagnosis and management. Anesthesiology 1997;86:1397.

Atlee J, Bosnjak Z. Mechanisms of cardiac arrhythmias during anesthesia. Anesthesiology 1990;72:347.

Atlee J, et al. Transesophageal atrial pacing for intraoperative sinus bradycardia or AV junctional rhythm: feasibility as prophylaxis in 200 anesthetized adults and hemodynamic effects of treatment. J Cardiothorac Vasc Anesth 1993;7:436.

Creswell L, et al. Hazards of post-operative atrial arrhythmias. Ann Thorac Surg 1993;56:539.

Feeley GW. Management of perioperative arrhythmias. J Cardiothorac Vasc Anesth 1997;11S1:10.

Mason J. A comparison of seven anti-arrhythmia drugs in patients with ventricular tachyarrhythmias. N Engl J Med 1993;329:452.

Purdy R, et al. Handbook of Cardiac Drugs. Boston: Little, Brown, 1995.

Pharmacology of Vasodilators, Vasopressors, and Inotropes

Ansell J, et al. Amrinone induced thrombocytopenia. Arch Intern Med 1984; 144:949.

Badner N, et al. An amrinone bolus prior to weaning from cardiopulmonary bypass improves cardiac function in mitral valve surgery patients. J Cardiothorac Vasc Anesth 1994;8:410.

Baim D, et al. Evaluation of a new bipyridine inotropic agent—milrinone—in patients with severe congestive heart failure. N Engl J Med 1983;309:748.

Benotti J, et al. Hemodynamic assessment of amrinone: a new inotropic agent. N Engl J Med 1978;299:1373.

Fowler M, Alderman E. Dobutamine and dopamine after cardiac surgery: greater augmentation of myocardial blood flow with dobutamine. Circulation 1984;70:I-103.

Gallagher J, et al. Prophylactic nitroglycerin infusion during coronary bypass surgery. Anesthesiology 1986;64:785.

Gray R, et al. Low cardiac output status after open heart surgery. Hemodynamic effects of dobutamine, dopamine and norepinephrine plus phentolamine. Chest 1981;80:16.

Groden D. Vasodilator therapy for congestive heart failure. Arch Intern Med 1993;153:445.

Halpern N, et al. Post-operative hypertension: a multi-center, randomized comparison between intravenous nicardipine and sodium nitroprusside. Crit Care Med 1992;20:1637.

Kikura M, et al. The effect of milrinone on hemodynamics and left ventricular function after emergence from cardiopulmonary bypass. Anesth Analg 1997;85:16.

Loeb H, et al. Superiority of dobutamine over dopamine for augmentation of cardiac output in patients with chronic low output cardiac failure. Circulation 1977;65:375.

MacGregor D, et al. Hemodynamics and renal effects of dopexamine and dobutamine in patients with reduced cardiac output coronary artery bypass grafts. Chest 1994;106:835.

Patel C, et al. The use of sodium nitroprusside in post-coronary bypass surgery: a plea for conservatism. Chest 1986;89:663.

Purdy R, et al. Handbook of Cardiac Drugs (2nd ed). Boston: Little, Brown, 1995.

Thompson B, Cockrill B. Renal-dose dopamine? A siren song? Lancet 1994;344:7.

Reoperative Surgery

Loop F, et al. Reoperation for coronary atherosclerosis. Ann Surg 1990; 212:378.

Owen E, et al. The third time coronary artery bypass graft. Is the risk justified? J Thorac Cardiovasc Surg 1990;100:31.

Weaning the Failing Heart from Cardiopulmonary Bypass

Bailey J, et al. Pharmacokinetics of amrinone during cardiac surgery. Anesthesiology 1991;75:961.

Baim D, et al. Evaluation of a new bipyridine inotropic agent—milrinone—in patients with severe congestive heart failure. N Engl J Med 1983;309:748.

Butterworth J. Selecting an inotrope for the cardiac surgery patient. J Cardiothorac Vasc Anesth 1993;7:26.

De Hert S, et al. Comparison of two different loading doses of milrinone for weaning from cardiopulmonary bypass. J Cardiothorac Vasc Anesth 1995;9:264.

Glower D, et al. Linearity of the Frank Starling relationship in the intact heart: the concept of pre-load recruitable stroke work. Circulation 1985;71:994.

Hardy J, Belisle S. Inotropic support of the heart that fails to successfully wean from cardiopulmonary bypass: the Montreal Heart Institute experience. J Cardiothorac Vasc Anesth 1993;7:33.

Mangano D. Biventricular function after myocardial revascularization in humans: deterioration and recovery patterns during the first 24 hours. Anesthesiology 1985;62:571.

Nugent M. Anesthesia and myocardial ischemia: the gains of the past have largely come from control of myocardial oxygen demand; the breakthrough of the future will involve optimizing myocardial oxygen supply. Anesth Analg 1992;75:1.

Pagel P, et al. Left ventricular diastolic function in the normal and diseased heart. Perspectives for the anesthesiologist part I. Anesthesiology 1993;79:836.

Pagel P, et al. Left ventricular diastolic function in the normal and diseased heart. Perspectives for the anesthesiologist part II. Anesthesiology 1993;79:1104.

Prielipp R, et al. Pharmacodynamics and pharmacokinetics of milrinone administration to increase oxygen delivery in critically ill patients. Chest 1996;109:1291.

Ventricular Assist Devices

Bregman D, Kaskel P. Advances in percutaneous intra-aortic balloon pumping. Crit Care Clin 1986;2:221.

Champsaur G, et al. Use of the Abiomed BVS System 5000 as a bridge to cardiac transplantation. J Thorac Cardiovasc Surg 1990;100:122.

Elberry J, et al. Effects of the left ventricular assist device on right ventricular function. J Thorac Cardiovasc Surg 1990;99:809.

Frazier OH, et al. First use of the hemopump, a catheter mounted ventricular assist device. Ann Thorac Surg 1990;49:299.

Frazier OH, et al. Multi-centered clinical evaluation of the Heart Mate 1000 IP left ventricular assist device. Ann Thorac Surg 1992;53:1080.

Göl MK, et al. Vascular complications related to percutaneous insertion of intra-aortic balloon pumps. Ann Thorac Surg 1994;58:1476.

Guyton RA, et al. Post-cardiotomy shock: clinical evaluation of the BVS 5000 bi-ventricular support system. Ann Thorac Surg 1993;56:346.

McCarthy PM, et al. Pre-peritoneal insertion of the Heart Mate 1000 IP implantable left ventricular assist device. Ann Thorac Surg 1994; 57:634.

Naunheim KS, et al. Intra-aortic balloon pumping in patients requiring cardiac operations. Risk analysis and long-term follow-up. J Thorac Cardiovasc Surg 1992;104:1654.

Symbas P, et al. Pulmonary artery balloon counter-pulsation for treatment of intra-operative right ventricular failure. Ann Thorac Surg 1985;39:437.

Right Ventricular Failure

Bastien O, et al. Evolution of right ventricular performance after CABG. Intensive Care Med 1988;14:499.

Boldt J, et al. Right ventricular function in patients with reduced left ventricular function undergoing myocardial revascularization. J Cardiothorac Vasc Anesth 1994;6:24.

Bondy R, et al. Reversal of refractory right ventricular failure with amrinone. J Cardiothorac Vasc Anesth 1991;5:255.

D'Ambra M, et al. Prostaglandin E: a new therapy for refractory right heart failure and pulmonary hypertension after mitral valve replacement. J Thorac Cardiovasc Surg 1988;89:567.

Dupuis J, et al. Amrinone and dobutamine as primary treatment of low cardiac output syndrome following coronary artery surgery: a comparison of their effects on hemodynamics and outcome. J Cardiothorac Vasc Anesth 1992;6:542.
Hurford W, Zapol W. The right ventricle and critical illness: a review of anatomy, physiology and clinical evaluation of its function. Intensive Care Medicine 1988;14:448.
Mangano D. Biventricular function after myocardial revascularization in humans: deterioration and recovery patterns during the first 24 hours. Anesthesiology 1985;62:571.
Skillington P, et al. Pulmonary artery balloon counter-pulsation for intraoperative right ventricular failure. Ann Thorac Surg 1991;51:658.

Nitric Oxide

Bigatello L, et al. Prolonged inhalation of low concentrations of nitric oxide in patients with severe adult respiratory distress syndrome. Effects on pulmonary hemodynamics and oxygenation. Anesthesiology 1994;80:161.
Frostell C, et al. Inhaled nitric oxide: a selective pulmonary vasodilator reversing hypoxic pulmonary vasoconstriction. Circulation 1991;83:2038.
Girard C, et al. Inhaled nitric oxide for right ventricular failure after heart transplantation. J Cardiothorac Vasc Anesth 1993;7:481.
Hemida M, et al. Role of nitric oxide in systemic response to dobutamine, epinephrine, and amrinone. J Cardiothorac Vasc Anesth 1995;9:627.
Loh E, et al. Cardiovascular effects of inhaled nitric oxide in patients with left ventricular dysfunction. Circulation 1994;90:2780.
Rich G, et al. Inhaled nitric oxide: selective pulmonary vasodilation in cardiac surgical patients. Anesthesiology 1993;78:1028.
Wessel D, et al. Delivery and monitoring of inhaled nitric oxide in patients with pulmonary hypertension. Crit Care Med 1994;22:930

Aprotinin and Antifibrinolytics

Dietrich W, et al. Influence of high dose aprotinin treatment on blood loss and coagulation patterns in patients undergoing myocardial revascularization. Anesthesiology 1990;73:1119.
Goldstein D, et al. Safety and efficacy of aprotinin under conditions of deep hypothermia and circulatory arrest. J Thorac Cardiovasc Surg 1995; 110:1615.
Horrow J, et al. Prophylactic tranexamic acid decreases bleeding after cardiac operations. J Thorac Cardiovasc Surg 1990;99:70.
Karski J, et al. Prevention of post-bypass bleeding with tranexamic and epsilon aminocaproic acid. J Cardiothorac Vasc Anesth 1993;7:431.
Lemmer J, et al. Aprotinin for coronary bypass surgery: efficacy, safety, and influence on early saphenous vein graft patency. J Thorac Cardiovasc Surg 1994;107:543.

Levy J, et al. Aprotinin reduces the incidence of strokes following cardiac surgery. Circulation 1996;94:I-535.

Murkin J, et al. Aprotinin significantly decreases bleeding and transfusion requirements in patients receiving aspirin and undergoing cardiac operations. J Thorac Cardiovasc Surg 1994;107:554.

Royston D. High dose aprotinin therapy: a review of the first five years' experience. J Cardiothorac Vasc Anesth 1992;6:76.

Royston D. Intraoperative coronary thrombosis: can aprotinin be incriminated? J Cardiothorac Vasc Anesth 1994;8:137.

Shore-Lesserson L, et al. Tranexamic acid reduces transfusions and mediastinal drainage in repeat cardiac surgery. Anesth Analg 1996;83:18.

Smith PK, Muhlbaier LH. Aprotinin: safe and effective only with the full dose regimen. Ann Thorac Surg 1996;62:1575.

Vander Salm T, et al. Reduction of bleeding after heart operation through the prophylactic use of EACA. J Thorac Cardiovasc Surg 1996;112:1098.

Heparin Anticoagulation

Anderson E. Heparin resistance prior to cardiopulmonary bypass. Anesthesiology 1986;64:504.

Brister S, et al. Thrombin generation during cardiac surgery. Is heparin the ideal anti-coagulant? Thrombosis and Haemostasis 1993;70:259.

Cines D, et al. Immune endothelial cell injury in heparin associated thrombocytopenia. N Engl J Med 1987;316:581.

Dietrich W, et al. The influence of pre-operative anti-coagulation on heparin response during cardiopulmonary bypass. J Thorac Cardiovasc Surg 1991;102:505.

Doherty D, et al. "Heparin-free" cardiopulmonary bypass: first reported use of heparinoid (org. 10172) to provide anti-coagulation for cardiopulmonary bypass. Anesthesiology 1990;73:562.

Fitch J. Con: heparin is not the best anti-coagulant for cardiopulmonary bypass. J Cardiothorac Vasc Anesth 1996;10:819.

Gravlee G, et al. Heparin management protocol for cardiopulmonary bypass influences postoperative heparin rebound but not bleeding. Anesthesiology 1992;76:393.

Hirsch J, et al. Guide to anti-coagulant therapy part I: heparin. Circulation 1994;89:1449.

Sabbagh A, et al. Fresh frozen plasma: a solution to heparin resistance during cardiopulmonary bypass. Ann Thorac Surg 1984;37:466.

Shorten G, Comunale M. Heparin-induced thrombocytopenia. J Cardiothorac Vasc Anesth 1996;10:521.

Stow E, Rinder C. Pro: heparin is the best anti-coagulant for cardiopulmonary bypass. J Cardiothorac Vasc Anesth 1996;10:817.

Warkentin T, et al. A 14 year study of heparin induced thrombocytopenia. Am J Med 1996;101:502.

Young J, et al. Adequate anti-coagulation during cardiopulmonary bypass determined by activated clotting time and the appearance of fibrin monomers. Ann Thorac Surg 1978;26:281.

Protamine

Frater R. Administration of protamine through the left atrium. J Thorac Cardiovasc Surg 1985;90:154.

Horrow J. Protamine: a review of its toxicity. Anesth Analg 1985;64:348.

Levy J, et al. Prospective evaluation of risk of protamine reactions in NPH insulin-dependent diabetics. Anesth Analg 1986;65:739.

Lowenstein E, Zapol W. Protamine reactions, explosive mediator release and pulmonary vasoconstriction. Anesthesiology 1990;73:373.

Lowenstein E, et al. Catastrophic pulmonary vasoconstriction associated with protamine reversal of heparin. Anesthesiology 1983;59:470.

Metz S, et al. Methylene blue does not neutralize heparin after cardiopulmonary bypass. J Cardiothorac Vasc Anesth 1996;10:474.

Michelsen L, et al. Heparinase I (Neutralase) reversal of systemic anticoagulation. Anesthesiology 1996;85:339.

Morel D, et al. C5A in thromboxane generation associated with pulmonary vaso and broncho-constriction during protamine reversal of heparin. Anesthesiology 1987;66:597.

Pharo G, Horrow J . Suspected protamine allergy: diagnosis and management for coronary artery surgery. Anesth Analg 1994;78:181.

Cardiopulmonary Bypass

Aranki S, et al. Single clamp technique: an important adjunct to myocardial and cerebral protection in coronary operations. Ann Thorac Surg 1994;58:296.

Baraka A, et al. Effect of alpha stat versus pH stat strategy on oxyhemoglobin dissociation and whole body oxygen consumption during hypothermic cardiopulmonary bypass. Anesth Analg 1992;74:32.

Buckberg G. Normothermic blood cardioplegia. Alternative or adjunct? J Thorac Cardiovasc Surg 1994;107:860.

Cremer J, et al. Systemic inflammatory response syndrome after cardiac operations. Ann Thorac Surg 1996;61:1714.

Diehl J, et al. Efficacy of retrograde coronary sinus cardioplegia in patients undergoing myocardial revascularization. A prospective randomized trial. Ann Thorac Surg 1988;45:595.

Fremes S, et al. A clinical trial of blood and crystalloid cardioplegia. J Thorac Cardiovasc Surg 1984;88:726.

Gill R. Neuropsychologic dysfunction after cardiac surgery: what is the problem? J Cardiothorac Vasc Anesth 1996;10:91.

Gu Y, et al. Heparin-coated circuits reduce the inflammatory response to cardiopulmonary bypass. Ann Thorac Surg 1993;55:1917.

Hayashida N, et al. Tepid antegrade and retrograde cardioplegia. Ann Thorac Surg 1995;59:721.

Hickey P, et al. Pulsatile and non-pulsatile cardiopulmonary bypass: a review of a counterproductive controversy. Ann Thorac Surg 1983;36:720.

Lichtenstein S, et al. Warm heart surgery. J Thorac Cardiovasc Surg 1991;101:269.

Mills N, Ochsner J. Massive air embolisms during cardiopulmonary bypass: causes, prevention and management. J Thorac Cardiovasc Surg 1980;80:708.

Murkin J, et al. Cerebral auto-regulation and flow metabolism coupling during cardiopulmonary bypass. Influence of $PaCO_2$. Anesth Analg 1987;66:825.

Murkin J, et al. A randomized study of the influence of perfusion technique and pH management strategy in 316 patients undergoing coronary artery bypass surgery. Neurologic and cognitive outcomes. J Thorac Cardiovasc Surg 1995;110:349.

Patel R, et al. Alpha stat acid base regulation during cardiopulmonary bypass improves neuropsychiatric outcome in patients undergoing coronary artery bypass grafts. J Thorac Cardiovasc Surg 1996;111:1267.

Prough D, et al. Response of cerebral blood flow to changes in carbon dioxide tension during hypothermic cardiopulmonary bypass. Anesthesiology 1986;64:576.

Royston D, Stammers A. Extracorporeal systems. J Cardiothorac Vasc Anesth 1997;11:3.

Spanier T, et al. Activation of coagulation and fibrinolytic pathways in patients with left ventricular assist devices. J Thorac Cardiovasc Surg 1996;112:1090.

Stammers A. Historical aspects of cardiopulmonary bypass: from antiquity to acceptance. J Cardiothorac Vasc Anesth 1997;11:266.

Urshel J, et al. Catheter-induced pulmonary artery rupture in the setting of cardiopulmonary bypass. Ann Thorac Surg 1993;56:588.

Transesophageal Echocardiography

Bergquist B, et al. Transesophageal echocardiography and myocardial revascularization. I. Accuracy of intraoperative real time interpretation. Anesth Analg 1996;82:1132.

Bergquist B, et al. Transesophageal echocardiography and myocardial revascularization. II. Influence on intraoperative decision making. Anesth Analg 1996;82:1139.

Bryden K, Hall R. Con: transesophageal echocardiography is not a cost effective monitor during cardiac surgery. J Cardiothorac Vasc Anesth 1997;11:250.

Byran A, et al. Transesophageal echocardiography and adult cardiac operations. Ann Thorac Surg 1995;59:773.

Cahalan M, et al. Training in transesophageal echocardiography. In the lab or on the job? Anesth Analg 1995;81:217.

Chung F, et al. Transesophageal echocardiogram may fail to diagnose perioperative myocardial infarction. Can J Anaesth 1991;38:98.

Hartman G, et al. High reproducibility in the interpretation of intraoperative transesophageal echocardiographic evaluation of aortic atheromatous disease. Anesth Analg 1996;82:539.

Konstadt S, Oka Y. Intraoperative echocardiography. J Cardiothorac Vasc Anesth 1996;10:697.

Konstadt S, et al. Ascending aorta how much does transesophageal echocardiography see? Anesth Analg 1994;78:240.

Leung J, et al. Prognostic importance of post-bypass regional wall motion abnormalities in patients undergoing coronary artery bypass graft surgery. Anesthesiology 1989;71:16.

Matsumato M, et al. Application of transesophageal echocardiography to continuous intraoperative monitoring of the left ventricular performance. Am J Cardiol 1980;46:95.

Murphy P. Pro: intraoperative transesophageal echocardiography is a cost-effective strategy for cardiac surgical procedures. J Cardiothorac Vasc Anesth 1997;11:246.

Poterack K. Who uses transesophageal echocardiography in the operating room? Anesth Analg 1995;80:454.

Sheikh K, et al. Intraoperative transesophageal Doppler color flow imagery used to guide patient selection and operative treatment of ischemic mitral regurgitation. Circulation 1991;84:594.

Troianos C, et al. Transesophageal echocardiographic diagnosis of aortic dissection during cardiac surgery. Anesthesiology 1991;75:179.

Repair of the Ascending Thoracic Aorta and Deep Hypothermic Circulatory Arrest

Bellinger D, et al. Developmental and neurologic status of children after heart surgery with hypothermic circulatory arrest or low flow cardiopulmonary bypass. N Engl J Med 1995;332:549.

Coselli J, et al. Determinants of brain temperature for safe circulatory arrest during cardiovascular operations. Ann Thorac Surg 1988;45:638.

Coselli J, et al. Aortic arch operations: current treatment and results. Ann Thorac Surg 1995;59:19.

Greeley WJ. Con: deep hypothermic circulatory arrest must be used selectively and discretely. J Cardiothorac Vasc Anesth 1991;5:638.

Grey D, et al. Surgical treatment of aneurysm of the ascending aorta with aortic insufficiency. J Thorac Cardiovasc Surg 1983;86:864.

Michenfelder J. Hypothermia plus barbiturates: apples plus oranges? Anesthesiology 1978;49:157.

Murphy D, et al. Recognition and management of ascending aortic dissection complicating cardiac surgical operations. J Thorac Cardiovasc Surg 1983;85:247.

Pressler V, McNamara J. Thoracic aortic aneurysm: natural history and treatment. J Thorac Cardiovasc Surg 1980;79:489.

Roberts W. Aortic dissection: anatomy, consequences and causes. Am Heart J 1981;101:195.

Still R, et al. Intraoperative aortic dissection. Ann Thorac Surg 1992;53:374.

Takamoto S, et al. Simple hypothermic retrograde cerebral perfusion during aortic arch replacement. J Thorac Cardiovasc Surg 1992;104:1106.

Usui A, et al. Retrograde perfusion through a superior vena cava cannula protects the brain. Ann Thorac Surg 1992;53:47.

Valvular Repair and Replacement

Carabello B, Crawford F. Medical progress: valvular heart disease. N Engl J Med 1997;337:32.

Enriquez-Sarano M, et al. Valve repair improves the outcome of surgery for mitral regurgitation. Circulation 1995;91:1022.

Joyce F, et al. Treatment of hypertrophic cardiomyopathy by mitral valve repair and septal myectomy. Ann Thorac Surg 1994;57:1025.

Kosakai Y, et al. Cox Maze procedure for chronic atrial fibrillation associated with mitral valve disease. J Thorac Cardiovasc Surg 1994;108:1049.

Scott W, et al. Determinants of operative mortality for patients undergoing aortic valve replacement. Discriminant analysis of 1479 operations. J Thorac Cardiovasc Surg 1988;89:400.

Sheikh HK, et al. The utility of transesophageal echocardiography and Doppler color flow imagery in patients undergoing cardiac valve survey. J Am Coll Cardiol 1990;15:363.

Anesthesia for Automatic Implantable Cardioverter-Defibrillator Placement, Arrhythmia Surgery, and Pacemakers

Cox J, et al. The surgical treatment of atrial fibrillation. Development of a definitive surgical procedure. J Thorac Cardiovasc Surg 1991;101:569.

Donovan K, et al. The hemodynamic importance of maintaining atrial ventricular synchrony during cardiac pacing in critically ill patients. Crit Care Med 1991;19:320.

Ferguson T, et al. Direct operation versus ICD therapy for ischemic ventricular tachycardia. Ann Thorac Surg 1994;58:1291.

Kelly J, Royster R. Non-invasive transcutaneous cardiac pacing. Anesth Analg 1989;69:229.

Pinosky M, et al. Intravenous sedation for placement of automatic implantable cardioverter defibrillator. J Cardiothorac Vasc Anesth 1996;10:764.

Platia E, et al. Treatment of malignant ventricular arrhythmias with endocardial resection and implantation of the automatic cardioverter defibrillator. N Engl J Med 1986;314:213.

Trappe H, et al. Cardioverter defibrillator implantation in the catheterization laboratory: initial experience in 48 patients. Am Heart J 1995;129:259.

Winkle R, et al. Long-term outcome with the automatic implantable cardioverter defibrillator. J Am Coll Cardiol 1989;13:1353.

Transplantation

Adatia I, et al. Inhaled nitric oxide in the treatment of postoperative graft dysfunction after lung transplantation. Ann Thorac Surg 1994;57:1311.
Copeland J, et al. Successful coronary artery bypass grafting for high risk left main coronary artery atherosclerosis after cardiac transplantation. Ann Thorac Surg 1990;49:106.
Girard C, et al. Inhaled nitric oxide for right ventricular failure after heart transplantation. J Cardiothorac Vasc Anesth 1993;7:481.
Reitz B, et al. Heart lung transplantation: successful therapy for patients with pulmonary vascular disease. N Engl J Med 1983;306:557.
Vincent J, et al. Prostaglandin E_1 infusion for right ventricular failure after cardiac transplantation. J Thorac Cardiovasc Surg 1992;103:33.

Emergency Angioplasty

Grines CL, et al. A comparison of immediate angioplasty with thrombolytic therapy for acute myocardial infarction. N Engl J Med 1993;328:673.
The Gusto IIb Investigators. A clinical trial comparing primary coronary angioplasty with tissue plasminogen activator for acute myocardial infarction. N Engl J Med 1997;336:1621.
Stark KS, et al. Myocardial salvage after failed coronary angioplasty. J Am Coll Cardiol 1990;15:78.
Talley JD, et al. Failed elective percutaneous transluminal angioplasty requiring coronary artery bypass surgery: in hospital and late clinical outcome at five years. Circulation 1990;82:1203.
Zijlstra F, et al. A comparison of immediate coronary angioplasty with intravenous streptokinase in acute myocardial infarction. N Engl J Med 1993;328:680.

Defects in Adult Heart Structure

Abraham K, et al. Tetralogy of Fallot in adults: a report on 147 patients. Am J Med 1979;66:811.
Bolooki H. Emergency cardiac procedures in patients in cardiogenic shock due to complications of coronary artery disease. Circulation 1989;79:I137.
Daggett W, et al. Improved results of surgical management of post-infarction ventricular septal defect. Ann Surg 1982;196:269.

Moore C, et al. Post-infarction ventricular septal rupture: the importance of location of infarction and right ventricular function in determining survival. Circulation 1986;74:45.

Perloff J. Congenital heart disease in adults: a new cardiovascular subspecialty. Circulation 1991;84:1881.

Reynan K. Frequency of primary tumors of the heart. Am J Cardiol 1996;77:107.

Cardiac Surgery and Neurologic Injury

Engleman R, et al. What is the best perfusion temperature for coronary revascularization? J Thorac Cardiovasc Surg 1996;112:1622.

Martin T, et al. Prospective, randomized trial of retrograde warm blood cardioplegia: myocardial benefit and neurologic threat. Ann Thorac Surg 1994;57:298.

Mora C, et al. The effect of temperature management during cardiopulmonary bypass on neurologic and neuropsychological outcomes in patients undergoing coronary revascularization. J Thorac Cardiovasc Surg 1996;112:514.

Murkin J. The role of CPB management in neuro behavioral outcomes after cardiac surgery. Ann Thorac Surg 1995;159:1308.

Nussmeier N. Adverse neurologic events: Risks of intracardiac versus extracardiac surgery. J Cardiothorac Vasc Anesth 1996;10:31.

Nussmeier N, Arlund C. Neuropsychiatric complications after cardiopulmonary bypass: cerebral protection by a barbiturate. Anesthesiology 1986;64:165.

Roach G, et al. Adverse cerebral outcomes after coronary bypass surgery. N Engl J Med 1996;338:1857.

Swain J. Cardiac surgery and the brain. N Engl J Med 1993;329:1119.

Tuman K, et al. Differential effects of advanced age on neurologic and cardiac risks of coronary artery operation. J Thorac Cardiovasc Surg 1992;104:1510.

Wong B, et al. Central nervous system dysfunction after warm or hypothermic cardiopulmonary bypass. Lancet 1992;339:1383.

Perioperative Hemorrhage and Tamponade

Chernow B. Blood conservation in critical care, the evidence accumulates. Crit Care Med 1993;21:481.

Chuttani K, et al. Diagnosis of cardiac tamponade after cardiac surgery: relative value of clinical, echocardiographic and hemodynamic signs. Am Heart J 1994;127:913.

Horrow J, Ellison N. Effective hemostasis in cardiac surgery. Can J Anaesth 1992;39:309.

Lambert C, et al. The treatment of post-perfusion bleeding using epsilon-aminocaproic acid, cryoprecipitate, fresh frozen plasma and protamine sulphate. Ann Thorac Surg 1978;28:440.

NIH Consensus Conference. Perioperative red blood cell transfusion. JAMA 1988;260:2700.

NIH Consensus Conference. Platelet transfusion therapy. JAMA 1987;257:1777.

Schoebrechts B, et al. Usefulness of transesophageal echocardiography in patients with acute hemodynamic deterioration late after cardiac surgery. Chest 1993;104:1631.

Woodman R, Harkin L. Bleeding complications associated with cardiopulmonary bypass. Blood 1990;76:1680.

Postoperative Care

Boldt J, et al. Influence of PEEP ventilation immediately after cardiopulmonary bypass and right ventricular function. Chest 1988;94:566.

Chuttani K, et al. Diagnosis of cardiac tamponade after cardiac surgery: relative value of clinical, echocardiographic, and hemodynamic signs. Am Heart J 1994;127:913.

Engleman R, et al. Fast track recovery of the coronary bypass patient. Ann Thorac Surg 1994;58:1742.

Guiteras Val P, et al. Diagnostic criteria and prognosis of perioperative myocardial infarction following bypass surgery. J Thorac Cardiovasc Surg 1983;86:878.

Hass G, et al. Acute pancreatitis after cardiopulmonary bypass. Am J Surg 1985;149:508.

Higgins T. Pro: early endotracheal extubation is preferable to late extubation in patients following coronary artery surgery. J Cardiothorac Vasc Anesth 1992;6:488.

Higgins T, et al. Propofol versus midazolam for intensive care unit sedation after coronary artery bypass grafts. Crit Care Med 1994;22:1415.

Higgins T, et al. Immediate post-operative care of the cardiac surgical patient. J Cardiothorac Vasc Anesth 1996;10:643.

Hilberman M, et al. Acute renal failure following cardiac surgery. J Thorac Cardiovasc Surg 1979;77:880.

Johnson D, et al. Respiratory function after cardiac surgery. J Cardiothorac Vasc Anesth 1996;10:571.

Mangano D, et al. Post-operative myocardial ischemia. Therapeutic trials using intensive analgesia following surgery. Anesthesiology 1992;76:342.

Smith R, et al. Ventricular dysrhythmias in patients undergoing coronary artery bypass graft surgery: incidence, characteristics and prognostic significance. Am Heart J 1992;123:73.

Tuman K, et al. Morbidity and duration of ICU stay after cardiac surgery. A model for preoperative risk assessment. Chest 1992;102:36.

Wasnick J, Hoffman W (eds). Postoperative Critical Care of the Massachusetts General Hospital (2nd ed). Boston: Little, Brown, 1992.

Anesthesia for Minimally Invasive Coronary Bypass Surgery

Greenspan A, et al. Minimally invasive direct coronary artery bypass: surgical techniques and anesthetic considerations. J Cardiothorac Vasc Anesth 1996;10:507.

Hensley F. Minimally invasive myocardial revascularization surgery: here to stay? J Cardiothorac Vasc Anesth 1996;10:445.

Jacobsohn E, et al. Online contrast echo cardiographic assessment of myocardial perfusion: its role in minimally invasive coronary artery bypass procedures. J Cardiothorac Vasc Anesth 1997;11:517.

Murry C, et al. Ischemic pre-conditioning slows energy metabolism and delays ultra structural damage during a sustained ischemic episode. Circ Res 1990;66:913.

Pfister A, et al. Coronary artery bypass without cardiopulmonary bypass. Ann Thorac Surg 1992;54:1085.

Uppal R, et al. Right thoracotomy for reoperative right coronary artery bypass procedures. Ann Thorac Surg 1994;57:123.

Wasnick J. Minimally invasive direct coronary artery bypass procedure and pacing pulmonary artery catheter. J Cardiothorac Vasc Anesth 1996;10:975.

Wasnick J, et al. Anesthetic management of coronary artery bypass via mini-thoracotomy with video assistance. J Cardiothorac Vasc Anesth 1995;9:731.

Wasnick J, et al. Anesthesia and minimally invasive thoracoscopically assisted coronary artery bypass: a brief clinical report. J Cardiothorac Vasc Anesth 1997 (publication pending).

Index